Essentials of Schizophrenia

D1613452

Essentials of Schizophrenia

EDITED BY

JEFFREY A. LIEBERMAN, M.D.
T. SCOTT STROUP, M.D., M.P.H.
DIANA O. PERKINS, M.D., M.P.H.

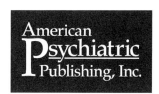

American Psychiatric Publishing, Inc.

Washington, DC
London, England

If you would like to buy between 25 and 99 copies of this or any other APPI title, you are eligible for a 20% discount; please contact APPI Customer Service at appi@psych.org or 800-368-5777. If you wish to buy 100 or more copies of the same title, please email us at bulksales@psych.org for a price quote.

Manufactured in the United States of America on acid-free paper
15 14 13 12 11   5 4 3 2 1
First Edition

Typeset in Adobe's Frutiger and Janson Text.

American Psychiatric Publishing, Inc.
1000 Wilson Boulevard
Arlington, VA 22209-3901
www.appi.org

Library of Congress Cataloging-in-Publication Data
Lieberman, Jeffrey A., 1948–
    Essentials of schizophrenia / edited by Jeffrey A. Lieberman, T. Scott Stroup, Diana O. Perkins. — 1st ed.
        p. ; cm.
    Includes bibliographical references and index.
    ISBN 978-1-58562-401-0 (pbk. : alk. paper) 1. Schizophrenia. I. Stroup, T. Scott, 1960– II. Perkins, Diana O., 1958– III. Title.
    [DNLM: 1. Schizophrenia. WM 203]
    RC514.L54 2012
    616.89'8—dc22

                                                                          2011011090

British Library Cataloguing in Publication Data
A CIP record is available from the British Library.

*To our patients for their courage and for their assistance
in the search for the causes of and cure for their illness.*

*To my family in gratitude for their love, support, and patience—
J.A.L.*

To Thelma and Meg with love—T.S.S.

*With appreciation to my husband, Clark,
for his intellectual and emotional support,
and to my children, Chris, Nick, and Katie,
for their tolerance and love—D.O.P.*

CONTENTS

CONTRIBUTORS

Jean Addington, Ph.D.
Professor, Department of Psychiatry, University of Calgary, Calgary, Alberta, Canada

Mary F. Brunette, M.D.
Medical Director, Bureau of Behavioral Health, Bureau of Behavioral Health, New Hampshire Department of Health and Human Services; Associate Professor of Psychiatry, Dartmouth Medical School, Concord, New Hampshire

Lisa Dixon, M.D., M.P.H.
Professor and Director, Division of Services Research, Department of Psychiatry, University of Maryland School of Medicine; Deputy Director and Associate Director of Research, VA Capitol Health Care Network MIRECC, Baltimore, Maryland

Robert E. Drake, M.D., Ph.D.
Andrew Thomson Professor of Psychiatry and Professor of Community and Family Medicine, Dartmouth Medical School, Lebanon, New Hampshire; Director, Dartmouth Psychiatric Research Center, Concord, New Hampshire

Charles E. Eesley, Ph.D.
Assistant Professor, Department of Management Science & Engineering, Stanford University, Stanford, California

Nora R. Frohberg, M.D.
Assistant Professor of Clinical Psychiatry, Department of Psychiatry, University of Missouri; Staff Psychiatrist, Harry S. Truman Memorial Veterans Hospital, Columbia, Missouri

Shirley M. Glynn, Ph.D.
Research Psychologist, Semel Institute for Neuroscience and Human Behavior, UCLA Geffen School of Medicine, Los Angeles, California; VA Greater Los Angeles Healthcare System

Alan I. Green, M.D.
Raymond Sobel Professor of Psychiatry, Professor of Pharmacology and Toxicology, and Chairman, Department of Psychiatry, Dartmouth Medical School, Lebanon, New Hampshire

Dilip V. Jeste, M.D.
Estelle and Edgar Levi Chair in Aging, Distinguished Professor of Psychiatry and Neurosciences, Director, Sam and Rose Stein Institute for Research on Aging, and Chief, Geriatric Psychiatry Division, University of California, San Diego/VA Medical Center, San Diego, California

Richard S. E. Keefe, Ph.D.
Professor and Director, Schizophrenia Research Group, Department of Psychiatry and Behavioral Sciences, Duke University Medical Center, Duke University School of Medicine, Durham, North Carolina

Anzalee Khan, Ph.D.
Manhattan Psychiatric Center, Ward's Island, New York; Fordham University, New York, New York

John Lauriello, M.D.
Chancellor's Chair of Excellence and Professor of Psychiatry, Department of Psychiatry, University of Missouri School of Medicine, Columbia, Missouri; Medical Director, Missouri Psychiatric Center

Jeffrey A. Lieberman, M.D.
Chairman, Department of Psychiatry, College of Physicians and Surgeons of Columbia University; Director, New York State Psychiatric Institute; Psychiatrist-in-Chief, New York Presbyterian Hospital–Columbia University Medical Center, New York, New York

J. P. Lindenmayer, M.D.
Clinical Professor, Department of Psychiatry, New York University School of Medicine, New York, New York; Clinical Director, Psychopharmacology Research Unit, Manhattan Psychiatric Center–Nathan Kline Institute for Psychiatric Research, New York, New York

Stephen R. Marder, M.D.
Professor, Department of Psychiatry and Biobehavioral Sciences, David Geffen School of Medicine, University of California Los Angeles; Director, VISN 22 Mental Illness Research, Education, and Clinical Center (MIRECC), Veterans Affairs Medical Center, Los Angeles, California

Joseph P. McEvoy, M.D.
Associate Professor, Department of Psychiatry and Behavioral Sciences, Duke University Medical Center, Durham, North Carolina; Deputy Clinical Director, John Umstead Hospital, Butner, North Carolina

Susan R. McGurk, Ph.D.
Associate Professor of Psychiatry, Dartmouth Medical School, Lebanon, New Hampshire; Dartmouth Psychiatric Research Center, Concord, New Hampshire

Erick Messias, M.D., M.P.H., Ph.D.
Associate Professor of Psychiatry and Medical Director, Walker Family Clinic, Psychiatric Research Institute, University of Arkansas for Medical Sciences, Little Rock, Arkansas

Alexander L. Miller, M.D.
Clinical Professor, Department of Psychiatry, The University of Texas Health Science Center at San Antonio, San Antonio, Texas

Kim T. Mueser, Ph.D.
Professor of Psychiatry and of Community and Family Medicine, Dartmouth Medical School, Lebanon, New Hampshire; Dartmouth Psychiatric Research Center, Concord, New Hampshire

Douglas L. Noordsy, M.D.
Associate Professor of Psychiatry, Department of Psychiatry, Dartmouth Medical School, Lebanon, New Hampshire

David L. Penn, Ph.D.
Professor, Department of Psychology, University of North Carolina at Chapel Hill, Chapel Hill, North Carolina

Diana O. Perkins, M.D., M.P.H.
Professor and Medical Director of OASIS (Outreach and Support Intervention Services), Department of Psychiatry, University of North Carolina–Chapel Hill School of Medicine, Chapel Hill, North Carolina

Amy E. Pinkham, Ph.D.
Assistant Professor, Department of Psychology, Southern Methodist University, Dallas, Texas

T. Scott Stroup, M.D., M.P.H.
Director, Program for Intervention Effectiveness Research, New York State Psychiatric Institute, Department of Psychiatry, College of Physicians and Surgeons of Columbia University, New York, New York

Marvin S. Swartz, M.D.
Professor and Head, Division of Social and Community Psychiatry, Department of Psychiatry and Behavioral Sciences, Duke University Medical Center, Durham, North Carolina

DISCLOSURE OF COMPETING INTERESTS

The following contributors to this book have indicated a financial interest in or other affiliation with a commercial supporter, a manufacturer of a commercial product, a provider of a commercial service, a nongovernmental organization, and/or a government agency, as listed below:

Lisa Dixon, M.D., M.P.H.—*Principal Investigator:* Addressing Adherence in the Treatment of Schizophrenia and Other Severe Mental Illness, Ortho McNeil Janssen Scientific Affairs, December 2009–December 2010; convened a meeting to consider issues and policy/research recommendations regarding adherence and disparities in above by race and ethnicity

Robert E. Drake, M.D., Ph.D.—The Dartmouth Psychiatric Research Center receives support for research and educational materials on employment services from the following: *Grants:* National Institute on Drug Abuse; National Institute on Disability and Rehabilitation Research; National Institute of Mental Health, Robert Wood Johnson Foundation, Substance Abuse and Mental Health Services Administration; *Contracts:* Assistant Secretary for Planning and Evaluation–Department of Health and Human Services, Guilford Press, Hazelden Press, MacArthur Foundation, Oxford University Press, National Institute of Mental Health, Research Foundation for Mental Health, Gifts from Johnson & Johnson Corporate Contributions, Segal Foundation, Social Security Administration, Thomson Foundation, Vail Foundation, West Foundation

Alan I. Green, M.D.—*Research support:* Eli Lilly, Janssen, Lundbeck; *Service on Data Monitoring Committee:* Eli Lilly; *Stock ownership:* Johnson & Johnson, Mylan, Pfizer; Pending patent applications regarding treatment for substance abuse

Dilip V. Jeste, M.D.—AstraZeneca, Bristol-Myers Squibb, Eli Lilly, and Janssen donate medication for our National Institute of Mental Health–funded grant "Metabolic Effects of Newer Antipsychotics in Older Patients."

Richard S. E. Keefe, Ph.D.—*Research funding:* Allon, AstraZeneca, Department of Veterans Affairs, GlaxoSmithKline, National Institute of Mental Health, Novartis, Singapore Medical Research Council; *Consultant/ Advisory Board:* Abbott, Bioline, BrainCells, CHDI, Dainippon Sumitomo Pharma, Eli Lilly, EnVivo, Lundbeck, Memory Pharmaceuticals, Merck, NeuroSearch, Pfizer, Roche, Sanofi/Aventis, Shire, Solvay, Takeda, Wyeth; *Royalties:* Brief Assessment of Cognition in Schizophrenia (BACS), MATRICS Battery (BACS Symbol Coding); *Shareholder:* NeuroCog Trials Inc.; *Other:* Duke University holds the copyright for the ScoRS, and licenses are issued by NeuroCog Trials Inc. There is currently no license fee to use the ScoRS.

John Lauriello, M.D.—*Consultant:* Eli Lilly

Jeffrey A. Lieberman, M.D.—2010–2011: *Grant/Research support:* Allon*, GlaxoSmithKline*, Eli Lilly*, Merck*, Novartis*, Pfizer*, Hoffmann–La Roche Ltd.*, Sepracor (Sunovion)*, Targacept*; *Advisory Board:* Bioline*, Intracellular Therapies, Pierre Fabre*, PsychoGenics*; *Patent:* Repligen

2009–2010: *Grant/Research support:* Merck*; *Advisory Board:* Eli Lilly*; *Patent:* Repligen

(*Dr. Lieberman receives no direct financial compensation or salary support for participation in these research, consulting, or advisory board activities.)

J.P. Lindenmayer, M.D.—*Grant support:* AstraZeneca, Azur, Dainippon Sumitomo; Eli Lilly, Janssen, National Institute of Mental Health, Otsuka, Pfizer; *Consultant:* Eli Lilly, Janssen

Stephen R. Marder, M.D.—*Research:* GlaxoSmithKline, Novartis; *Advisory Board:* Bristol-Myers Squibb, Lundbeck, Otsuka, Pfizer, Roche, Sanofi/Aventis, Schering-Plough, Wyeth

Joseph P. McEvoy, M.D.—*Honoraria:* Eli Lilly; *Consultant:* Merck, Roche

Alexander L. Miller, M.D.—*Advisory Board:* Rules-Based Medicine (March 2010); *Investigator-initiated research grant:* Pfizer; *Consultant:* RBM Inc. (2010).

Douglas L. Noordsy, M.D.—*Consulting honoraria, speaking honoraria, and/or research support:* AstraZeneca, Bristol-Myers Squibb, Eli Lilly, Janssen, Merck, Novartis, Sunovion

Diana O. Perkins, M.D., M.P.H.—*Consultant:* Eli Lilly, Endo Pharmaceutical, Sunovion; *Advisory Board:* Genentech (CNS Advisory Board), Merck (Clinical Advisory Board)

The following contributors stated that they had no competing interests during the year preceding manuscript submission:

Jean Addington, Ph.D.	Erick Messias, M.D., M.P.H., Ph.D.
Mary F. Brunette, M.D.	Kim T. Mueser, Ph.D.
Nora R. Frohberg, M.D.	David L. Penn, Ph.D.
Shirley M. Glynn, Ph.D.	Amy E. Pinkham, Ph.D.
Anzalee Khan, Ph.D.	T. Scott Stroup, M.D., M.P.H.
Susan R. McGurk, Ph.D.	Marvin S. Swartz, M.D.

PREFACE

Schizophrenia and schizophrenia-spectrum disorders remain common and frequently disabling illnesses that pose enormous challenges for affected individuals, their families, mental health care providers, healthcare systems, and society at large. However, advances in the understanding of the causes of schizophrenia and its pathophysiology, and research on treatment approaches, provide hope for the future. Much research is being done to develop new methods of diagnostic assessment, new treatments, and ultimately the discovery of the causes and cures for schizophrenia. While we await these breakthroughs, there is much that can be done to improve the lives and outcomes of patients with mental illness by applying existing knowledge and making evidence-based treatments available.

Although recent research has clarified that the antipsychotic medications currently available have many shortcomings, we know ever more about how best to deploy these essential treatments. Increasingly we know that psychosocial treatments are critical to optimal outcomes, including recovery.

Research demonstrating that untreated psychosis and delays in seeking treatment are associated with poorer outcomes has led to new initiatives in Australia, the United States, and elsewhere to promote earlier detection of psychosis and to intervene promptly and comprehensively. This extremely practical work may have a tremendous yield.

The textbook we edited, *The American Psychiatric Publishing Textbook of Schizophrenia*, published in 2006, is a comprehensive resource on schizophrenia. This book, *Essentials of Schizophrenia*, focuses on the clinical essentials of schizophrenia, including epidemiology, manifestations of illness, comorbidities, and treatment strategies. We have assembled chapters by an eminent roster of experts who provide the latest clinically relevant information. We are grateful to these experts for their outstanding contributions. We hope that this volume will serve as an essential source of knowledge and resource for clinicians, trainees, and students who seek to help people with schizophrenia and their families.

Jeffrey A. Lieberman, M.D.
T. Scott Stroup, M.D., M.P.H.
Diana O. Perkins, M.D., M.P.H.

EPIDEMIOLOGY AND NATURAL HISTORY

DIANA O. PERKINS, M.D., M.P.H.

JEFFREY A. LIEBERMAN, M.D.

EPIDEMIOLOGY

Epidemiological studies inform us about the burden of a disease to society, and findings often generate hypotheses about disease risk and prognosis. In this section we review epidemiological studies investigating the rate at which schizophrenia develops over a given time in different populations *(incidence)*, and the total number of persons who have schizophrenia at a given time *(prevalence)*. Note that prevalence is influenced by incidence rates and also by factors that cause persons with schizophrenia to leave the population (e.g., death, recovery). We also discuss the results of ecological studies investigating environmental factors associated with differences in incidence and prevalence of schizophrenia.

INCIDENCE AND PREVALENCE

The incidence and prevalence of schizophrenia are highly variable in different populations. These variations give clues about the possible contribution of genetic and environmental factors to disease risk. As reported in a systematic review of more than 100 large-scale epidemiological studies from 32 countries, the median incidence rate for schizophrenia is 15.2 per 100,000 persons per year, with the lowest 10% of rates at 7.7 and the highest 90% of rates at 43 per 100,000 persons per year (McGrath et al. 2004). Thus, the incidence of schizophrenia has varied more than fivefold in different locations. Incidence variability occurs even at a local level. For example, in a study of schizophrenia incidence from 1997 to 1999 in England, the age-adjusted incidence in London was 20.1, in Nottingham 7.6, and in Bristol 7.2 per 100,000 persons per year (Kirkbride et al. 2006).

Thus, it is not surprising that the prevalence of schizophrenia also is highly variable. In a systematic review that included 19 studies, the median point prevalence of schizophrenia was 4.6 per 1,000 persons, with the 10th percentile 1.9 and the 90th percentile 10.0 per 1,000 persons (Saha et al. 2005). Perhaps the most meaningful way to look at the risk of developing schizophrenia is the *lifetime morbid risk*, which is the lifetime prevalence of schizophrenia including all persons in a birth cohort. The median lifetime morbid risk of schizophrenia is 7.2 per 1,000 persons, with the 10th percentile 3.1 and the 90th percentile 27.1 per 1,000 persons. It is therefore correct to say that about 0.7% of persons will develop schizophrenia in their lifetime but that this proportion varies in different populations from 0.3% to 2.7%. Thus, the often-mentioned lifetime prevalence of schizophrenia of 1% worldwide is a reasonable approximation but appears to be higher than is supported by recent epidemiological studies.

FACTORS ASSOCIATED WITH INCIDENCE AND PREVALENCE

Large-scale, well-conducted epidemiological studies have found several factors associated with incidence and prevalence of schizophrenia. For example, meta-analyses conclude that schizophrenia is about 1.4 times more common in males than in females (Aleman et al. 2003; McGrath et al. 2004). In addition a number of studies point to the involvement of environment in schizophrenia risk. Urban birth or living in an urban area is associated with an approximate 1.9-fold increased risk of schizophrenia in males and a 1.3-fold increased risk in females compared with nonurban populations (Kelly et al. 2010). First-generation immigrants have an approximate 2.7-fold and second-generation immigrants an approximate 4.5-fold increased risk of schizophrenia, with impact similar on males and females (Cantor-Graae and Selten

2005). Schizophrenia prevalence is higher in countries that are further from the equator, and schizophrenia incidence similarly varies for men but not for women (Saha et al. 2006).

Perinatal complications, especially maternal infections, severe maternal malnutrition, maternal exposure to severe stressful events, and birth complications, are environmental risk factors for schizophrenia (Verdoux 2004). While ecological studies examining the risk of schizophrenia in persons with prenatal exposure to viral epidemics have equivocal findings, follow-up studies using much stronger case-control designs provide evidence that risk of schizophrenia is about sevenfold higher in persons with in utero exposure to infectious agents (Brown and Derkits 2010). Several studies find the risk of schizophrenia is about doubled in individuals gestated during a famine (Brown and Susser 2008). Maternal exposure to severe stressful life events, such as war or the death of a close relative, is associated with about a 50% increase in schizophrenia risk (Khashan et al. 2008; Malaspina et al. 2008; van Os and Selten 1998). Obstetrical complications, especially those involving significant hypoxia, are associated with about a twofold increased risk of schizophrenia (Cannon et al. 2002). A more recent hypothesis regarding differences in schizophrenia risk associated with latitude and immigration is related to maternal vitamin D deficiency (Eyles et al. 2009; Mackay-Sim et al. 2004).

The above findings have generated important hypotheses regarding schizophrenia etiology. Most established is the *neurodevelopmental hypothesis of schizophrenia*, which purports that altered brain development early in life increases risk of later schizophrenia. Environmental exposures, including infectious agents or the maternal response to infectious agents, vitamin deficiencies, or maternal response to stressful life events, are hypothesized to alter the developmental trajectory of a genetically vulnerable brain. Because almost all of the environmental risk factors affect large populations, it is hypothesized that only a minority of exposed persons have the genetic background necessary ultimately needed to develop the disease.

NATURAL HISTORY

Most individuals who develop a schizophrenic psychotic disorder will have a chronic illness. The severity of positive, negative, cognitive, and mood symptoms is highly variable, as is the severity of social and vocational disability. Long-term outcome varies from sustained, complete recovery, to severe disability from chronic residual symptoms. In this section we discuss prognosis and factors that are associated with prognosis.

RECOVERY AND CHRONICITY

Not all individuals who develop schizophrenia develop chronic symptoms and functional impairment. Most patients will experience symptomatic remission from their first episode (Derks et al. 2010; Emsley et al. 2007; Henry et al. 2010; Lieberman et al. 2003), but almost all of these patients will later have symptomatic relapse and clinical deterioration. Definitions of sustained recovery are varied, but all require both remission of symptoms and good social and vocational function. Studies find that between 1% and 38% of the individuals meeting criteria for schizophrenia will enjoy a sustained symptomatic and functional recovery after one or more psychotic episodes (Harrison et al. 2001; Huber et al. 1980; Lauronen et al. 2005; Wiersma et al. 1998). These studies, despite methodological limitations, paint a consistent picture: as many as one of every five individuals who develop a schizophrenic psychotic disorder will have a sustained recovery, and a small proportion completely recover from a first episode without subsequent relapse.

The consistent finding that most patients recover from a first episode and that a substantial minority may have a relatively benign course may be surprising to clinicians who regularly treat individuals with schizophrenia. Functional disability and persistent or recurrent symptoms are common in most patients who require chronic treatment, and recovery is rarely observed. The reason for the discrepancy between the observations of clinicians and the results of these epidemiological studies is primarily that recovered patients often do not seek ongoing treatment and thus are not part of the population of individuals who require chronic treatment.

Long-term prospective and follow-back studies find a range of disability and symptom chronicity in individuals meeting criteria for a schizophrenic psychotic disorder. A significant minority—about 1 of every 10 patients—will have persistent, unremitting psychotic symptoms throughout the course of their illness (Wiersma et al. 1998). By the end of the first decade of illness, a consistent prognostic picture emerges: about one-third of patients will have a relatively good outcome, with no more than mild symptoms and functional impairments; the remaining two-thirds will have moderate to severe symptoms and functional impairments.

DEATH

The risk of premature death is increased in persons with schizophrenia. In a recent meta-analysis, the observed number of deaths in persons with schizophrenia was about three times higher than the expected number of deaths (given the person's age, ancestry, etc.) (Saha et al. 2007). The risk for death by suicide was about 13-fold higher, and risk for accidental death was about

2-fold higher. Because the greatest risk of suicide appears to be during recovery from a first psychotic episode, specialized treatment during this time is indicated to reduce risk of death by suicide.

The risk for death from natural causes, including cardiovascular disease, diabetes, and lung disease, is about twice the expected risk. The risk for these diseases may be in part genetically based; however, much of the risk may be related to lifestyle and social and environmental factors and thus is potentially preventable.

Independent of cancers associated with tobacco use, the overall cancer risk appears not to be elevated in persons with schizophrenia (Catts et al. 2008). Examination of risk of cancers that are related to tobacco use revealed a modest increased risk for lung cancer (~1.3-fold) but no difference in risk for bladder cancer. After adjustment for tobacco use, the risk of lung and bladder cancer was actually about 1.5-fold lower in persons with schizophrenia compared with the general population. The overall risk of cancer was significantly less (about 10% less than expected) in first-degree relatives of persons with schizophrenia. The reason for this relatively surprising finding is unclear but leads to speculation about genetic vulnerability factors for schizophrenia that may also be protective against cancer.

FACTORS ASSOCIATED WITH PROGNOSIS

The cause of the extreme heterogeneity in long-term outcome—from complete recovery to incapacitating symptoms and disability—is not known but is of obvious interest. Prognosis is very likely related in part to the extent and severity of the underlying disease pathology. Disease course also may be related to environmental factors, including the extent that treatment is optimal, the support and demands of the patient's community, and the availability of resources to support recovery. Evidence suggests that most patients with schizophrenia have a neuroprogressive component to their disease that potentially could be prevented by optimal treatment and support (Lieberman 2006).

To better predict prognosis and also to develop treatment strategies that could improve outcome, numerous studies have examined the relation between clinical, demographic, and treatment variables and outcome.

CLINICAL FEATURES AND ENVIRONMENT

Clinical features associated with a poor prognosis include poor premorbid social and school function, insidious onset, earlier age at onset, prominent negative symptoms, more severe cognitive impairments, and male sex (Tsang et al. 2010). Gradually emerging symptoms are also associated with poor prognosis, and abrupt onset precipitated by stressful events is associated with a good prognosis (van Os et al. 1994). These clinical features are often intercorrelated, suggesting that together they characterize a poor-prognosis illness. For example, some features, such as severe cognitive impairments and negative symptoms, may underlie others, such as poor premorbid social and school function.

There is a consistent finding of substantially better prognosis for individuals with schizophrenic psychotic disorders in developing countries than in developed countries, perhaps because of some social, cultural, or environmental factors that may improve prognosis (Jablensky and Sartorius 2008). Greater social support, less severe life stressors, and dietary factors are proposed explanations. The availability of family support is associated with better long-term clinical and functional outcomes in first-episode patients (Pharoah et al. 2006). Stressful life events may be associated with increased relapse risk in individuals with schizophrenia, with the effects of stress on dopamine, glutamate, and corticosteroid systems in the brain a theorized mechanism (Walker et al. 2008).

EFFECT OF ANTIPSYCHOTICS ON PROGNOSIS

Although antipsychotic drugs are an effective treatment of psychotic symptoms, debate continues over whether the introduction of antipsychotics has affected the course and ultimate prognosis of schizophrenic psychotic disorders. The evidence that addresses this issue includes comparisons of outcomes before and after the availability of antipsychotics, clinical studies that examined the effect of maintenance antipsychotic treatment on outcome, and studies that examined the relation of duration of psychosis before first treatment initiation to outcome. This body of research provides indirect support for the notion that antipsychotic medications positively influence prognosis.

The long-term outcomes of first-episode patients from prospective or follow-back studies conducted prior to the introduction of antipsychotics are significantly worse than the outcomes from studies conducted after the introduction of antipsychotics (Hegarty et al. 1994). Supporting the observation of improved prognosis since the introduction of antipsychotics is an analysis of outcomes from a cohort of patients that bridged the introduction of antipsychotics (Huber et al. 1980). In this study, patients who received antipsychotics for their first psychotic episode 1) were more likely to have a complete remission than were those who had their first episode before antipsychotics were available (27.9% vs. 14.6%) and 2) generally had less severe psychopathology at long-term follow-up (mean=22 years).

Epidemiological outcome studies generally do not report the relation of sustained recovery from a first psychotic episode and maintenance antipsychotic treatment. Studies do report that antipsychotic use is associated with reduced likelihood of relapse after recovery from a first episode (Robinson et al. 1999; Wunderink et al. 2007; Zarate and Tohen 2004). Recurrent episodes early in the course of illness are associated with increased likelihood of developing chronic residual positive and negative symptoms, suggesting that relapse may result in clinical deterioration (Lieberman et al. 2008).

In addition, there is good evidence that the shorter the duration of the first episode of psychosis prior to initiating antipsychotics, the greater the level of symptomatic and functional recovery (Perkins et al. 2005). The relation of duration of initial untreated psychosis and outcome is independent of premorbid function or mode of onset. Thus, antipsychotic medication may affect a progressive pathological process. These findings support the notion that relapse prevention through maintenance antipsychotic use may improve long-term outcomes.

CONCLUSION

The course of schizophrenia is highly heterogeneous, with outcomes ranging from complete recovery to chronic incapacity. Numerous factors are associated with outcome, and several treatment interventions may increase the likelihood of sustained recovery. First, antipsychotic treatment and other interventions should occur as close to psychosis onset as is possible. Second, long-term maintenance treatment is also associated with sustained recovery. Almost all patients, but not every patient, will require maintenance antipsychotic treatment to remain in recovery, but it is not currently possible to discern reliably those individuals who will have a benign course from those who will have a more severe course. Prevention of recurrent episodes is likely to be critical to preventing disease progression (Lieberman et al. 2008). Interventions that encourage family and social support may also impact prognosis. Although even more speculative, optimal prenatal care that includes appropriate vitamin supplementation and minimization of pre- and perinatal complications, including maternal infectious disease, exposure to stressful life events, and obstetrical complications, may influence disease risk as well as disease severity.

REFERENCES

Aleman A, Kahn RS, Selten JP: Sex differences in the risk of schizophrenia: evidence from meta-analysis. Arch Gen Psychiatry 60:565–571, 2003

Brown AS, Derkits EJ: Prenatal infection and schizophrenia: a review of epidemiologic and translational studies. Am J Psychiatry 167:261–280, 2010

Brown AS, Susser ES: Prenatal nutritional deficiency and risk of adult schizophrenia. Schizophr Bull 34:1054–1063, 2008

Cannon M, Jones PB, Murray RM: Obstetric complications and schizophrenia: historical and meta-analytic review. Am J Psychiatry 159:1080–1092, 2002

Cantor-Graae E, Selten JP: Schizophrenia and migration: a meta-analysis and review. Am J Psychiatry 162:12–24, 2005

Catts VS, Catts SV, O'Toole BI, et al: Cancer incidence in patients with schizophrenia and their first-degree relatives—a meta-analysis. Acta Psychiatr Scand 117:323–336, 2008

Derks EM, Fleischhacker WW, Boter H, et al: Antipsychotic drug treatment in first-episode psychosis: should patients be switched to a different antipsychotic drug after 2, 4, or 6 weeks of nonresponse? J Clin Psychopharmacol 30:176–180, 2010

Emsley R, Rabinowitz J, Medori R, et al: Remission in early psychosis: rates, predictors, and clinical and functional outcome correlates. Schizophr Res 89:129–139, 2007

Eyles DW, Féron F, Cui X, et al: Developmental vitamin D deficiency causes abnormal brain development. Psychoneuroendocrinology 34 (suppl 1):S247–S257, 2009

Harrison G, Hopper K, Craig T, et al: Recovery from psychotic illness: a 15- and 25-year international follow-up study. Br J Psychiatry 178:506–517, 2001

Hegarty JD, Baldessarini RJ, Tohen M, et al: One hundred years of schizophrenia: a meta-analysis of the outcome literature. Am J Psychiatry 151:1409–1416, 1994

Henry LP, Amminger GP, Harris MG, et al: The EPPIC follow-up study of first-episode psychosis: longer-term clinical and functional outcome 7 years after index admission. J Clin Psychiatry 71:716–728, 2010

Huber G, Gross G, Schuttler R, et al: Longitudinal studies of schizophrenic patients. Schizophr Bull 6:592–605, 1980

Jablensky A, Sartorius N: What did the WHO studies really find? Schizophr Bull 34:253–255, 2008

Kelly BD, O'Callaghan E, Waddington JL, et al: Schizophrenia and the city: a review of literature and prospective study of psychosis and urbanicity in Ireland. Schizophr Res 116:75–89, 2010

Khashan AS, Abel KM, McNamee R, et al: Higher risk of offspring schizophrenia following antenatal maternal exposure to severe adverse life events. Arch Gen Psychiatry 65:146–152, 2008

Kirkbride JB, Fearon P, Morgan C, et al Heterogeneity in incidence rates of schizophrenia and other psychotic syndromes: findings from the 3-center AeSOP study. Arch Gen Psychiatry 63:250–258, 2006

Lauronen E, Koskinen J, Veijola J, et al: Recovery from schizophrenic psychoses within the northern Finland 1966 Birth Cohort. J Clin Psychiatry 66:375–383, 2005

Lieberman JA: Neurobiology and the natural history of schizophrenia. J Clin Psychiatry 67(10):e14, 2006

Lieberman JA, Phillips M, Gu H, et al: Atypical and conventional antipsychotic drugs in treatment-naive first-episode schizophrenia: a 52-week randomized trial of clozapine vs chlorpromazine. Neuropsychopharmacology 28:995–1003, 2003

Lieberman JA, Drake RE, Sederer LI, et al: Science and recovery in schizophrenia. Psychiatr Serv 59:487–496, 2008

Mackay-Sim A, Féron F, Eyles D, et al: Schizophrenia, vitamin D, and brain development. Int Rev Neurobiol 59:351–380, 2004

Malaspina D, Corcoran C, Kleinhaus KR, et al: Acute maternal stress in pregnancy and schizophrenia in offspring: a cohort prospective study. BMC Psychiatry 8:71, 2008

McGrath J, Saha S, Welham J, et al: A systematic review of the incidence of schizophrenia: the distribution of rates and the influence of sex, urbanicity, migrant status and methodology. BMC Med 2:13, 2004

Perkins DO, Gu H, Boteva K, et al: Relationship between duration of untreated psychosis and outcome in first-episode schizophrenia: a critical review and meta-analysis. Am J Psychiatry 162:1785–1804, 2005

Pharoah F, Mari J, Rathbone J, et al: Family intervention for schizophrenia. Cochrane Database Syst Rev (4):CD000088, 2006

Robinson D, Woerner MG, Alvir JM, et al: Predictors of relapse following response from a first episode of schizophrenia or schizoaffective disorder. Arch Gen Psychiatry 56:241–247, 1999

Saha S, Chant D, Welham J, et al: A systematic review of the prevalence of schizophrenia. PLoS Med 2(5):e141, 2005

Saha S, Chant DC, Welham JL, et al: The incidence and prevalence of schizophrenia varies with latitude. Acta Psychiatr Scand 114:36–39, 2006

Saha S, Chant D, McGrath J: A systematic review of mortality in schizophrenia: is the differential mortality gap worsening over time? Arch Gen Psychiatry 64:1123–1131, 2007

Tsang HW, Leung AY, Chung RC, et al: Review on vocational predictors: a systematic review of predictors of vocational outcomes among individuals with schizophrenia: an update since 1998. Aust N Z J Psychiatry 44:495–504, 2010

van Os J, Selten JP: Prenatal exposure to maternal stress and subsequent schizophrenia: the May 1940 invasion of the Netherlands. Br J Psychiatry 172:324–326, 1998

van Os J, Fahy TA, Bebbington P, et al: The influence of life events on the subsequent course of psychotic illness. A prospective follow-up of the Camberwell Collaborative Psychosis Study. Psychol Med 24:503–513, 1994

Verdoux H: Perinatal risk factors for schizophrenia: how specific are they? Curr Psychiatry Rep 6(3):162–167, 2004

Walker E, Mittal V, et al: Stress and the hypothalamic pituitary adrenal axis in the developmental course of schizophrenia. Annu Rev Clin Psychol 4:189–216, 2008

Wiersma D, Nienhuis FJ, Slooff CJ, et al: Natural course of schizophrenic disorders: a 15-year followup of a Dutch incidence cohort. Schizophr Bull 24:75–85, 1998

Wunderink L, Nienhuis FJ, Sytema S, et al: Guided discontinuation versus maintenance treatment in remitted first-episode psychosis: relapse rates and functional outcome. J Clin Psychiatry 68:654–661, 2007

Zarate CA Jr, Tohen M: Double-blind comparison of the continued use of antipsychotic treatment versus its discontinuation in remitted manic patients. Am J Psychiatry 161:169-171, 2004

2

PSYCHOPATHOLOGY

J. P. Lindenmayer, M.D.

Anzalee Khan, Ph.D.

Schizophrenia is a serious mental illness characterized by positive, negative, and cognitive symptoms that affect almost all aspects of mental activity, including perception, attention, memory, and emotion. Symptoms are associated with various degrees of persistent social and functional impairments. Schizophrenia affects about 1% of the U.S. population (see Chapter 1, "Epidemiology and Natural History" in this book). It is estimated that people with schizophrenia occupy 10% of hospital beds in the United States, and approximately 30% of people with the disease are hospitalized at one point in their lives; 20% live in supervised housing (e.g., group homes). Schizophrenia and schizoaffective disorder together constitute the fifth leading cause of disability (World Health Organization 2008) and are responsible for more years of life lived with disability than all malignancies and HIV combined (Harrow et al. 1997; Moller et al. 1988).

The disorder begins usually in late adolescence and early adulthood. The median age at onset is about 23 years in men and 28 years in women. Onset is rare before 16 years and uncommon after 50 years. The disorder can have a relatively acute onset, over the course of 2–3 weeks, or an insidious one.

Most individuals experience a prodromal phase before the first episode during which certain signs and symptoms will be present, but the criteria for the disorder are not all fulfilled (McGorry et al. 1996).

DIAGNOSIS OF SCHIZOPHRENIA

The definitions and criteria used to establish the diagnosis of schizophrenia have undergone important and wide changes over the years despite the fact that the definition and descriptions of the symptoms themselves have remained rather stable.

Traditionally, American nosology was based on Bleuler's four "A's": disturbance in Affect, Association, Autism, and Ambivalence. These criteria resulted in a relatively broad concept of schizophrenia, which was elaborated in the second edition of *Diagnostic and Statistical Manual of Mental Disorders* (DSM-II; American Psychiatric Association 1968). DSM-III (American Psychiatric Association 1980) and DSM-III-R (American Psychiatric Association 1987) brought about a radical departure from this approach and introduced a much narrower concept with 1) a clear limitation of the number and type of symptoms, 2) a requirement for a specific duration of symptoms, and 3) the inclusion of a course criterion. This development was the result of critiques of the lack of reliability and validity of diagnosis (Beck et al. 1962; Spitzer and Fleiss 1974) and the important influence of Schneider's "first-rank symptoms" (Schneider 1959, 1974), which focused on specific allegedly pathognomonic symptoms of schizophrenia (e.g., thought broadcasting, thought insertion, auditory hallucinations of voices commenting on one's activity). In addition, the work of the Washington University School (Feighner et al. 1972) introduced the requirement of duration of at least 6 months before the diagnosis could be established. The definition of schizophrenia in DSM-III was largely based on Schneiderian first-rank symptoms and a required duration of 6 months, including prodromal and residual periods of illness. This definition resulted in a much narrower concept of schizophrenia, somewhat closer to the British and European concept of the disorder.

There was a further narrowing with the introduction of DSM-IV (American Psychiatric Association 1994), and its text revision, DSM-IV-TR (American Psychiatric Association 2000), which include specific negative symptoms. Criterion A in DSM-IV includes four positive symptoms and one negative symptom; at least two of these have to be present for this criterion to be fulfilled. The criterion for duration of acute phase symptoms was extended from 1 week to 1 month. If delusions (criterion A) are judged to be bizarre, only this single symptom is required to satisfy criterion A for schizophrenia. Similarly, the diagnosis of schizophrenia can be made with only hallucinations within criterion A, if these consist of voices keeping up a running commentary on the person's behavior or thoughts or if two or three voices are conversing with each other. The greatest difference between DSM-III-R and DSM-IV criteria for schizophrenia is in the description of characteristic symptomatology. The criterion for duration of acute-phase symptoms is extended from 1 week to 1 month. Hallucinations are no longer required to be prominent. DSM-IV (and DSM-IV-TR) uses the term *disorganized speech* instead of incoherence or marked loosening of associations for schizophrenic thought disorder. DSM-IV includes negative symptoms, such as affective flattening, alogia, and avolition, in criterion A. For criterion B, the requirement for a decrease in social/occupational functioning is broadened. Criterion C requires continuous signs of the disorder for at least 6 months, whereas criterion D delineates schizophrenia from schizoaffective and mood disorders.

This definition of schizophrenia remains somewhat different in the International Classification of Diseases, 10th Revision (ICD-10; World Health Organization 1992). ICD-10 takes a more cross-sectional approach without including the decline in social/occupational functions as required by DSM-IV. The requirement for duration of symptoms is reduced to only 1 month, in contrast to 6 months in DSM-IV. Among the positive symptoms, Schneiderian symptoms are well represented, and only one is required for the diagnosis of schizophrenia, reflecting the pathognomonic importance ICD-10 continues to give to the Schneiderian first-rank symptoms. Negative symptoms such as marked apathy, paucity of speech, and blunting or incongruity of emotional responses are given more prominence as well. The ICD-10 definition is narrower than the DSM-IV definition regarding positive symptoms in that it requires predominantly Schneiderian first-rank symptoms.

Although ICD-10 includes a prodromal phase in schizophrenia, the criterion of greater than 1 month's duration of symptoms does not include the prodromal phase. Conversely, DSM-IV acknowledges the prodromal phase, which may be present during the 6-month diagnostic period and is part of the evolving disorder.

In terms of affective symptoms, DSM-IV criteria for schizophrenia allow for the presence of affective symptoms if the symptoms are relatively brief, whereas ICD-10 specifies that they must follow the psychotic symptoms. The subtypes of ICD-10 and DSM-IV are undifferentiated, residual, disorganized (hebephrenic in ICD-10), catatonic, and paranoid schizophrenia (see section "Subtypes of Schizophrenia" and Table 2–1 later in this chapter). In addition, ICD-10 contains simple and postschizophrenic depression as further subtypes.

DIAGNOSTIC ASSESSMENT TOOLS

The diagnostic classifications most often used in clinical practice are DSM-IV-TR and ICD-10. The Research Diagnostic Criteria (RDC; Spitzer et al. 1978) are mostly used in research. The reliability of diagnostic assessments and of the characteristic symptoms of schizophrenia can be improved by the use of structured interview instruments. Among these are the Present State Examination (PSE; Wing 1970), Schedule for Affective Disorders and Schizophrenia (SADS; Endicott and Spitzer 1978), Diagnostic Interview Schedule (DIS; Robbins et al. 1981), Structured Clinical Interview for DSM-IV (SCID; First et al. 1997), and Comprehensive Assessment of Symptoms and History (CASH; Andreasen 1985).

In the following sections, we discuss the characteristic symptoms of schizophrenia, their differential diagnosis, their assessment, and some of their neurocognitive correlates. The symptoms are grouped into five syndromal domains—1) positive symptoms, 2) negative symptoms, 3) cognitive symptoms, 4) excitement symptoms, and 5) anxiety/depression symptoms—based on our own analyses of extensive psychometric data (Lindenmayer et al. 1994, 1995).

DEVELOPMENT OF THE SYNDROMAL CONCEPT OF SCHIZOPHRENIA

Schizophrenia is a disorder with a significant heterogeneous presentation of symptoms both in individual patients and over the course of the illness. Crow (1980, 1985), in a seminal contribution, described type I and type II schizophrenia, which he considered dichotomous syndromes with relatively independent underlying pathophysiological processes. Crow postulated that the negative syndrome (type II schizophrenia) would be stable because it was hypothesized to reflect structural brain abnormalities (e.g., enlarged ventricles) and dopaminergic hypofunction leading to lesser antipsychotic responsiveness and to poor outcome. Type II reflected an underlying degenerative process or a developmental impairment. In contrast, patients with positive schizophrenia (type I schizophrenia) had normal brain structures, good response to treatment, and better outcomes. Andreasen and Olsen (1982) further elaborated the syndromal concept of schizophrenia by contributing definitive psychopathological descriptions of the two domains. They proposed that positive-symptom patients and negative-symptom patients can be classified into two distinct categories. However, this dichotomous typological approach was later found not to be valid because many patients could not be classified as belonging to either category and in fact showed features of both syndromes (Andreasen et al. 1990; Kay 1990).

A heuristically fruitful approach is to consider the positive and negative syndromes as representing different psychopathological dimensions rather than coexclusive subtypes of schizophrenia (Kay 1990). The two syndromes differ in their association with premorbid functioning, family history of illness, cognitive profile, and neurological signs.

Another important reason for the development and renewed research interest in the characteristics of positive and negative syndromes was the development of rating scales for the assessment of schizophrenia symptoms, which used the subdivision into positive and negative symptoms (see Andreasen 1982; Fenton and McGlashan 1992; Kay et al. 1987; Moller et al. 1994): Brief Psychiatric Rating Scale (BPRS; Overall and Gorham 1962), an 18-item symptom scale that includes a more narrow set of schizophrenia symptoms; and the Scale for the Assessment of Positive Symptoms (SAPS) and the Scale for the Assessment of Negative Symptoms (SANS) (Andreasen 1982), consisting of 35 and 29 items, respectively. The SAPS includes five subscales of symptoms (hallucinations, delusions, bizarre behavior, positive formal thought disorder, and inappropriate affect), whereas the SANS includes five areas of negative symptoms (affective flattening or blunting, alogia, avolition-apathy, anhedonia-asociality, attention).

Similarly, Kay and colleagues (1987) created the Positive and Negative Syndrome Scale (PANSS), consisting of three subscales measuring 7 positive, 7 negative, and 16 general psychopathology symptoms. Both scales have developed precise operationalized item descriptions with defined levels of severity. They have shown excellent reliability and internal and external validity, resulting in their wide use in research and treatment studies.

The traditional positive-negative distinction of schizophrenic phenomenology is incomplete and must be enlarged to include other, in part nonoverlapping, syndromal domains, such as cognitive and affective symptoms. A number of studies have examined the symptom presentation of large samples of patients with schizophrenia using factor analysis of symptoms assessed with the newer symptom scales. These studies have resulted in a number of expanded syndromal models of schizophrenia.

Most factor analyses based on the SAPS and the SANS have suggested a clustering of schizophrenia symptoms into three factors (Andreasen et al. 1995; Liddle 1987; Peralta et al. 1992): 1) positive or psychotic cluster (hallucinations, delusions, catatonic symptoms), 2) negative cluster (anhedonia, avolition, poverty of speech, blunted affect), and 3) disorganization cluster (disorganized speech, inappropriate affect, bizarre behavior). Using the PANSS,

Lindenmayer et al. (1994) proposed a five-factor model of schizophrenia, consisting of a positive factor (delusions, hallucinatory behavior, grandiosity, unusual thought content, suspiciousness/persecution), a negative factor (blunted affect, emotional withdrawal, poor rapport, passive/apathetic social withdrawal, lack of spontaneity, active social avoidance), an excitement factor (excitement, hostility, uncooperativeness, poor impulse control), a cognitive factor (conceptual disorganization, difficulty with abstract thinking, disorientation, poor attention, preoccupation), and a depression/anxiety factor (anxiety, guilt feelings, tension, depression). This model has proved to be very robust across various phases of the illness, cross-culturally and longitudinally, as well as stable after antipsychotic treatments (Lindenmayer et al. 1995; Marder et al. 1997; Peralta et al. 1992; Toomey et al. 1997; White et al. 1997). In addition, it is heuristically plausible that each psychopathological syndromal dimension relates to an underlying pathophysiological abnormality, which in turn may be associated to one or more liability genes. This approach also has the advantage of accommodating the apparent continuity of some clinical manifestations seen in disorders represented in the schizophrenia spectrum concept. The syndromal approach furthermore allows for the evaluation of treatment interventions on each one of the psychopathological domains separately and to define comorbidity phenomena more appropriately.

Refining the negative syndrome concept further, Carpenter and colleagues (1988, 1991) called attention to the differences between primary negative symptoms and secondary negative symptoms. Primary negative symptoms are thought to be expressions of the avolitional aspects of schizophrenia, to fluctuate less over the course of the illness, to be less responsive to situational changes, and to rarely remit (Carpenter and Kirkpatrick 1988). Secondary negative symptoms are reversible and often caused by drug effects (e.g., extrapyramidal symptoms), depression, or absence of stimulation. Carpenter and Kirkpatrick (1988) also proposed referring to primary negative symptoms as "deficit symptoms."

In the next sections, we describe in detail positive symptoms, negative symptoms, cognitive symptoms, excitement symptoms, and symptoms of depression and anxiety in schizophrenia.

POSITIVE SYMPTOMS

CONCEPT OF POSITIVE SYMPTOMS

Positive symptoms of schizophrenia are symptoms that are in excess of or distortions of normal functions—specifically additions to normal thoughts, emotions, or behaviors (Weiden et al. 1999). Because of their relatively easier recognition and easier quantitative assessment, positive symptoms, more than negative symptoms, have been used in the past in diagnostic classificatory systems. Positive symptoms can be present throughout the different phases of the disorder, from the prodromal phase to the acute psychotic phase and, to a lesser degree, the more stable postpsychotic or residual phase. Positive symptoms are generally the targets of treatment with antipsychotic medications and are considered to be treatment responsive.

DELUSIONS

Delusions are false beliefs about which a person is firmly convinced and is impervious to outside contradictory evidence. Delusions must be distinguished from a person's religious or cultural beliefs. Generally, the latter are also held by the group or community of people who form the individual's religious or cultural group and do not interfere with day-to-day functioning as delusions often do in patients with schizophrenia.

Delusional perception may be an important starting point for the development of a system of delusional ideas. An abnormal significance, usually in the sense of self-reference, despite the absence of any emotional or logical reason, is attributed to a normal perception (Fish 1984). For example, an individual with schizophrenia observes that the traffic light is switching from green to red and concludes that it means to him personally that an outside force is telling him to curb his homosexual interests. Such primary delusional experiences will then be expanded and elaborated into a group of secondary delusions. At times, these delusions will be highly systematized and complex, centering on one or two themes. Systematized delusions are usually seen in patients who are cognitively intact and who function quite well outside an acute episode.

Delusions in their mildest form may be questioned by the individual and persist for weeks to months (Andreasen 1984). The presence of bizarre delusions, which are entirely inconsistent with shared social realism and are illogical to most people, are recognized by DSM-IV-TR as being sufficient as a characteristic symptom (Cluster A) to qualify for schizophrenia, underlining the weight this symptom is attributed in the diagnosis of schizophrenia. Examples of bizarre delusions include an individual reporting his heart is missing or that aliens are seeking that individual to rule their planet.

Differential Diagnosis of Delusions

Other psychotic disorders. Delusions found in other psychotic disorders are at times not easy to differentiate from those found in schizophrenia. These conditions include delusional disorder, shared psychotic disorder (folie à deux), and acute psychotic disorder. Delusions in these disorders are usually nonbizarre and center on one or two themes. These delusions may have been started by a small and/or real slight in the person's life and then become elaborated and embedded in a paranoid delusional system. These individuals often get involved in extensive letter writing campaigns, litigiousness, and legal actions to seek redress of perceived delusional wrongs.

These disorders are chronic except for acute psychotic disorder, which has a duration of less than 6 months. The person's functioning is usually not markedly impaired, but hostility and violence may at times be associated. There are no hallucinatory experiences or marked thought disorders, and affect is usually well preserved. Delusions of jealousy may be included in which there are unconfirmed and unfounded thoughts that a person is being disloyal or treacherous within a relationship. The delusions are usually accompanied by attempts to find evidence to support the delusional belief. Individuals with delusions of jealousy are not satisfied until evidence is obtained, which can sometimes lead to violent episodes with a significant other (Soyka et al. 1991).

Capgras syndrome.   Named for its discoverer, the French psychiatrist Jean Marie Joseph Capgras (1873–1950), this syndrome is characterized by a belief that people in one's life (e.g., family members, doctors, close friends) have been replaced by exact doubles. Those afflicted may even believe that they themselves are represented somewhere by a double they never see. The persons who are not replaced are always identified accurately. Capgras syndrome is also referred to as delusional misidentification, illusion of doubles, illusion of negative doubles, misidentification syndrome, nonrecognition syndrome, phantom double syndrome, and subjective doubles syndrome. In about 35% of patients diagnosed with the Capgras syndrome or related substitution delusions, the syndrome has an organic etiology (Alexander et al. 1979; Ellis et al. 1997).

Organic delusional syndrome.   DSM-IV-TR places organic delusional syndrome (ICD-9-Clinical Modification [CM]; World Health Organization 1978) under psychotic disorder due to general medical condition with delusions. The psychotic disturbance is identifiable from history, physical examination, or laboratory results. The delusions are the unequivocal physiological corollary of a general medical condition. Whereas multiple delusions can be present in these syndromes, they are accompanied typically by disorientation, confusion, and memory impairments, which determine the correct diagnosis. In addition, hallucinatory experiences often complete the clinical picture.

Affective disorder with psychotic features. Delusions in manic or depressive states are usually mood-congruent—that is, they are consistent with the underlying mood, both for the manic state (inflated worth, power, wealth) and for the depressive state (guilt, death, deserving punishment).

Types of Delusions

Persecutory delusions. Individuals afflicted with persecutory delusions believe they are being conspired or discriminated against, threatened, or intentionally victimized. The conspiracy or victimization can be by someone familiar to them (e.g., a family member, friend, doctor, or nurse), someone in the media (e.g., a television personality), a powerful external organization (e.g., the FBI, KGB, or CIA), religious figures such as the devil, or extraterrestrial forces. Persecutory delusions are among the most common symptoms of schizophrenia, although they can also be seen in delusional disorder, psychotic depression, and organic delusional syndromes. Particularly, delusions with mood incongruent or idiosyncratic content are seen in persons with schizophrenia. Individuals sometimes report opposite influences, resulting in a persecutory delusional conviction of being controlled by opposing outside forces, such as God or the devil, matter and antimatter, the sun and the moon, or positive and negative electron charges. Individuals may be convinced that there are sophisticated electronic devices secretly hidden in all areas of their surroundings that spy on them and monitor their every movement. The delusions can be systematized and can lead to inappropriate or irresponsible actions jeopardizing the safety of the individual or others.

EXAMPLE

Mr. A felt that he was under constant government surveillance through planted microphones and hidden cameras in the ceiling and was receiving through electronic devices irritating high-frequency tones affecting his arms and legs. These tones were interfering with his functioning and his relationships with others. He believed that all were involved in this plot, which ultimately was designed to kill him because he was a spy.

Delusions of reference. Individuals with delusions of reference attach a personal meaning to the actions, remarks, and statements of other people, and to objects or events when in fact there is none. A common example is an individual's belief that a television program is specifically directed at him or her. There is a conviction of certitude that the individual's observation is absolutely correct without the need of any corroboration by others or any other supporting evidence. In contrast, when a nondelusional individual is unsure that the remark, action, or statement is referring to him or her, the person will be suspicious and will be able to acknowledge that the idea is misguided.

The content of a delusion of reference is often idiosyncratic and can be derogatory, persecutory, or enhancing of one's self-worth.

Delusions of being controlled.   Individuals with delusions of control feel that an outside force or agency is controlling or manipulating their thoughts, feelings, or parts of their body. These delusions are also referred to as delusions of passivity and are often associated with somatic hallucinations. Patients may use them as delusional explanations of abnormal somatic sensations.

EXAMPLE

A person with schizophrenia responded to the question: Is somebody influencing your mind or your head? "Yes, they have a weapon that the CIA and the Defense Department use. They use microwaves. They send them inside your head. They convert these from analog to digital. They pick up your thoughts and they change you to another person."

Thought insertion.   Individuals with thought insertion believe that some of their thoughts are not their own but have been implanted by an outside agency. Often, there is a persecutory theme and a sense that their thoughts are controlled or manipulated by an outside agency. The condition differs from the symptoms of obsessive-compulsive patients, where patients may be distraught by recurrent intrusive thoughts but are certain that these thoughts originate from their own mind and not by an outside force. In schizophrenia, individuals misplace their own intentions and attribute them to an agency or to someone else (Frith et al. 1992).

Thought withdrawal and thought broadcasting.   The individual believes that thoughts have been taken out of his or her mind. Further, the individual can often trace the initial experience of a thought and then the incident of that thought being removed. In thought broadcasting, one's thoughts are passively transmitted to others, often through electronic or telepathic means.

Delusions of sin or guilt.   Individuals with delusions of sin or guilt believe that they have committed a terrible crime. These delusions can manifest themselves as a minor error in the past that the individual believes may lead to a major disaster or divine retribution that can also affect his or her family. They may also be associated with grandiose ideas that the committed sin will destroy the whole world and also may be associated with delusions of nihilism. The content of these delusions usually is bizarre and mostly mood incongruent. In contrast, delusions of sin and guilt that are seen in severe depressive episodes with psychotic symptoms are usually comprehensible and ego-syntonic (i.e., referring to a person's personality aspects, thoughts, or behaviors that are viewed by the person as acceptable). In persons with psychotic depression, these mood-congruent delusions are usually associated with vegetative symptoms of depression, ideas of hopelessness, worthlessness, and possibly suicidal ideation.

EXAMPLE

An individual with schizophrenia believed that he had killed millions of Jews during World War II, although he was born after 1945. He stated that he felt he was worse than Hitler; in fact, he believed he was the greatest killer in the world and deserved punishment for his deeds.

Grandiose delusions. Individuals who experience delusions of grandiosity believe they have extraordinary powers, wealth, fame, or talents. They may think they are religious saviors, world leaders, or famous persons. Grandiose delusions in the extreme can affect behavior, be acted upon, and lead to irresponsible or dangerous and even deadly actions (e.g., believing that one has the ability to fly and stepping out of a window). Grandiose delusions are also seen in individuals with mania with psychosis. Other manic features, such as elated mood, hyperactivity and expansiveness, flight of ideas, and accelerated speech, will help in the differential diagnosis.

EXAMPLE

An individual displaying grandiose delusions answered to a question regarding whether he had any special talents: "I am very famous. I am known in London and Paris as an inventor; I have invented candy bars, which bear my name. They are writing a book about me."

Somatic delusions. Somatic delusions consist of preoccupations that a body part is diseased or malfunctions without objective medical evidence. The delusion can involve a false belief in a medical condition or physical deformity. These delusions are at times associated with kinesthetic hallucinations representing abnormal somatic perceptions supporting the delusional somatic belief. Somatic delusions must be differentiated from hypochondriacal preoccupations, which are exaggerated fears of somatic illness and tend not to be bizarre as in the case of schizophrenic somatic delusions. Further, hypochondriacal preoccupations are not attributed to external forces. In contrast to the hypochondriacal individual, the person with schizophrenia reacts to rather significant but delusionally held medical morbidity remarkably calmly.

EXAMPLE

An individual with schizophrenia answered to a question regarding his health: "Not good. I have my nostrils clogged, which is affecting my brain. A spear flew into my nose, made out of plastic, and went into my brain and has affected my mood; it made me down and depressed."

HALLUCINATORY EXPERIENCES

A hallucination is defined as a sensory perception in the absence of any externally generated stimulus or perception. Certain abnormal sensory perceptions are reported as distinct from actual hallucinations and could be called "prehallucinatory experiences." They include hypersensitivity to sound, light, smells, misperceptions of movements, and changes in the perception of people's faces or bodies. These abnormal perceptions are often seen during the prodromal phase of schizophrenia.

Auditory Hallucinations

Auditory hallucinations are the most common type of hallucinations observed in individuals with schizophrenia. Auditory hallucinations are usually voices that often comment on the person's everyday activities, that may be threatening, or that, in rare cases, command the individual to execute an action (Andreasen et al. 1995; Mueser et al. 1990). Less frequently, the hallucinations are sounds other than voices. Voices may be heard from inside one's head or may appear to come from the outside. They may be perceived as being as clear as the voice of the interviewer, or less frequently, they are muffled and difficult to understand. Usually, the sentence structure of the voices is clear, although at times, when the voices consist of insults or accusations, they may be just short, monosyllabic words. Often voices are accusatory, hostile, or unfriendly. They consist of a string of sentences, may be continuous, and may occur every day. Occasionally, as with delusional beliefs of powerful opposite forces, patients may report "good" and "bad" voices. The response to auditory hallucinations may vary. In acute stages of the illness, patients may be terrified. They may be seen to respond in an audible fashion to auditory hallucinations or, if in distress about them, to scream or yell at them. In more chronic stages of the illness patients will display little affect or emotional responses to what would appear to the interviewer to be rather terrifying voices. The execution of commands transmitted by auditory hallucinations is rare, although some patients will follow the instructions that can lead to suicidal or homicidal actions.

Auditory hallucinations are reported by 50%–70% of patients with schizophrenia (Andreasen and Flaum 1991; Hoffman et al. 2003; Sartorius et al. 1974). Patients with schizophrenia rarely present auditory hallucinations in isolation. The hallucinations are usually associated with delusional interpretations, which may be attempts at explaining abnormal perceptions or, conversely, be elaborations of a delusional paranoid system. In fact, single auditory hallucinations (elementary hallucination) should alert the clinician to look for another, nonschizophrenia diagnosis. Auditory hallucinations in individuals with psychotic depression tend to consist of short sentences and are mood congruent.

Auditorization of thoughts refers to instances when individuals report that they hear their thoughts aloud in their head. They can clearly describe this phenomenon and at times are able to differentiate these loud thoughts from ordinary silent thoughts. It is possible that auditorization of thoughts is a precursor of auditory hallucinations.

Visual Hallucinations

Individuals with visual hallucinations observe people, shapes, colors, and objects that are not physically present. Visual hallucinations are less frequent in individuals with schizophrenia compared with those with delirium. Visual hallucinations tend to be associated with delusional interpretation of threatening or persecutory themes, or, in the context of religious delusions, they are seen as visions of religiously meaningful figures. The major differential diagnosis is with visual hallucinations encountered in organic and delirious states. The latter hallucinations are more elementary in nature, often represent animals, and may be accompanied by tactile hallucinations. The presence of significant cognitive impairment (e.g., disorientation) will help to rule in an organic etiology.

Somatic and Tactile Hallucinations

Somatic and tactile hallucinations involve physical sensations, for example, of being touched by another person, object, or animal, or a perception that one's body has been altered in some way. These hallucinations are also known as *haptic* or *kinesthetic hallucinations* and consist of the perception of heat, cold, or electricity shocks. The individual can also experience somatic passivity, in which the patient believes that an outside agent has caused him or her to be a passive receiver of unwanted bodily sensations, for example a burning sensation in the brain or a sensation of being raped.

Olfactory Hallucinations

Olfactory hallucinations are sensations, such as unusual smells, that no one else around the individual experiences. Often, olfactory hallucinations are related to gustatory hallucinations, in which the individual may describe unusual tastes like sweet, salty, bitter, or odd flavors (Carter 1992). These hallucinations are often associated with a persecutory theme. Olfactory hallucinations can also be seen in temporal lobe epilepsy ("uncinate fits"), in which they are usually accompanied by an altered state of consciousness with altered perception and occurring in a paroxysmal context.

BIZARRE BEHAVIOR

Some individuals with schizophrenia behave in unusual and eccentric ways or transgress social mores. For example, they may talk to themselves, walk backward, laugh suddenly without explanation, make unnatural faces, mimic behaviors, masturbate in public, engage in repetitive behaviors, express manneristic speech patterns, or maintain a rigid posture for an extensive period of time. Bizarre behavior is generally found in individuals with disorganized or catatonic schizophrenia.

Clothing and Appearance

Some individuals with schizophrenia may dress in an uncommon manner or modify their appearance in an eccentric fashion but more often neglect their appearance, which results in disheveled clothing, an unkempt look, and lack of personal hygiene. Patients often may overdress during warm weather.

Social and Sexual Behavior

Individuals' social and sexual behavior may at times represent a deviation from the norm. For example, masturbating in public, mimicking the behaviors of others, and spontaneous laughter or sudden outbursts may occur.

Motor Behavior

Bizarre motor behavior can involve unusual mannerisms, grimacing, or rocking movements. Stereotyped and ritualistic movements can be observed. Catatonic motor behavior is an extreme form of bizarre behavior that can include maintaining a rigid or unnatural posture with an awkward, stilted, disorganized appearance, and resisting efforts to be moved or engaging in purposeless and unstimulated motor activity. Waxy flexibility, a rare form of catatonic motor behavior, consists of maintenance of postures that the examiner has induced in the individual. An important differential diagnostic issue in assessing stereotyped movements is the recognition of involuntary movements caused by tardive dyskinesia. These neurological involuntary movements may look purposeless, repetitive, and stereotypical, but they have characteristic features and are usually located in the extremities or lingual and perioral areas.

Inappropriate Affect

This affective dysfunction is at times incorrectly classified under flat affect; however, it reflects not an absence of affect, but rather incongruity of affect. Affect expression is misplaced and does not correspond to the ideational content the person is expressing at the time. Sudden and unexpected discharges of affect may occur. The patient may smile while talking about a sad topic or may unexpectedly burst out in anger when discussing a minor psychological insult.

NEGATIVE SYMPTOMS

CONCEPT OF NEGATIVE SYMPTOMS

Negative symptoms are a frequent and persistent characteristic of schizophrenia. They can emerge as early as during the prodromal stage of the disorder, long before the presentation of the first psychotic episode (Hafner et al. 1995). It is generally accepted that there are primary and secondary negative symptoms (Carpenter and Kirkpatrick 1988; Tandon and Greden 1989). *Primary negative symptoms* are deficit symptoms that may precede psychosis onset and usually persist between the episodes. These symptoms include primary anhedonia, flattening and narrowing of affect, poverty of speech, avolition, and reduced social activity (Carpenter and Kirkpatrick 1988).

Secondary negative symptoms are "nondeficit" symptoms and are hypothesized to correlate with psychotic episodes, depression or demoralization, and medication side effects (Carpenter et al. 1991). Secondary negative symptoms usually respond to treatment of the underlying cause.

COURSE OF NEGATIVE SYMPTOMS

Studies generally show that negative symptoms are more stable than positive symptoms over time and are less likely to improve over the course of illness (Addington and Addington 1991; Crow 1981; Hull et al. 1997; Kay et al. 1986; Lindenmayer et al. 1984; Pfohl and Winokur 1982). In a longitudinal study of symptoms, Arndt and colleagues (1995) found that negative symptoms were already prominent at the time of the individuals' first episode and remained relatively stable for approximately 2 years in which the individuals were followed. Hafner et al. (1999), exploring five SANS measures of negative symptoms, found that in a sample of 115 first episodes of schizophrenia, alogia, attention, affect, abulia, and anhedonia persisted over a 5-year period. Similarly, Amador and colleagues (1999) presented evidence for a high degree of stability of primary negative symptoms over an approximate 4-year follow-up period. Negative symptoms are often associated with impairment of general intellectual ability and executive function, including verbal fluency and performance on tasks such as the Wisconsin Card Sorting Test, measuring general reasoning ability.

SPECIFIC NEGATIVE SYMPTOMS

Blunted or Flat Affect

Blunted or flat affect is characterized by an absence and diminution of emotional reaction to stimuli. Some affected individuals show fewer emotions (e.g., anger, pleasure, sadness), whereas others exhibit a total lack of facial expression (Salem and Kring 1999). However, despite this lack of affect these individuals report sensations of positive and negative emotions (Kring and Neale 1996). An important differential diagnosis is pseudoparkinsonism (masked facies) induced by antipsychotic medication.

The individual shows decreased spontaneous movements and may maintain the same posture, with fewer shifts in body position for some time when sitting. Movements of limbs when walking are reduced. There is also a paucity of expressive gestures. The individual is unable to show emotion by the use of gestures when responding to stimuli. For example, there is a reduction in the use of hand gestures in conjunction with speech to emphasize or enhance the meaning of accompanying speech. The individual avoids direct eye contact or may appear to be staring when responding verbally. The individual lacks vocal inflections and is unable to show emotions by varying the tone of voice. Speech is characterized by a monotonic quality, and words are not emphasized (Andreasen 1983).

Poor Rapport

Signs of poor rapport include avoidance of eye contact, lack of responsiveness to questions, and reduced verbal and nonverbal communication of personal information with others. Individuals with poor rapport show a lack of interpersonal empathy, a reduced interaction in conversation, and a lack or total avoidance of interactions with others.

Passive/Apathetic Social Withdrawal

Individuals with passive or apathetic social withdrawal have fewer social interactions with others, which can eventually result in a lack of speech (alogia). There is a reduction in social activity and a decrease in interest in forming close relationships. The individual's interaction with others may be brief and superficial. There may be few or no friends, and most of their time is spent isolated from others. This has also been referred to as *asociality* or *apathy*.

Reduced sexual interests and activities.   There is a lack of, or impairment in, sexual interests and activities. Individuals may report minimal sexual drive or express a lack of enjoyment from sexual activities (Andreasen 1983).

Inability to feel intimacy and closeness.   The individual is unable to form a close relationship with others, and there is an inability to recognize others' emotional needs (Mueser et al. 1996). This results in a lack of mutuality in relationships.

Stereotyped Thinking

Individuals with stereotyped thinking show repetitive or barren thoughts that may infringe and interfere with their thinking. The individual maintains rigid beliefs that may appear unreasonable or excessive. Conversations revolve around a recurrent theme, and the individual is unable to shift to a new topic. There is an impoverishment in the amount of nuances and intermediate positions between extreme statements. At the extreme, the individual's conversation is limited to only a few topics or to repetitive and rigid demands or statements that severely impair the amount and content of conversation.

Alogia

Alogia refers to deficient fluency or productivity of thought and speech associated with avolition or apathy. Individuals with alogia demonstrate a restriction in the amount of spontaneous speech and respond to questions with brief, concrete, and unembellished answers. In some instances, the individual does not respond to questions or responses are monosyllabic. Leading questions are constantly needed by the interviewer to proceed with the conversation. Harvey and colleagues (1997) suggest that poverty of speech is more common and more severe in geriatric patients with schizophrenia, perhaps as a result of cognitive and biological factors.

Poverty of content of speech.   The individual's speech is adequate in amount but expresses little information because it is vague, excessively abstract or concrete, repetitive, or stereotyped.

Increased latency of response.   The individual takes a longer time to respond to questions than normal and may appear distant or preoccupied when asked a question.

Avolition and Apathy

Avolition and apathy appear as a distinctive lack of energy, drive, or interest in initiating activities and a lack of persistence in pursuing activities as well as social interactions. An individual with avolition and apathy shows a lack of motivation in completing tasks and a lack of initiative or goals. He or she has few interests and reduced investment in personal activities. When asked about current world events, the individual may only be partially aware of events and know only limited details about them. The individual participates in few or no activities or only engages in passive activities such as watching television.

EXAMPLE

Individuals with chronic schizophrenia on an inpatient psychiatric unit in New York City were exposed to both ample television and newspaper coverage of the World Trade Center attack in New York on September 11, 2001. During group discussions in the aftermath of the tragedy it became clear that patients took relatively little notice of the event, that their emotional response was limited, and that there were few spontaneous verbal expressions about this event.

An important differential diagnostic concern is anhedonia found in states of depression. Anhedonia associated with depression is accompanied by the usual symptoms of depression, such as ideas of hopelessness, worthlessness, and helplessness, together with the vegetative signs of depression.

Grooming and hygiene.   The individual displays a lack of interest in grooming and hygiene. This trait is characterized by sloppy, obsolete, blemished attire, and infrequent daily hygienic activities such as washing hands, combing one's hair, and brushing one's teeth.

Impersistence at work or school.   The individual has difficulty seeking or maintaining employment or does not complete tasks in school or work.

Physical anergia.   The individual has a tendency to be physically inert. When encouraged, the individual participates briefly and then reverts to immobility. The individual shows a lack of drive or spontaneous activity.

DEFICIT STATES OF SCHIZOPHRENIA

The concept of *deficit schizophrenia* was introduced to distinguish a relatively homogeneous subgroup of individuals within schizophrenia. Deficit schizophrenia is characterized by persistent primary negative symptoms such as restricted affect, diminished emotional range, poverty of speech, curbing of interests, and reduced sense of purpose and social drive. Kirkpatrick and colleagues (2001) found that deficit schizophrenia exists among 15% of first-episode individuals and among 25%–30% of those with chronic schizophrenia. The clinical features of schizophrenic deficit states refer to the cohesive and idiopathic set of signs and symptoms as presented in the Schedule for Deficit Syndromes (Kirkpatrick et al. 1989).

COGNITIVE SYMPTOMS: CONCEPTUAL DISORGANIZATION/ FORMAL THOUGHT DISORDER

Schizophrenic thought disorder is often included under the rubric of positive symptoms, although recent research suggests that it represents an independent dimension of symptomatology in schizophrenia (Andreasen and Olsen 1982; Kay 1990; Liddle 1987; Lindenmayer et al. 1994; Peralta et al. 1992; Thompson and Meltzer 1993). This discrete dimension has been variably called "disorganization factor," "cognitive factor," or "thought disorder factor."

DEFINITIONS AND CLASSIFICATION

Disturbance of thinking is a cardinal and almost constant symptom of schizophrenia. It describes a persistent underlying disturbance of conscious thought and is recognized largely by its effects on speech and writing. Bleuler (1911/ 1950) believed that "peculiar association disturbances" were fundamental features of schizophrenia.

There is abundant literature on the formal thought and language pathology in schizophrenia. It can be grouped into pathology of word use and pathology of sentence use. According to Oppenheimer (1971), "A word evolves from the lowest level of its meaningless sound quality to the highest level of its metaphorical meaning. Between these levels are, in descending order, connotation, denotation, and verbalization" (p. 228). In schizophrenia there can be deficits in any one of these levels of word formation, such as desymbolization of words, expansions of the meaning of a word, conceptual contaminations, and neologisms. In pathological use of sentences, individuals may not be able to exclude words or ideas that belong to different semantic categories, resulting in a disorganized structure of the sentence appearing as loosening of associations. Adherence to the appropriate mental set or context of a sentence may be incomplete and results in tangentiality.

Thought disorders have been grouped into two categories by Andreasen (1982) and Cutting and Murphy (1988): 1) intrinsic disturbance of thinking (e.g., concreteness) and 2) disordered language and speech (e.g., derailment or tangentiality).

Mechanisms of Thought Disorder

Thought disorder is not a unitary concept; it can be better conceptualized in terms of its multidimensional makeup (Cuesta and Peralta 1999). Recent attempts to understand the cognitive underpinnings of thought disorder in schizophrenia have focused on abnormalities in attention, on problems in the use of contextual cues, and on impairments of executive functions. Finally, the role of impairments in executive functions underlying thought disorder is illustrated in detail in Chapter 4, "Neurocognitive Impairments," of this book.

Measurement of Thought Disorder

Careful listening to the word productions and sentence construction of individuals with schizophrenia allows for assessing thought disorder. Difficulty in abstract thinking and concrete thinking can be measured with proverb interpretations and similarities. Proverb interpretation challenges the individual's ability in abstract-symbolic thinking, in shifting of sets, and in the ability to generalize. The task of establishing similarities reveals difficulties in classification and categorization. Object-sorting tasks can be used to assess overinclusion; an overinclusive reply would include too many or unsuitable items within a group of items. The thought disorder index evaluates the verbal productions of schizophrenic patients in an unstructured interaction (Hurt et al. 1983).

The assessment of thought, language, and communication (Andreasen 1979a, 1979b) offers a clinical rating for a series of different types of thought disorders. In addition, the SAPS (Andreasen 1982), the SANS (Andreasen 1982), and the PANSS (Kay et al. 1987), frequently used to assess symptoms in schizophrenia research, provide for some measures of thought disorder.

Types of Thought Disorders

Derailment (Loosening of Associations)

Derailment occurs when an individual's speech shows loss of logical or meaningful connections between words or sentences. The relationship between sentences may be indirect or may not be present at all. The individual is also unaware of the lack of association between sentences.

Example

An individual with schizophrenia responded to the request to interpret the proverb "Don't cry over spilt milk": "I believe you should release the tension now of all milk on the ground. I think you should cry over spilt milk. I think you should release yourself after all that milk is on the ground. You should let it out in tears. You know you hold it inside and you could explode a lot, all of these little things kept inside."

Tangentiality

Tangentiality is a disruption in the associative thought process in which one tends to deviate readily and gradually from the topic under discussion to other topics, which arise in the course of associations, but connections are still recognizable by the listener.

EXAMPLE

An individual with schizophrenia complained about a clinician whom she felt made homosexual advances toward her: "She was a pervert homosexual, and she said I was her red painted lady in the closet, and that I knew nothing about this world. But I went to the library and found the red Bible and read up on it, in a hurry. And it was a lie."

Incoherence

Incoherence refers to sentence patterns that are unintelligible and incomprehensible because of total loss of logical connections. At times there are periods of coherent parts that are incorporated in an incoherent sentence. Incoherence can also occur at a semantic level, in which words are substituted in a phrase or sentence and the meaning is distorted. Conjunctions and adjectives can also be deleted (Andreasen 1984). In extreme situations, incoherence can also be referred to as *word salad*.

EXAMPLE

An individual is asked, "How do you feel today?" He responds, "I'm feeling that people say doctors are wrong. In Europe, there was a meeting. The president of the United States, it was AIDS. But in Iraq the man pulled it out with the money under the train tracks. Save yourself, help yourself." The individual is unable to join the associated concepts of each sentence into one coherent response that would convey a comprehensible meaning to the listener. He shifts sets inappropriately, and there is no relationship among sentences. He is unable to include any logical causality.

Illogicality

Individuals who show illogicality respond to questions without a logical rationalization. Examples are non sequiturs, in which the individual formulates an illogical response to a logical question, and faulty inductive inferences, in which the individual makes conclusions based on incoherent assertions (Andreasen 1984).

Circumstantiality

Circumstantiality refers to a disturbance in the thought process, in which the individual gives an unwarranted amount of details, which are frequently tangential, elaborate, and irrelevant, and finds it difficult to make a direct statement or give a direct answer to a question. Circumstantial speech eventually returns to the original topic.

EXAMPLE

In the following example, a man with schizophrenia uses circumstantiality and tangentiality in response to a question about his overall life philosophy. "You have to be modern and you have to be sophisticated, you have to have a girlfriend, you have to go to church. You have to have your name in the Bible. You go out with your wife or fiancée. And you have to learn, should be married, and be a good neighbor."

Clanging

Clanging consists of usage of the sound of a word or its phonetic resemblance (clang equivalence) rather than its meaning, which is substituted for the correct word. Some individuals speak only in rhymes, and others will engage in repetitive speech (Capleton 1996) as a substitute for logical associations.

EXAMPLE

An individual with schizophrenia explained: "We are liberal Jewish; however, we speak British, not Yiddish."

Neologism

Neologism is another well-recognized pathology of word use, in which a new nonsensical word is created that often is a condensation or combination of two different words. This is in contrast to the creative use of neologisms in everyday language, which elicits in the listener amusement or understanding.

EXAMPLE

An individual who considered himself to be overweight, reported to have an "altership." Asked about its meaning, he explained: "It is me at 177 pounds; then I will be Sonny Boy, a rock star."

Difficulty in Abstract Thinking

Difficulty in abstract thinking is reflected in impairment of symbolic ability to think beyond concrete and egocentric thinking, which leads to difficulties in proverb interpretation and in generalizations. There may be the inverse tendency to be overly abstract and to use stilted or manneristic language. In mental status exams, proverb interpretations are commonly used to evaluate an individual's ability to think abstractly.

EXAMPLE

In interpreting the proverb "Don't cry over spilt milk," an individual with schizophrenia stated: "Don't cry over spilt milk are the decisions we make about the decision-making process. The essence of men making decisions." Another example of overly abstract, stilted speech: "The barrister comported himself utterly brusque when I previously inspected his interface with his patron."

Echolalia

Some schizophrenia patients exhibit echolalia by repeating words, phrases, fragments, or sounds that were presented to them. Related to this is *echopraxia*, in which the individual repeats or imitates observed gestures or physical expressions.

Thought Blocking

Thought blocking refers to cessation or complete interruption in the flow of the stream of thought. It can be interrupted suddenly, and there is a disruption in the flow of conversation. Thought blocking can be recognized when disruptions in speech are abrupt, prominent, and continual. The individual may describe it as a sudden and inclusive "draining of the brain."

POOR ATTENTION

Individuals with schizophrenia often present with poor concentration, distractibility from internal or external stimuli, and difficulties in shifting focus to new stimuli. Individuals will exhibit impaired attention, particularly in the acute psychotic phase. Scanning the environment during a clinical interview rather than focusing on the interviewer's questions may be seen during the interview. It may be difficult for the individual to follow a more complex set of questions, and he or she may lose track of an interviewer's question. In another situation, the individual may not be able to respond to a new topic being introduced and will continue to talk about the previous topic, totally oblivious to the new inquiry.

EXCITEMENT SYMPTOMS: HOSTILITY AND AGGRESSION

Symptoms contributing to this domain of psychopathology of schizophrenia are hostility, excitement, uncooperativeness, and poor impulse control. We address in this section predominantly the symptoms of hostility and aggression.

Hostility and aggression in schizophrenia involve verbal and nonverbal expressions of anger and resentment, including sarcasm, passive-aggressive behavior, verbal abuse and assaultiveness, irritability, suspicion, and uncooperativeness (Volavka 2002). Hostility/aggression in schizophrenia is difficult to predict (Monahan et al. 2000; Steadman et al. 1998; Wallace et al. 1998) and can be both a trait and state phenomenon.

The probability of violent behavior among individuals with mental disorders is greater than that of the general population. There is an increased risk of violence among individuals with schizophrenia based on examination of criminal records (Hodgins 1992; Wessely et al. 1994), results of a twin study (Coid et al. 1993), and data from persons who committed homicide (Eronen et al. 1996). Although individuals with mental disorders certainly do not carry out most violent crimes, they are at increased jeopardy for committing them (Citrome and Volavka 1999). Evidence exists for an increased incidence of hostile and aggressive behavior in schizophrenia, estimated at 2–10 times that of the general population (Hafner and Boker 1982; Wessely 1997). Results of the Epidemiologic Catchment Area project reported that the probabilities of violent behavior in schizophrenia were 5.3 times greater for males and 5.9 times greater for females than in individuals with no diagnosed mental disorder (Regier et al. 1990).

Causes of Aggressive Behavior in Schizophrenia

Causes of aggressive behavior are complex and multifactorial. Some important underlying causes are the presence of comorbid substance abuse, substance dependence, and intoxication (Citrome and Volavka 2001; Steadman et al. 1998). In addition, the disease process itself produces hallucinations and delusions, which may provoke violence (Citrome and Volavka 1999). Krakowski and Czobor (1997), in a study examining psychosis and ward turmoil in schizophrenic inpatients, reported that persistent violence, in contrast to episodic violence, was associated with frontal lobe neurocognitive deficits. Episodic violence was associated with significant florid positive symptoms and tended to abate as positive symptoms improved. Such episodic violence can be related to delusional perceptions that other people are persecuting the individual, against which the individual has to defend him- or herself with a preemptive aggressive act. Environmental factors that are associated with aggressive behavior include a chaotic or unstable home or hospital situation, which may encourage maladaptive aggressive behaviors (Owen et al. 1998).

Assessment

Aggression can be clinically assessed by means of the Overt Aggression Scale (Yudofsky et al. 1986) or the excitement factor of the PANSS, which also includes hostility, uncooperativeness, and poor impulse control. In most studies aggression is measured by using data from different sources (Swanson et al. 2000). Steadman and colleagues (2000) have proposed an actuarial tool for assessing the risk of violence, which has been evaluated in psychiatric inpatients (Monahan et al. 2000).

DIFFERENTIAL DIAGNOSIS

One of the most important differential diagnoses of violent behaviors in individuals with schizophrenia is substance abuse and withdrawal. Substance abuse enhances the probability of aggressive behavior more than schizophrenia alone (Swanson 1994). Aggressive and violent behavior can be triggered by alcohol, cocaine, phencyclidine (PCP), or amphetamine intoxication (Smith and Hucker 1994; Swanson 1994). Additionally, withdrawal from abused substances can lead to hostility and aggressive behavior (Citrome and Volavka 1999; Verhayden et al. 2003). Other less frequent differential diagnostic considerations are medical conditions. Brain injuries, brain tumors, and rarely temporal lobe epilepsies or metabolic disturbances may lead to aggressive behavior in individuals who do not have a prior history of continuous aggressive tendencies.

DEPRESSION, SUICIDE AND SELF-INJURY, AND ANXIETY

DEPRESSION

Symptoms that contribute to the depressive domain of psychopathology in schizophrenia are anxiety, depression, guilt feelings, and tension. Although not uncommon, these symptoms tend to be associated with specific phases of the illness.

Depressive Symptoms in the Course of Schizophrenia

Bottlender and colleagues (2000) found depressive symptoms to be frequent among individuals in a first episode. The ability to distinguish schizophrenia from depression is most difficult early in the course of schizophrenic illness. The prodrome of schizophrenia can resemble depression, and some of the symptoms required in DSM-IV-TR for a major depressive episode (e.g., anhedonia, attention difficulties, psychomotor abnormalities) are common in schizophrenia as well (Andreasen and Flaum 1991). Other differential diagnostic issues to consider include schizoaffective disorder, negative symptoms of schizophrenia, and symptoms of pseudoparkinsonism due to antipsychotic medication effects. Siris (1995) reviewed 30 studies of depression in schizophrenia and found incidence rates ranging from 7% to 65%, with a modal rate of 25% (Hirsch and Jolley 1989; Johnson 1988).

Symptoms of depression can be present in all phases of schizophrenia: during first episodes (Koreen et al. 1993), chronic illness (Leff 1990), relapse, and remission in individuals receiving maintenance antipsychotics (Van Putten 1975). Depression can precede psychosis as prepsychotic depression (Green et al. 1990; McGlashan and Carpenter 1976; Roth 1970), or depression in the course of schizophrenia can be assessed as a result of recovery from an acute psychotic episode (postpsychotic depression). Traditional research has regarded the presence of affective symptoms during the course of schizophrenia to be a favorable predictive factor (Roth 1970; Valliant 1964). Subsequent research, however, has reported that depression in the course of chronic schizophrenia may also display a distinct morbidity and mortality profile that includes poor outcome, reduced social adjustment (Carpenter et al. 1988), increased rates of relapse (Birchwood et al. 1993), treatment noncompliance (Hogarty et al. 1995; Van Putten 1974), and increased risk of suicide (Drake et al. 1986; Miles 1977; Roy et al. 1983; Westermeyer et al. 1991).

Postpsychotic Depressive Disorder

Postpsychotic depression represents both a reaction to the realization of the damage the illness has caused and a reaction of distress to the symptoms of the illness. It occurs in approximately 25% of psychotic patients (Jeczmien et al. 2001) and is characterized by significant anhedonia. McGlashan and Carpenter (1976) were the first to present postpsychotic depressive disorder of schizophrenia as a syndrome in itself, which was subsequently included in DSM-IV as a diagnostic entity for further study.

Siris (1990) has argued that postpsychotic depression has been used to describe clinically diverse types of patients. In one group of individuals, depressive symptoms are clearly present during an acute psychotic episode and resolve as the positive symptoms resolve, although sometimes more slowly (also referred to as "revealed depression"). In other individuals, significant depressive symptoms appear after the acute episode has resolved. The main clinical symptoms are depressed affect and generalized motor slowness (Jeczmien et al. 2001). Also, Cutler and Siris (1991) reported that approximately one-quarter of people with schizophrenic and postpsychotic depression experience panic attacks, indicating that symptoms of anxiety may be part of the clinical profile of postpsychotic depressive disorder. Further studies (Shuwall and Siris 1994) indicated that in postpsychotic depression, the presence of psychosis and anxiety is linked with a higher level of suicidal ideation regardless of the level of depression.

Differentiating Depressive Symptoms From Negative Symptoms

Several studies have suggested that depression may be associated with negative symptoms (Fitzgerald et al. 2002; Kulhara et al. 1989; Norman et al. 1998; Sax et al. 1996). Overlapping features of depressive symptoms and negative symptoms include reduced social and personal interests, reduced pleasure, diminished energy, and loss of motivation, together with psychomotor retardation (Andreasen and Olsen 1982; Bermanzohn and Siris 1992; Carpenter et al. 1985; Crow 1980; Hausmann and. Fleischhacker 2002; Lindenmayer and Kay 1989; Romney and Candido 2001; Siris 2000). Distinguishing features of depressive symptoms are distinct sad mood, disturbance in sleep and appetite, guilt, hopelessness, or suicidal thoughts suggesting depression, while blunted affect suggests negative symptoms (Barnes et al. 1989; Kibel et al. 1993; Kuck et al. 1992; Lindenmayer et al. 1991; Müller et al. 2001; Norman and Malla 1991).

Is Schizoaffective Disorder a Subtype of Schizophrenia?

The term *schizoaffective disorder* was used to describe individuals showing an overlap of features of schizophrenia and affective disorder (Norman and Malla 1991). More recently, schizoaffective disorder has been classified distinctively according to different diagnostic systems (Barnes et al. 1989; Kibel et al. 1993; Kuck et al. 1992). Operationalized criteria such as those in ICD-10 (World Health Organization 1992) specify schizophrenic depressive symptoms (called *postschizophrenic depression*), whereby the individual has some schizophrenic symptoms with prominent depressive symptoms that are distressing and fulfill at least one criterion of a depressive episode. In DSM-IV-TR, schizoaffective disorder refers to individuals in whom a full affective syndrome co-occurs with the complete psychotic syndrome but who also have considerable episodes of psychosis in the absence of an affective syndrome.

In spite of these specific definitions, discussion persists as to whether schizoaffective disorder should be considered a subtype of schizophrenia, a subtype of affective disorder, a distinct entity with dimensions between schizophrenia and affective disorder, a co-occurrence of two distinct diatheses, or an erroneous concept altogether (Siris 2000).

DSM-5 is projected to be released in 2013, The proposed revisions for the diagnostic concept are not very different from DSM -IV. The five characteristic symptoms in Section A continue to be the same, with a requirement of a 1-month period of acute symptoms as before, as is the requirement for the persistence of the disturbance for at least 6 months. The main revision, resulting from a systematic review focusing on subtypes within schizophrenia and within psychotic disorders as a whole, includes the elimination of the DSM-IV subtypes. The rationale for the deletion is that there are fundamental limitations in statistical methods, measurement, and design suggesting that the face-value interpretations of reported subtypes are largely undermined if not unfounded, and that their use in DSM should be discontinued.

Measurement of Depression in Schizophrenia

The Calgary Depression Rating Scale for Schizophrenia (CDSS) is the standard assessment instrument for measuring depression in schizophrenia, because of its proven reliability and validity (Addington et al. 1990, 1991; Müller et al. 2005).

SUICIDE AND SELF-INJURY

Suicide

The occurrence of suicide attempts during the course of schizophrenia is a serious complication of the illness. Older studies estimated that 9%–24% of individuals with schizophrenia die by suicide (Caldwell and Gottesman 1992; Siris et al. 1993), but a more recent examination of the lifetime risk of suicide in schizophrenia estimated that the figure is about 5% (Palmer et al. 2005). An estimated 3,600 people with schizophrenia commit suicide each year in the United States alone (Meltzer 1999), a rate more than 20 times higher than in the general population (Allebeck 1989; Black 1988; Meltzer et al. 2000). It has been reported that up to 40% of patients diagnosed with schizophrenia will have at least one suicide attempt in the course of their illness (Meltzer et al. 2000; Planansky and Johnston 1971).

Given the clinical relevance of suicide attempts in the course of schizo-phrenia, several studies have investigated the clinical variables associated with suicidal behavior. Male gender, younger age, unemployment, presence of depressive symptoms (particularly hopelessness), a positive family history for suicide attempts, comorbid substance abuse, lack of a supportive environ-ment, and a longer duration of untreated psychosis have been associated with increased suicide risk in individuals with schizophrenia (Black et al. 1988; Breier and Astrachan 1984; Caldwell and Gottesman 1990; Heila et al. 1997; Siris 2001). Substance and drug use is another important risk factor for sui-cidal behavior. Heila and colleagues (1997) reported that substance use, par-ticularly alcohol use, is a specific risk factor in older males with schizophre-nia. Social dysfunction is an additional risk factor. Continually depressed mood—specifically hopelessness and psychomotor instability—was signifi-cantly associated with suicide in a prospective study examining 104 individ-uals with schizophrenia, 15 of whom committed suicide (Drake et al. 1986).

Gupta and colleagues (1998), in a study investigating 336 individuals with schizophrenia or schizoaffective disorder, found that 98 with a history of attempted suicide had exhibited a significantly higher mean number of lifetime depressive episodes compared with 238 individuals with no prior suicidal history. Kaplan and Harrow (1996) have provided prospective evidence that poor overall function, poor social and work function, and poor quality of life are predictive risk factors for later suicide.

Self-Injury

The National Mental Health Association (Contero and Lader 1998) describes self-injury, including self-mutilation, self-harm, or self-abuse, as the deliberate, repetitive, impulsive, nonlethal harming of oneself. Self-injury includes 1) cutting, 2) scratching, 3) picking at scabs or interfering with wound healing, 4) burning, 5) punching self or objects, 6) infecting oneself, 7) inserting objects in body openings, 8) bruising or breaking bones, 9) some forms of hair-pulling, as well as other various forms of bodily harm. These behaviors are relatively uncommon in individuals with schizophrenia but can lead to significant dangers in individuals' health when they do occur. Examples of self-injurious behaviors include burning the skin with an iron or cigarette, cutting off a finger, enucleating an eye, or cutting the skin with a knife or razor in a ritualistic manner.

Genital self-mutilation is a rare, severe form of self-injurious behavior. It is usually seen in schizophrenia as being the result of delusions and hallucinations (Becker and Hartmann 1997; Martin and Gattaz 1991; Mishra and Kar 2001). Specific risk factors of genital self-mutilation include command hallucinations, religious delusions (Bhargava et al. 2001), substance abuse, and social isolation (Tobias et al. 1988).

ANXIETY

Although anxiety is common during the prodromal and the acute psychotic phase, it is less prominent during the chronic stages of the illness. During the prodromal phase, even before the presentation of delusional or hallucinatory manifestations, anxiety can be a very common feature. Anxiety can arise as a component of psychosis. For example, an individual with schizophrenia may become hypervigilant as a reaction to delusional perception and hallucinations. The sudden onset of hallucinations can generate marked depression and anxiety. An important differential diagnosis is the iatrogenic anxiety of akathisia induced by antipsychotic treatment. The timing of onset of the predominant motor restlessness in the legs associated with the antipsychotic treatment may help clarify the diagnosis.

It has been reported that approximately 45% of people with schizophrenia may also have an anxiety disorder (Pallanti et al. 2003). Studies have shown that alcohol abuse in schizophrenia can produce anxiety symptoms (Drake and Wallach 1989; Strakowski et al. 1994). Similarly, marijuana use in schizophrenia is associated with increased symptoms of anxiety (Ziedonis and Nickou 2001, p. 198).

As with depression, anxiety is occasionally an early precursor of a psychotic relapse (Docherty et al. 1978). Jorgensen (1998) examined anxiety as one of several warning signs of recurrence of psychotic symptoms in 131 patients with schizophrenia. Results showed that delusional formation correlated with anxiety and early signs of psychosis.

DIFFERENTIAL DIAGNOSIS OF SCHIZOPHRENIA

The diagnosis of schizophrenia is not easy to establish, particularly when individuals present with a first psychotic episode. It should be emphasized that no single feature (e.g., family history, cross-sectional symptomatology) can determine a diagnosis of schizophrenia. A comprehensive history of symptom development, family history, careful clinical interview exploring all symptom dimensions, and review of any physical signs, together with laboratory assessments, will be necessary to arrive at an accurate diagnosis. In terms of symptom presentation, formal thought disorders and affect disorders are characteristic features of schizophrenia. At times, the diagnosis may not be clear in the beginning of the disorder, and there may be need for an extended observation period to examine the stability and course of symptoms. The following psychiatric illnesses must be excluded before diagnosing schizophrenia:

SCHIZOPHRENIFORM DISORDER

DSM-IV-TR requires the duration for schizophreniform disorder to be at least 1 month but less than 6 months (American Psychiatric Association 2000, p. 317). Hence, schizophreniform disorder is likely to be diagnosed in individuals who have an abrupt rather than insidious onset and who have good premorbid adjustment. The most important distinctions between the two disorders are mode of onset and duration of symptoms.

SCHIZOAFFECTIVE DISORDER

Schizoaffective disorder is characterized by an uninterrupted period of illness during which there is at some time a major depressive episode, a manic episode, or a mixed episode that meets the respective full criteria together with symptoms that meet criterion A for schizophrenia for at least 1 month (DSM-IV-TR). Schizoaffective disorder differs from schizophrenia in that both the required affective symptoms and the features of schizophrenia are prominent and co-occur (Tsuang et al. 1985). Patients with schizoaffective disorder may also have a relatively abrupt onset of illness and do not meet the social/occupational dysfunction criteria required for a diagnosis of schizophrenia as specified in DSM-IV-TR. DSM-IV-TR specifies that during the episode of illness there have to be delusions and hallucinations for at least 2 weeks that occur in the absence of prominent mood symptoms. Both bipolar and depressive schizoaffective subtypes have been defined.

AFFECTIVE DISORDERS

Mood disorders such as bipolar disorder and major depressive disorder with psychotic features are diagnosed when there are psychotic symptoms that occur only during periods of diagnosable mood disturbance. For example, bipolar individuals with mania may display a wide variety of psychotic symptoms such as hallucinations, paranoid delusions, and formal thought disorder (Csernansky 2002). Inflated self-esteem and grandiose ideas may expand into delusions of grandiosity, and irritability and suspiciousness into delusions of persecution. Individuals with schizophrenia will usually have delusions with mood-incongruent and bizarre content, whereas patients with major depressive episodes or bipolar manic episodes may experience hallucinations, and/ or delusions that are usually mood congruent.

DELUSIONAL DISORDER

Delusional or paranoid disorder can be frequently confused with schizophrenia. The age at onset of delusional disorder is later than that for schizophrenia, and there is typically less deterioration in occupational and social functioning. Another distinction is that in delusional disorder, there is a well-articulated, nonbizarre delusional system with only one or two themes. Thus, the diagnosis of delusional disorder does not include hallucinations, disorganized behavior, or negative symptoms (Csernansky 2002).

BRIEF PSYCHOTIC DISORDER

Brief psychotic disorder has a rapid onset, generally following a major stressor. Individuals with brief psychotic disorder are characterized by one (or more) positive symptoms such as delusions, hallucinations, disorganized speech, or grossly disorganized or catatonic behavior. Symptoms of brief psychotic disorder occur shortly after or in response to a psychotic stressor such as trauma. A distinctive feature of brief psychotic disorder from schizophrenia is that symptoms can only last from 1 day to 1 month and that the individual shows a full return to premorbid level of functioning.

SCHIZOTYPAL PERSONALITY DISORDER

Schizotypal personality disorder is characterized by social and interpersonal deficits evidenced by reduced competence for relationships, cognitive distortions, and unconventional behavior. Individuals with this disorder may have bizarre forms of thinking and perceiving and often seek isolation from others. Schizotypal personality disorder generally begins in early adulthood and presents in a variety of contexts, as indicated by some of the following symptoms (American Psychiatric Association 2000): ideas of reference (excluding delusions of reference), odd beliefs or magical thinking that influences behavior and is inconsistent with subcultural norms, odd thinking and speech, suspiciousness or paranoid ideation, inappropriate or constricted affect, lack of close friends or confidants other than first-degree relatives, and excessive social anxiety. In contrast to schizophrenia, schizotypal personality disorder does not involve delusions or hallucinations, and there is no deterioration in social and occupational functioning.

BODY DYSMORPHIC DISORDER

The main characteristic feature of body dysmorphic disorder (BDD) is a preoccupation with an alleged deficiency in one's physical body shape. Individuals with BDD may display disproportionate distress about an insignificant imperfection or have persistent, anxiety-provoking feelings concerning a minor flaw. Underlying this distress is a persistent distortion of one's body scheme, which may take on delusional proportions. Distress is most regularly focused on head and face but may also involve any other body part. Individuals with BDD do not experience hallucinations and disorganized thinking. They do not assign the cause of their distorted body image to outside malevolent forces as patients with schizophrenia often do.

PSYCHOTIC DISORDERS DUE TO MEDICAL CONDITIONS

It is important to differentiate psychosis caused by head trauma, brain tumors, multiple sclerosis, Huntington's disease, or Wilson's disease from schizophrenia. In these disorders, cognitive symptoms such as disorientation, short-term memory loss, and confusion will predominate the clinical picture. A full neurological and medical examination will assist with the diagnosis. Also, adverse effects to medications can manifest as psychotic symptoms. For example, symptoms of psychosis can occur during treatment with L-dopa, anticholinergics, and corticosteroids (Guggenheim and Babigian 1974; Rudick et al. 1997).

SUBSTANCE-INDUCED PSYCHOTIC DISORDERS

The main characteristic of substance-induced psychotic disorders is the presence of prominent hallucinations and delusions, which are thought to be directly related to the physiological effects of a substance. There has to be evidence, based on history, physical examination, and laboratory findings, that the disorder arises in the context of substance withdrawal or intoxication. Usually, the disorder lasts as long as there is use of the substance (onset during intoxication) or can begin after the individual has stopped using substances (onset during withdrawal). Hallucinogens such as lysergic acid diethylamide (LSD) and stimulants such as methamphetamine, amphetamine, cocaine, and PCP can generate visual and auditory hallucinations. Alcohol hallucinations, which tend to be visual and kinesthetic, differ from those seen in schizophrenia in that they occur only after extended use of alcohol and usually last for a short period of time (Csernansky 2002). Generally individuals with substance-induced psychotic disorders are aware that their hallucinations are not real, which is characteristically not the case with individuals with schizophrenia (Csernansky 2002).

SUBTYPES OF SCHIZOPHRENIA

The subtypes of schizophrenia are distinguished by the prevalent symptomatology. Initially, Kraepelin (1919) divided "dementia praecox" into three clinical subtypes: hebephrenic, catatonic, and paranoid. He later expanded on these three subtypes to include several other categories, yet emphasized that the subgrouping of different clinical descriptions was of restricted clinical value (pp. 89–180). Currently, there are various subtypes of schizophrenia as specified by the particular diagnostic system. Table 2–1 presents the most dominant subtypes occurring in schizophrenia patients, which include paranoid, disorganized (hebephrenic), catatonic, undifferentiated, and residual schizophrenia. However, DSM-5, to be released in 2013, will most likely eliminate the DSM-IV subtypes because of insufficient underlying consistent research data (see subsection "Is Schizoaffective Disorder a Subtype of Schizophrenia?" earlier in this chapter).

TABLE 2–1.   Subtypes of schizophrenia (DSM-IV-TR and ICD-10)

Paranoid schizophrenia	Primarily marked by delusions of persecution and/or grandeur and frequent auditory hallucinations.
	Generally does not include the degree of disorganization of speech/behavior seen in other subtypes.
	Individuals are tense, suspicious, and guarded.
	Associated features include anxiety, anger, aloofness, and argumentativeness.
	Onset often later compared with other schizophrenia subtypes; little or no impairment in neurocognitive functions (American Psychiatric Association 2000).
	DSM-IV-TR: includes a preoccupation with one or more paranoid delusions, which may be systematized, or frequent auditory hallucinations along with no prominent symptoms of disorganized speech, disorganized behavior, or flat/inappropriate affect.
	ICD-10: similar to DSM-IV-TR but excludes paranoia and involutional paranoid state.
Disorganized or hebephrenic schizophrenia	Primarily marked by inappropriate affect, disorganized speech, and maladaptive behavior.
	Disorganized (hebephrenic) behavior can lead to significant interference with activities of daily living.
	DSM-IV-TR: includes disorganized speech, disorganized behavior, and flat/inappropriate affect and excludes catatonia and delusions and hallucinations that are systematized into a lucid theme.
	ICD-10: similar to DSM-IV-TR but adds that the disorganized/hebephrenic subtype should normally be diagnosed for the first time only in adolescents or young adults, with a period of 2–3 months of observation ensuring sustained characteristic features.
	ICD-10 also indicates that the premorbid personality of these individuals includes timid and solitary behavior.

TABLE 2–1.	Subtypes of schizophrenia (DSM-IV-TR and ICD-10) *(continued)*
Undifferentiated schizophrenia	Incorporates a combination of symptoms from other subtypes. Individuals should meet criterion A of DSM-IV-TR (American Psychiatric Association 2000, p. 312) and should not have symptoms of catatonia or paranoid and disorganized schizophrenia. ICD-10, although following DSM-IV-TR criteria, includes the stipulation that undifferentiated schizophrenia should not satisfy the criteria for residual schizophrenia (described below) or postschizophrenia depression.
Residual schizophrenia	A state in which the individual is not currently suffering from severe delusions, hallucinations, or disorganized speech and behavior but lacks motivation and interest in day-to-day living. DSM-IV-TR: includes an absence of prominent delusions, hallucinations, disorganized speech, and grossly disorganized or catatonic behavior. It also specifies the existence of negative symptoms or two or more of the symptoms specified in criterion A (American Psychiatric Association 2000, p. 312) present in an attenuated form (e.g., odd beliefs). ICD-10 adds as a requirement an absence of dementia or other organic brain disease or disorder and chronic depression or institutionalism that could explain the negative impairments.
Catatonic schizophrenia	Primarily marked by motor disturbances ranging from immobility to excessive meaningless activity. Dominated by psychomotor symptoms. DSM-IV-TR includes two or more and ICD-10 specifies at least one of the following behaviors: stupor (marked reduction or suspended sensibility) or mutism, excitement not influenced by external stimuli, bizarre postures, meaningless resistance toward instructions or attempts to be moved, rigidity, waxy flexibility, and echolalia or echopraxia. Differential diagnosis includes brain disease, metabolic instability, substance abuse, or mood disorders such as bipolar disorder.

CONCLUSION

Schizophrenia is a disorder with a significant heterogeneous presentation of a variety of symptoms that can affect virtually all areas of psychological functioning and which are best understood to represent separate psychopathological syndromal domains. These major symptom domains include positive, negative, cognitive, excitement, and depression/anxiety symptoms and are found in each patient with schizophrenia to a variable extent. Each of these domains will affect patients' instrumental, social, and occupational functioning to various degrees and can lead to significant overall functional impairment.

REFERENCES

Addington J, Addington D: Positive and negative symptoms of schizophrenia: their course and relationship over time. Schizophr Res 5:51–59, 1991

Addington D, Addington J, Schissel B: A depression rating scale for schizophrenics. Schizophr Res 3:247–251, 1990

Addington A, Addington J, Maticka-Tyndale E, et al: Reliability and validity of a depression rating scale for schizophrenics. Schizophr Res 6:201–208, 1991

Alexander MP, Stuss DT, Benson DF: Capgras syndrome: a reduplicative phenomenon. Neurology 29:334–339, 1979

Allebeck P: Schizophrenia: a life-shortening disease. Schizophr Bull 15:81–89, 1989

Amador XF, Kirkpatrick B, Buchanan RW, et al: Stability of the diagnosis of deficit syndrome in schizophrenia. Am J Psychiatry 156:637–639, 1999

American Psychiatric Association: Diagnostic and Statistical Manual of Mental Disorders, 2nd Edition. Washington, DC, American Psychiatric Association, 1968

American Psychiatric Association: Diagnostic and Statistical Manual of Mental Disorders, 3rd Edition. Washington, DC, American Psychiatric Association, 1980

American Psychiatric Association: Diagnostic and Statistical Manual of Mental Disorders, 3rd Edition, Revised. Washington, DC, American Psychiatric Association, 1987

American Psychiatric Association: Diagnostic and Statistical Manual of Mental Disorders, 4th Edition. Washington, DC, American Psychiatric Association, 1994

American Psychiatric Association: Diagnostic and Statistical Manual of Mental Disorders, 4th Edition, Text Revision. Washington, DC, American Psychiatric Association, 2000

Andreasen N: Thought, language, and communication disorders, I: clinical assessment, definition of terms, and evaluation of their reliability. Arch Gen Psychiatry 36:1315–1321, 1979a

Andreasen N: Thought, language, and communication disorders, II: diagnostic significance. Arch Gen Psychiatry 36:1325–1330, 1979b

Andreasen NC: Negative symptoms in schizophrenia: definition and reliability. Arch Gen Psychiatry 39:784–788, 1982

Andreasen NC: Scale for the Assessment of Negative Symptoms (SANS). Iowa City, University of Iowa, 1983

Andreasen NC: Scale for the Assessment of Positive Symptoms (SAPS). Iowa City, University of Iowa, 1984

Andreasen NC: The Comprehensive Assessment of Symptoms and History (CASH). Iowa City, University of Iowa, 1985

Andreasen NC, Flaum M: Schizophrenia: the characteristic symptoms. Schizophr Bull 17:27–49, 1991

Andreasen NC, Olsen S: Negative v positive schizophrenia: definition and validation. Arch Gen Psychiatry 39:789–794, 1982

Andreasen NC, Swayze VW, Flaum M, et al: Ventricular enlargement in schizophrenia evaluated with computed tomographic scanning: effects of gender, age, and stage of illness. Arch Gen Psychiatry 47:1008–1015, 1990

Andreasen NC, Arndt S, Alliger R, et al: Symptoms of schizophrenia: methods, meanings, and mechanisms. Arch Gen Psychiatry 52:341–351, 1995

Arndt S, Andreasen NC, Flaum M, et al: A longitudinal study of symptom dimensions in schizophrenia: prediction and patterns of change. Arch Gen Psychiatry 52:352–360, 1995

Barnes TR, Curson DA, Liddle PF, et al: The nature and prevalence of depression in chronic schizophrenic inpatients. Br J Psychiatry 154:486–491, 1989

Beck AT, Ward CH, Mendelson M: A study of consistency of clinical judgments and ratings. Am J Psychiatry 119:351–357, 1962

Becker H, Hartmann U: [Genital self-injury behavior: phenomenologic and differential diagnosis considerations from the psychiatric viewpoint]. Fortschr Neurol Psychiatr 65:71–78, 1997

Bermanzohn PC, Siris SG: Akinesia: a syndrome common to parkinsonism, retarded depression, and negative symptoms of schizophrenia. Compr Psychiatry 33:221–232, 1992

Bhargava CS, Sethi S, Vohra AK: Klingsor syndrome: a case report. Indian J Psychiatry 43:349–350, 2001

Birchwood M, Mason R, Macmillan F, et al: Depression, demoralization and control over psychotic illness: a comparison of depressed and non-depressed patients with a chronic psychosis. Psychol Med 23:387–395, 1993

Black DW: Mortality in schizophrenia: the Iowa record-linkage study: a comparison with general population mortality. Psychosomatics 29:55–60, 1988

Black DW, Winokur G, Nasrallah A: Effect of psychosis on suicide risk in 1,593 patients with unipolar and bipolar affective disorders. Am J Psychiatry 145:849–852, 1988

Bleuler E: Dementia Praecox or the Group of Schizophrenias (1911). Translated by Zitkin J. New York, International Universities Press, 1950

Bottlender R, Strauss A, Moller HJ: Prevalence and background factors of depression in first admitted schizophrenic patients. Acta Psychiatr Scand 101:153–160, 2000

Breier A, Astrachan BM: Characterization of schizophrenic patients who commit suicide. Am J Psychiatry 141:206–209, 1984

Caldwell CB, Gottesman II: Schizophrenics kill themselves too: a review of risk factors for suicide. Schizophr Bull 16:571–589, 1990

Caldwell CB, Gottesman II: Schizophrenia: a high-risk factor for suicides: clues to risk reduction. Suicide Life Threat Behav 22:479–493, 1992

Capleton RA: Cognitive function in schizophrenia: association with negative and positive symptoms. Psychol Rep 78:123–128, 1996

Carpenter WT Jr, Kirkpatrick B: The heterogeneity of the long-term course of schizophrenia. Schizophr Bull 14:645–652, 1988

Carpenter WT, Heinrichs DW, Alphs LD: Treatment of negative symptoms, Schizophr Bull 11:440–452, 1985

Carpenter WT Jr, Buchanan RW, Brier A, et al: Psychopathology and the question of neurodevelopmental or neurodegenerative disorder. Schizophr Res 5:192–194, 1991

Carter JL: Visual, somatosensory, olfactory and gustatory hallucinations: the interface of psychiatry and neurology. Psychiatr Clin North Am 15:347–358, 1992

Citrome L, Volavka J: Schizophrenia: violence and comorbidity. Curr Opin Psychiatry 12:47–51, 1999

Citrome L, Volavka J: Aggression and violence in patients with schizophrenia, in Schizophrenia and Comorbid Conditions: Diagnosis and Treatment. Edited by Hwang MY, Bermanzohn PC. Washington, DC, American Psychiatric Press, 2001, pp 149–185

Coid B, Lewis SW, Revely AM: A twin study of psychosis and criminality. Br J Psychiatry 162:87–92, 1993

Contero K, Lader W: Self-injury. November 1998. Available at: http://www.nmha.org/infoctr/factsheets/selfinjury.cfm. Accessed May 23, 2005.

Crow TJ: Molecular pathology of schizophrenia: more than one disease process? Br Med J 280:66–68, 1980

Crow TJ: Positive and negative symptoms and the role of dopamine. Br J Psychiatry 139:251–254, 1981

Crow TJ: The two-syndrome concept: origins and current status. Schizophr Bull 11:471–486, 1985

Csernansky JG: Schizophrenia: A New Guide for Clinicians. New York, Marcel Dekker, 2002

Cuesta MJ, Peralta V: Thought disorder in schizophrenia: testing models through confirmatory factor analysis. Eur Arch Psychiatry Clin Neurosci 249:55–61, 1999

Cutler JL, Siris SG: "Panic-like" symptomatology in schizoaffective patients with postpsychotic depression: observations and implications. Compr Psychiatry 32:465–473, 1991

Cutting J, Murphy D: Schizophrenic thought disorder: a psychological organic interpretation. Br J Psychiatry 152:310–319, 1988

Docherty JP, Van Kammen DP, Siris SG, et al: Stages of onset of schizophrenic psychosis. Am J Psychiatry 135:420–426, 1978

Drake RE, Wallach MA: Substance abuse among the chronic mentally ill. Hosp Community Psychiatry 40:1041–1046, 1989

Drake RE, Gates C, Cotton PG: Suicide among schizophrenics: a comparison of attempters and completed suicides. Br J Psychiatry 149:784–787, 1986

Ellis HD, Young AW, Quayle AH, et al: Reduced autonomic responses to faces in Capgras delusion. Proc Biol Sci 264:1085–1092, 1997

Endicott J, Spitzer RL: A diagnostic interview: the Schedule for Affective Disorders and Schizophrenia. Arch Gen Psychiatry 35:837–844, 1978

Eronen M, Hakola P, Tiihonen J: Mental disorders and homicidal behavior in Finland. Arch Gen Psychiatry 53:497–501, 1996

Feighner JP, Robbins E, Guze SB, et al: Diagnostic criteria for psychiatric research. Arch Gen Psychiatry 26:57–63, 1972

Fenton WS, McGlashan TH: Testing systems for assessment of negative symptoms in schizophrenia. Arch Gen Psychiatry 49:179–184, 1992

First MB, Spitzer RL, Gibbon M, et al: Structured Clinical Interview for DSM-IV Axis I Disorders (SCID-1). Washington, DC, American Psychiatric Association, 1997

Fish F: Schizophrenia, 3rd Edition. Edited by Hamilton M. Baltimore, MD, Williams & Wilkins, 1984

Fitzgerald PB, Rolfe TJ, Berwer K, et al: Depressive, positive, negative and parkinsonian symptoms in schizophrenia. Aust N Z J Psychiatry 36:340–346, 2002

Frith CD, Friston KJ, Liddle PF, et al: PET imaging and cognition in schizophrenia. J R Soc Med 85:222–224, 1992

Green MF, Nuechterlein KH, Ventura J, et al: The temporal relationship between depressive and psychotic symptoms in recent onset schizophrenia. Am J Psychiatry 147:179–182, 1990

Guggenheim FG, Babigian HM: Catatonic schizophrenia: epidemiology and clinical course: a 7-year register study of 798 cases. J Nerv Ment Dis 158:291–305, 1974

Gupta S, Black DW, Arndt S, et al: Factors associated with suicide attempts among patients with schizophrenia. Psychiatr Serv 49:1353–1355, 1998

Hafner H, Boker W: Crimes of Violence by Mentally Abnormal Offenders. Cambridge, UK, Cambridge University Press, 1982

Hafner H, Nowotny B, Loftler W, et al: When and how does schizophrenia produce social deficits? Eur Arch Psychiatry Clin Neurosci 246:17–28, 1995

Hafner H, Loffler W, Maurer K, et al: Depression, negative symptoms, social stagnation, and social decline in the early course of schizophrenia. Acta Psychiatr Scand 100(2):105–118, 1999

Harrow M, Sands JR, Silverstein ML, et al: Course and outcome for schizophrenia versus other psychotic patients: a longitudinal study. Schizophr Bull 23:287–303, 1997

Harvey PD, Lombardi J, Leibman M, et al: Age related differences in formal thought disorder in chronically hospitalized schizophrenic patients: a cross sectional study across nine decades. Am J Psychiatry 154:205–210, 1997

Hausmann A, Fleischhacker WW: Differential diagnosis of depressed mood in patients with schizophrenia: a diagnostic algorithm based on a review. Acta Psychiatr Scand 106:83–96, 2002

Heila H, Isometsa ET, Henriksson KV, et al: Suicide and schizophrenia: a nationwide psychological autopsy study on age and sex specific clinical characteristics of 92 suicide victims with schizophrenia. Am J Psychiatry 154:1235–1242, 1997

Hirsch SR, Jolley AG: The dysphoric syndrome in schizophrenia and its implications for relapse. Br J Psychiatry Suppl 5:46–50, 1989

Hodgins S: Mental disorder, intellectual deficiency, and crime: evidence from a birth cohort. Arch Gen Psychiatry 49:476–483, 1992

Hoffman RE, Hawkins KA, Gueorguieva R, et al: Transcranial magnetic stimulation of left temporoparietal cortex and medication-resistant auditory hallucinations. Arch Gen Psychiatry 60:49–56, 2003

Hogarty GE, McEvoy JP, Ulrich RF, et al: Pharmacotherapy of impaired affect in recovering schizophrenic patients. Arch Gen Psychiatry 52:29–41, 1995

Hull JW, Smith TE, Anthony DT, et al: Patterns of symptom change: a longitudinal analysis. Schizophr Res 24:17–18, 1997

Hurt SW, Holzman PS, Davis JM: Thought disorders: the measurement of its changes. Arch Gen Psychiatry 40:1281–1285, 1983

Jeczmien P, Levkovitz Y, Weizman A, et al: Postpsychotic depression in schizophrenia. Isr Med Assoc J 3:589–592, 2001

Johnson DAW: The significance of depression in the prediction of relapse in chronic schizophrenia. Br J Psychiatry 152:320–323, 1988

Jorgensen P: Schizophrenic delusions: detection of warning signals. Schizophr Res 32:17–22, 1998

Kaplan KJ, Harrow M: Positive and negative symptoms as risk factors for later suicidal activity in schizophrenics vs depressives. Suicide Life Threat Behav 26:105–121, 1996

Kay SR: Positive-negative assessment in schizophrenia: psychometric issues and scale comparison. Psychiatr Q 61:163–168, 1990

Kay SR, Sevy S: Pyramidical model of schizophrenia. Schizophr Bull 16:537–545, 1990

Kay SR, Opler LA, Fiszbein A: Significance of positive and negative syndromes in chronic schizophrenia. Br J Psychiatry 149:439–448, 1986

Kay SR, Fisz-Bein A, Opler LA: The positive and negative syndrome scale (PANSS) for schizophrenia. Schizophr Bull 13:261–274, 1987

Kibel DA, Laffont I, Liddle PF: The composition of the negative syndrome of chronic schizophrenia, Br J Psychiatry 62:744–750, 1993

Kirkpatrick B, Buchanan RW, McKenney PD, et al: The Schedule for the Deficit Syndrome: an instrument for research in schizophrenia. Psychiatry Res 30:119–123, 1989

Kirkpatrick B, Buchanan RW, Ross DE, et al: A separate disease within the syndrome of schizophrenia. Arch Gen Psychiatry 58:165–171, 2001

Koreen AR, Siris SG, Chakos M, et al: Depression in first-episode schizophrenia. Am J Psychiatry 150:1643–1648, 1993

Kraepelin E: Dementia Praecox and Paraphrenia. Translated by Barclay RM. New York, Robert E Krieger Publishing Company, 1919

Krakowski M, Czobor P: Violence in psychiatric patients: the role of psychosis, frontal lobe impairment, and ward turmoil. Compr Psychiatry 38:230–236, 1997

Kring AM, Neale JM: Do schizophrenic patients show a disjunctive relationship among expressive, experiential, and psychophysiological components of emotion? J Abnorm Psychol 105:249–257, 1996

Kuck J, Zisook S, Moranville JT, et al: Negative symptomatology in schizophrenic outpatients. J Nerv Ment Dis 180:510–515, 1992

Kulhara P, Avasthi A, Chadda R, et al: Negative and depressive symptoms in schizophrenia. Br J Psychiatry 154:207–211, 1989

Leff J: Depressive symptoms in the course of schizophrenia, in Depression in Schizophrenia. Edited by DeLisi LE. Washington, DC, American Psychiatric Press, 1990, pp 1–23

Liddle PF: The symptoms of chronic schizophrenia: a re-examination of the positive-negative dichotomy. Br J Psychiatry 151:145–151, 1987

Lindenmayer JP, Kay SR: Depression, affect, and negative symptoms in schizophrenia. Br J Psychiatry 5 (suppl 7):108–114, 1989

Lindenmayer JP, Kay SR, Opler L: Positive and negative subtypes in acute schizophrenia. Compr Psychiatry 2594:445–464, 1984

Lindenmayer JP, Kay SR, Freidman C: Negative and positive syndromes after the acute phase: a prospective follow-up. Compr Psychiatry 27:276–286, 1986

Lindenmayer JP, Grochowski S, Kay SR: Schizophrenic patients with depression: psychopathological profiles and the relationship with negative symptoms. Compr Psychiatry 32:528–533, 1991

Lindenmayer JP, Bernstein-Hyman R, Grochowski S: Five-factor model of schizophrenia: initial validation. J Nerv Ment Dis 182:631–638, 1994

Lindenmayer JP, Bernstein-Hyman R, Grochowski S, et al: Psychopathology of schizophrenia: initial validation of a 5-factor model. Psychopathology 28:22–31, 1995

Marder SR, Davis JM, Chouinard G: The effects of risperidone on the five dimensions of schizophrenia derived by factor analysis: combined results of the North American trials. J Clin Psychiatry 58:538–546, 1997

Martin T, Gattaz WF: Psychiatric aspects of male genital self-mutilation. Psychopathology 24:170–178, 1991

Maziade M, Roy MA, Martinez M, et al: Negative, psychotism, and disorganized dimensions in patients with familial schizophrenia or bipolar disorder: continuity and discontinuity between the major psychosis. Am J Psychiatry 152:1458–1463, 1995

McGlashan TH, Carpenter WT: Postpsychotic depression in schizophrenia. Arch Gen Psychiatry 33:231–239, 1976

McGorry PD, Edwards J, Mihalopoulos C, et al: EPPIC: an evolving system of early detection and optimal management. Schizophr Bull 22:305–326, 1996

Meltzer HY: Suicide and schizophrenia: clozapine and the InterSePT study. J Clin Psychiatry 60 (suppl 12):47–50, 1999

Meltzer HY, Anand R, Alphs L: Reducing suicide risk in schizophrenia: focus on the role of clozapine. CNS Drugs 14:355–365, 2000

Miles CP: Conditions predisposing to suicide. J Ment Dis 164:231–246, 1977

Mishra B, Kar N: Genital self amputation for urinary symptoms relief or suicide? Indian J Psychiatry 43:342–344, 2001

Moller HJ, Schmid-Bode W, Cording-Tommel C, et al: Psychopathological and social outcome in schizophrenia versus affective/schizoaffective psychoses and prediction of poor outcome in schizophrenia: results from a 5-8 year follow-up. Acta Psychiatr Scand 77:379–389, 1988

Moller HJ, Van Praag HM, Aufdembrinke B, et al: Negative symptoms in schizophrenia: considerations for clinical trials: working group on negative symptoms in schizophrenia. Psychopharmacology (Berl) 115:221–228, 1994

Monahan J, Steadman HJ, Appelbaum PS, et al: Developing a clinically useful actuarial tool for assessing violence risk. Br J Psychiatry 176:312–319, 2000

Mueser KT, Yarnold PR, Levinson DF, et al: Prevalence of substance abuse in schizophrenia: demographic and clinical correlates. Schizophr Bull 16:31–56, 1990

Mueser KT, Doonan R, Penn DL, et al: Emotion recognition and social competence in chronic schizophrenia. J Abnorm Psychol 105:271–275, 1996

Müller MJ, Szegedi A, Wetzel H, et al: Depressive factors and their relationships with other symptom domains in schizophrenia, schizoaffective disorder and psychotic depression. Schizophr Bull 27:9–28, 2001

Müller MJ, Brening H, Gensch C, et al: The Calgary Depression Rating Scale for schizophrenia in a healthy control group: psychometric properties and reference values. J Affect Disord 88(1):69–74, 2005

Norman RMG, Malla AK: Dysphoric mood and symptomatology in schizophrenia. Psychol Med 21:897–903, 1991

Norman RMG, Malla AK, Cortese L, et al: Aspects of dysphoria and symptoms of schizophrenia, Psychol Med 28:1433–1441, 1998

Oppenheimer H: Clinical Psychiatry: Issues and Challenges. New York, Harper & Row, 1971

Overall JE, Gorham DR: The brief psychiatric rating scale. Psychol Rep 10:799–812, 1962

Owen C, Tarantello C, Jones M, et al: Violence and aggression in psychiatric units. Psychiatr Serv 49:1452–1457, 1998

Pallanti S, Quercioli L, Hollander E: Assessment and characterization of social anxiety in schizophrenia (S53C), in 2003 New Research Program and Abstracts, American Psychiatric Association 156th Annual Meeting, San Francisco, CA, May 17–22, 2003

Palmer BA, Pankratz S, Bostwick JM: The Lifetime Risk of Suicide in Schizophrenia: a reexamination. Arch Gen Psychiatry 62:247–253, 2005

Peralta V, De Leon J, Cuesta MJ: Are there more than two syndromes in schizophrenia? A critique of the positive-negative dichotomy. Br J Psychiatry 161:335–343, 1992

Pfohl B, Winokur G: The evolution of symptoms in institutionalized hebephrenic/catatonic schizophrenics. Br J Psychiatry 141:567–572, 1982

Planansky K, Johnston R: The occurrence and characteristics of suicidal preoccupation and acts in schizophrenia. Acta Psychiatr Scand 47:473–483, 1971

Regier DA, Farmer ME, Rae DS: Comorbidity of mental disorders with alcohol and other drug abuse: results from the Epidemiologic Catchment Area (ECA) Study. JAMA 264:2511–2518, 1990

Robbins LN, Helzer JE, Croughan J, et al: National Institute of Mental Health Diagnostic Interview Schedule: its history, characteristics, and validity. Arch Gen Psychiatry 38:381–389, 1981

Romney DM, Candido CL: Anhedonia in depression and schizophrenia: a reexamination. J Nerv Ment Dis 189:735–740, 2001

Roth S: The seemingly ubiquitous depression following acute schizophrenic episodes: a neglected area of clinical discussion. Am J Psychiatry 127:91–98, 1970

Roy A, Thompson R, Kennedy S: Depression in chronic schizophrenia. Br J Psychiatry 142:465–470, 1983

Rudick RA, Cohen JA, Weinstock-Guttman B, et al: Management of multiple sclerosis. N Engl J Med 337:1604–1611, 1997

Salem JE, Kring AM: Flat affect and social skills in schizophrenia: evidence for their independence. Psychiatry Res 87:159–167, 1999

Sartorius N, Shapiro R, Jablensky A: The international pilot study of schizophrenia. Schizophr Bull 1:21–35, 1974

Sax KW, Strakowski SM, Keck PEJ, et al: Relationship among negative, positive, and depressive symptoms in schizophrenia and psychotic depression. Br J Psychiatry 168:68–71, 1996

Schneider K: Clinical Psychopathology. Translated by Hamilton MW. New York, Grune & Stratton, 1959

Schneider K: Primary and secondary symptoms in schizophrenia, in Themes and Variations in European Psychiatry. Edited by Hirsch SR, Shepard M. Bristol, UK, John Wright, 1974, pp 40–46

Shuwall M, Siris SG: Suicidal ideation in postpsychotic depression. Compr Psychiatry 35:132–134, 1994

Siris SG: Depressive symptoms in the course of schizophrenia, in Depression in Schizophrenia. Edited by DeLisi LE. Washington, DC, American Psychiatric Press, 1990, pp 3–23

Siris SG: Depression and schizophrenia, in Schizophrenia. Edited by Hirsch SR, Weinberger DR. Oxford, England, Blackwell Science, 1995, pp 128–145

Siris SG: Depression in schizophrenia: perspective in the era of "atypical" antipsychotic agents. Am J Psychiatry 157:1379–1389, 2000

Siris SG: Suicide and schizophrenia. J Psychopharmacol 15:127–135, 2001

Siris SG, Mason SE, Shuwall MA: Histories of substance abuse, panic and suicidal ideation in schizophrenic patients with histories of post-psychotic depressions. Prog Neuropsychopharmacol Biol Psychiatry 17:609–617, 1993

Smith J, Hucker S: Schizophrenia and substance abuse. Br J Psychiatry 165:13–21, 1994

Soyka M, Naber G, Volcker A: Prevalence of delusional jealousy in different psychiatric disorders: an analysis of 93 cases. Br J Psychiatry 158:549–553, 1991

Spitzer RL, Fleiss JL: A re-analysis of the reliability of psychiatric diagnosis. Br J Psychiatry 125:341–347, 1974

Spitzer RL, Endicott J, Robins E: Research Diagnostic Criteria for a Selected Group of Functional Disorders. New York, New York State Psychiatric Institute, 1978

Steadman HJ, Mulvey EP, Monahan J, et al: Violence by people discharged from acute psychiatric inpatient facilities and by others in the same neighborhoods. Arch Gen Psychiatry 55:1–9, 1998

Steadman HJ, Silver E, Monahan J, et al: A classification tree approach to the development of actuarial violent risk assessment tools. Law Hum Behavior 24:83–100, 2000

Strakowski SM, Tohen M, Flaum M, et al: Substance abuse in psychotic disorders: associations with affective syndromes: DSM-IV Field Trial Work Group. Schizophr Res 14:73–81, 1994

Swanson J: Mental disorder, substance abuse and community violence: an epidemiological approach, in Violence and Mental Disorder: Developments in Risk Assessment. Edited by Monahan J, Steadman H. Chicago, IL, University of Chicago Press, 1994, pp 101–136

Swanson JW, Swartz MS, Borum R, et al: Involuntary outpatient commitment and reduction of violent behaviour in persons with severe mental illness. Br J Psychiatry 176:324–331, 2000

Tandon R, Greden J: Cholinergic hyperactivity and negative schizophrenic symptoms. Arch Gen Psychiatry 46:745–753, 1989

Thompson PA, Meltzer HY: Positive, negative, and disorganization factors from the Schedule for Affective Disorders and Schizophrenia and the Present State Examination: a three-factor solution. Br J Psychiatry 163:344–351, 1993

Tobias CR, Turns DM, Lippmann S, et al: Evaluation and management of self-mutilation. South Med J 81:1261–1263, 1998

Toomey R, Kremen WS, Simpson JC, et al: Revisiting the factor structure for positive and negative symptoms: evidence from a large heterogeneous group of psychiatric patients. Am J Psychiatry 154:371–377, 1997

Tsuang MT, Kendler KK, Gruenberg AM: A DSM-III schizophrenia: is there evidence for familial transmission? Acta Psychiatr Scand 71:77–83, 1985

Valliant GE: Prospective prediction of schizophrenic remission. Arch Gen Psychiatry 11:509–518, 1964

Van Putten T: Why do schizophrenic patients refuse to take their drugs? Arch Gen Psychiatry 31:67–72, 1974

Van Putten T: Why do patients with manic-depressive illness stop their lithium? Compr Psychiatry 16:179–183, 1975

Verheyden SL, Maidment R, Curran HV: Quitting ecstasy: an investigation of why people stop taking the drug and their subsequent mental health. J Psychopharmacol 17:371–378, 2003

Volavka J: Neurobiology of Violence, 2nd Edition. Washington, DC, American Psychiatric Publishing, 2002

Wallace C, Mullen P, Burgess P, et al: Serious criminal offending and mental disorder: case linkage study. Br J Psychiatry 172:477–484, 1998

Weiden P, Scheifler P, Diamond R, et al: Breakthroughs in Antipsychotic Medications. New York, WW Norton, 1999

Wessely S: The epidemiology of crime, violence and schizophrenia. Br J Psychiatry 170 (suppl 32):8–11, 1997

Wessely S, Castle D, Douglas AJ, et al: The criminal careers of incident cases of schizophrenia. Psychol Med 24:483–502, 1994

Westermeyer JF, Harrow M, Marengo JT: Risk for suicide in schizophrenia and other psychotic and nonpsychotic disorders. J Nerv Ment Dis 179:259–266, 1991

White L, Harvey PD, Opler L, et al: Empirical assessment of the factorial structure of clinical symptoms in schizophrenia: a multisite, multimodel evaluation of the factorial structure of the Positive and Negative Syndrome Scale. The PANSS Study Group. Psychopathology 30:263–274, 1997

Wing J: A standard form of psychiatric Present-State Examination and a method for standardizing the classification of symptoms, in Psychiatric Epidemiology: An International Symposium. Edited by Hare EH, Wing JK. London, Oxford University Press, 1970, pp 93–108

World Health Organization: International Classification of Diseases, 9th Revision, Clinical Modification. Ann Arbor, MI, Commission on Professional and Hospital Activities, 1978

World Health Organization: International Statistical Classification of Diseases and Related Health Problems, 10th Revision. Geneva, World Health Organization, 1992

World Health Organization: The Global Burden of Disease: 2004. Geneva, World Health Organization, 2008

Yudofsky SC, Silver JM, Jackson W, et al: The Overt Aggression Scale for the objective rating of verbal and physical aggression. Am J Psychiatry 143:35–39, 1986

Ziedonis D, Nickou C: Substance abuse in patients with schizophrenia, in Schizophrenia and Comorbid Conditions: Diagnosis and Treatment. Edited by Hwang MY, Bermanzohn PC. Washington, DC, American Psychiatric Press, 2001, pp 187–221

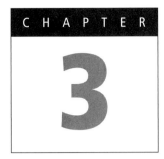

CHAPTER 3

PRODROME AND FIRST EPISODE

DIANA O. PERKINS, M.D., M.P.H.

JEFFREY A. LIEBERMAN, M.D.

In this chapter, we review the clinical features that characterize the prodrome and first-episode phases of schizophrenia. We also discuss the current understanding of optimal treatment of the first episode. In particular, recognition and treatment of psychosis soon after illness onset may improve outcomes; however, treatment delay continues to be a public health concern. Pharmacological treatment continues to be the cornerstone of treatment, but other modalities, including individual, group, and family therapies, may increase the likelihood of full recovery.

PRODROME

CLINICAL CHARACTERISTICS

Changes in perception, thought process, and thought content that are psychotic-like, but with less than full psychotic intensity, herald the development of psychosis for about 80% of schizophrenia patients (Perkins et al. 2000).

Examples include misperceptions (e.g., seeing things out the corner of one's eye, hearing knocking or whistling noises), subdelusional changes in thought process and content (e.g., becoming very suspicious of others, intrusive irrelevant thoughts), and disorganization of thought process (e.g., difficulty following conversations, frequent use of the wrong word). Individuals may experience problems with easy distractibility and poor attention; depressed, anxious, irritable, or labile moods; and negative symptoms (e.g., diminished motivation, drive, and interest in activities) that worsen over time. These symptoms often impair ability to function at school or work or in social situations, and the functional difficulties are often what bring the person to clinical attention (Addington et al. 2002). Much of the decline in social and occupational function associated with schizophrenia occurs during the prodrome, prior to the onset of frank psychosis (Häfner and an der Heiden 1999).

PROSPECTIVE RECOGNITION: PSYCHOSIS RISK SYNDROME

Several research groups have developed relatively similar clinical criteria to define a "psychosis risk syndrome." In North American research, the Criteria of Prodromal States (COPS) is the most widely used (Woods et al. 2009). These criteria include the presence of attenuated psychotic symptoms that have developed or worsened recently (in the past year) (Table 3–1). On the basis of these research definitions of a psychosis risk syndrome, efforts to prospectively identify individuals in the prodromal stage, prior to the onset of a full psychotic syndrome, have met with limited success. *These studies report that about a third of persons meeting research criteria for psychosis risk syndrome will develop a psychotic disorder within the ensuing 1–2 years* (Cannon et al. 2008; Woods et al. 2009; Yung et al. 2008).

TREATMENT APPROACHES

The evidence base for indicated prevention of psychosis includes only four small clinical trials, one with an antipsychotic alone (Woods et al. 2003), one with cognitive-behavioral psychotherapy alone (Morrison et al. 2004), and one with both psychotherapy and an antipsychotic (McGorry et al. 2002), and a trial using omega-3 fatty acids (fish oil supplements) (Amminger et al. 2010). Over a 1- to 2-year follow-up period, these interventions demonstrated similar levels of psychotic disorder risk reduction, from about 30% in the control group to about 10% in the intervention group. With treatment discontinuation, benefits were not sustained for antipsychotic and psychotherapy interventions, as a total of about one-third of the individuals developed a psychotic disorder (Morrison et al. 2007; Phillips et al. 2007).

TABLE 3–1.	Examples of psychosis risk syndrome symptoms
Attenuated delusions	A college freshman is noticing "connections" between seemingly unrelated events that have become "too personal to ignore" beginning last semester and now occurring almost daily.
	A high school student starts to sit in the back of the class because if she sits in the front she has an uncomfortable feeling that other students are watching her.
	A 16-year-old asks his grandmother if he can leave the store and go wait in the car because he has "a sense" that others are staring and even whispering to each other about him. He knows that this is likely his "imagination," but he is uncomfortable nonetheless.
Attenuated hallucinations	On a daily basis a 22-year-old cashier sees shadows, movements, and sometimes formed figures (like an animal) out of the corner of his eye, but when he turns to look nothing is there.
	A 13-year-old hears beeping sounds that can last for minutes, several times a week, and more rarely a momentary (a second or two) faint, unintelligible voice.
	Several times a week a 15-year-old high school sophomore experiences "voices," lasting less than a minute, that sound like her, who comment on what she is doing. She isn't sure if she is really "hearing" the voices as much as experiencing thoughts that seem somehow different from her own thoughts, "because they were saying things" that she was "not conscious of thinking, like talking to myself."
Attenuated disorganization	A 20-year-old college junior seeks psychiatric treatment because she feels that her "abilities have deteriorated," especially with difficulty communicating—she rambles, confuses words (i.e., say "done" when meaning to say "down"), has jumbled speech, and often loses track of what she is saying. She exhibits tangential thinking during her evaluation.
	A formerly high-achieving high school junior is having academic difficulties due to distractibility in class and difficulty following what the teachers are saying. She also has difficulty following conversations with friends and cannot tolerate crowds because "all the noise is confusing."

Treatment recommendations for patients with psychosis risk syndrome symptoms include education about psychosis risk and regular monitoring for development of psychosis. Because cannabis use may exacerbate subsyndromal psychotic symptoms (Corcoran et al. 2008) and may be an environmental risk factor for the development of psychosis (McLaren et al. 2010), promotion of abstinence in cannabis use is an obvious intervention, although it is unknown if abstinence is effective in reducing psychosis risk. Omega-3 fatty acids have shown promise (Amminger et al. 2010) and are a low-risk option, but additional research is clearly needed before benefits are proven. Psychotherapy and psychosocial interventions that address presenting symptoms and functional impairments are also low-risk interventions with potential benefits. Use of antipsychotic medications is controversial, given their side-effect risks, and these medications are generally not recommended unless psychosis develops.

TREATMENT OF THE FIRST EPISODE

EMERGENCE OF PSYCHOSIS (FIRST EPISODE)

Schizophrenic psychotic disorders, including schizophrenia, schizoaffective disorder, and schizophreniform disorder, usually begin in adolescence or early adulthood. The diagnosis of schizophrenia requires hallucinations, delusions, or disorganization, but it is often the other associated impairments in cognitive function and the severity of negative symptoms that most contribute to social and vocational impairments (Milev et al. 2005). The clinical progression of schizophrenia occurs during the initial decade of illness, followed by relative clinical stability (an der Heiden and Häfner 2000).

THE PROBLEM OF TREATMENT DELAY

Considerable delay often occurs between the onset of psychotic symptoms and treatment initiation (i.e., duration of untreated psychosis). In most communities, an average of a year or more elapses from the time psychosis first occurs to first treatment (Perkins et al. 2005). The reasons for treatment delays are not well understood, but lack of recognition of the symptoms of psychosis as a mental illness (rather than "bad behavior") by the patient, family, and health care providers may be involved (Judge et al. 2008).

For several reasons, treatment delay is currently one of the most serious deficiencies in the clinical management of schizophrenia. First, emerging psychosis often derails normal development, and early intervention may minimize functional losses during this crucial time for psychosocial development. Second, psychosis is associated with behavioral disturbances that later may be viewed as embarrassing or that are criminal and have legal consequences. Third, the onset of psychosis is a period when individuals are at increased risk for aggressive behaviors toward others, property, or themselves. Although little systematic study of this issue has been done, it stands to reason that the sooner psychosis is appropriately treated, the lower the risk for psychosis-related aggressive behaviors. Perhaps most important is that duration of untreated psychosis has emerged as an independent predictor of likelihood and extent of recovery from an initial first episode and thus may be a potentially modifiable prognostic factor (Perkins et al. 2005). Clinical progression is associated with neuroprogression, as evidenced by loss of brain tissue, suggesting that biological changes in the brain drive clinical deterioration (Borgwardt et al. 2009).

General Principles

The first episode of schizophrenia is usually frightening, and first treatment contact may result from coercion. Initial treatment should not only address psychosis but also minimize subjective distress and focus on establishing a therapeutic alliance. Along with striving for positive symptom improvement or remission, interventions focus on maintaining the patient in treatment and addressing barriers to functional recovery.

While most (>80%) first-episode patients can achieve psychotic symptom remission (i.e., no symptoms at a psychotic level intensity), a much lower proportion will have a sustained remission, and even fewer will experience a sustained functional recovery (Derks et al. 2010; Emsley et al. 2007; Henry et al. 2010; Lieberman et al. 2003). Even with good positive symptom response, sustained functional recovery occurs in a minority of patients, with the highest symptomatic and functional recovery rates seen in specialized first-episode treatment programs. The groundbreaking Early Psychosis Prevention and Intervention Centre (EPPIC) program in Australia reported that at 7 years of follow-up, about 60% of patients were symptomatically recovered, but only a third had functional recovery, and only about 25% experienced both symptomatic remission and functional recovery (Henry et al. 2010). These figures speak to the responsiveness of first-episode psychosis, but also to the very high risk of relapse, which often derails efforts at functional recovery and may be associated with clinical deterioration mediated by neuroprogression (Lieberman 2007).

Relapse risk is very high, even in patients with good symptomatic recovery, but long-term maintenance treatment with antipsychotic drugs reduces the risk of relapse substantially. Without maintenance treatment more than 90%

of patients, including those with remission from their first episode (Alvarez-Jiménez et al. 2009; Gitlin et al. 2001; Wunderink et al. 2007), will relapse. Thus, maintenance antipsychotic treatment is a treatment cornerstone. Functional recovery should be a specific treatment target and may include strategies that address residual negative and cognitive symptoms, including cognitive remediation, as well as social skills training and vocational rehabilitation.

ANTIPSYCHOTIC CHOICE AND DOSING

All antipsychotics are effective at reducing or eliminating positive symptoms; however, there may be individual differences in both symptomatic response and the experience of side effects. Based on exhaustive reviews of the relevant literature, the Schizophrenia Patient Outcomes Research Team (PORT) concluded that there was no evidence that there are significant differences in short-term efficacy between first- and second-generation antipsychotics for first-episode psychosis and that evidence supporting long-term benefits of the second-generation drugs is inconclusive (Buchanan et al. 2010). A recent meta-analysis also reached the conclusion that there are no differences in efficacy between first- and second-generation drugs but that side-effect profiles of the drugs are distinct (Crossley et al. 2010). Among atypical antipsychotics there are no clear winners (Boter et al. 2009; McEvoy et al. 2007).

The dose of antipsychotic needed to achieve positive symptom remission in first-episode patients is typically lower than the dose needed in chronically ill patients, and use of lower doses often minimizes side-effect risk. Consistent with these studies, practice guidelines from the American Psychiatric Association and the Schizophrenia PORT guidelines recommend that patients in a first psychotic episode should be given doses that are about half of the dose used in chronically ill populations (Buchanan et al. 2010; Dixon et al. 2009, 2010; Lehman et al. 2004). Rapid dose escalation increases the risk of poorly tolerated side effects without the likelihood of more rapid or better symptom response. Finally, studies indicate that the initial response to antipsychotic treatment is a good indicator of ultimate response. When a patient does not show improvement in severity of psychosis within the first two weeks of treatment, the likelihood of a good response to that particular antipsychotic is low, and the treating clinician should consider alternative treatment options (Derks et al. 2010).

POSITIVE SYMPTOMS

Most patients (>80%) achieve positive symptom remission with antipsychotic treatment (Boter et al. 2009; Emsley et al. 2007; Lieberman et al. 2003). In specialized first-episode treatment programs that attempt to provide optimized pharmacological and psychosocial treatment, positive symptom remission in 94% of patients has been reported (Cassidy et al. 2010).

Residual positive symptoms are often addressed by sequential trials of different antipsychotics because patients may have profound individual differences in response to any given antipsychotic. Clozapine is indicated in first-episode patients with significant residual positive symptoms despite trials of two or more antipsychotics (Agid et al. 2007). Nonpharmacological strategies—specifically cognitive-behavioral therapy—have shown efficacy for residual positive symptoms in chronic schizophrenia and may be useful in first-episode schizophrenia (Dixon et al. 2009, 2010).

NEGATIVE SYMPTOMS

Negative symptoms significantly impact functional recovery, regardless of the etiology. Thus, patients should be evaluated for the presence of negative symptoms, and when these symptoms are present, the cause should be identified and addressed. Often negative symptoms are secondary to either antipsychotic side effects (e.g., impaired motivation and drive secondary to D_2 blockade; parkinsonian-related akinesia or apathy), depression (e.g., social withdrawal, anhedonia), or the effects of illness on self-esteem (e.g., poor motivation due to concerns about failure). Treatment thus should address the underlying cause. Decreasing the D_2 blockade by lowering the dose, choosing an antipsychotic with relatively low risk of parkinsonian side effects, or treating parkinsonian symptoms with anticholinergic medications may reduce or eliminate secondary negative symptoms. Psychotherapies and rehabilitation therapies may address depression and self-esteem. Residual primary negative (i.e., deficit syndrome) symptoms are difficult to treat, with no proven treatments but with preliminary evidence to support the use of glutamatergic drugs (Tuominen et al. 2006) and neurosteroids (Marx et al. 2009). Finally, positive symptoms, including paranoid delusions and disorganization, may also manifest as social withdrawal, and thus some negative symptoms may improve as positive symptoms are successfully treated.

NEUROCOGNITIVE SYMPTOMS AND SOCIAL SKILLS

Few treatments are consistently shown to successfully address neurocognitive and social impairments. Antipsychotic drugs have a moderately positive effect on cognition in first-episode schizophrenia, but there is no consistent evidence that any single drug or group of drugs has an advantage over any other (Davidson et al. 2009; Keefe et al. 2007). A promising intervention is *cognitive enhancement therapy* (CET), which targets neurocognitive and social cognitive deficits. The intervention includes computer "games" that challenge memory, problem solving, and attention, and group sessions that emphasize building social skills. In a 2-year controlled trial, patients randomly assigned to receive CET had significant improvements on measures of neurocognitive and social cognitive function, social adjustment, and negative symptom severity (Eack et al. 2009, 2010a). In addition, CET treatment was associated with greater preservation of regional gray matter volumes, with the magnitude of preservation significantly associated with clinical response (Eack et al. 2010b).

MOOD SYMPTOMS

Little systematic evidence is available to guide clinicians when confronted with residual mood lability, dysphoria, or anxiety in first-episode patients. While not systematically studied in schizophrenia, benzodiazepines are effective generally in treating anxiety, but risk of abuse may limit use if a substance use disorder is present. In spite of the lack of evidence demonstrating effectiveness, mood stabilizers, including anticonvulsants and lithium, are widely used in treating patients with schizophrenia. Some evidence indicates that they may reduce impulsivity and aggression (Huband et al. 2010).

Mood symptoms are common in first-episode patients, especially as psychosis resolves. The sparse available clinical trial data give mixed results for the value of antidepressants in patients with schizophrenia, even those whose symptoms meet full major depression syndrome criteria (Whitehead et al. 2003).

SUICIDE

The suicide risk is high in patients with schizophrenia, with about 5%–10% of patients eventually dying by suicide. More than half of these suicides occur within the first 5 years of illness (Verdoux et al. 2001). Although the presence of depression in the presenting psychotic episode or in the postpsychotic period is an important risk factor for suicide, patients with schizophrenia may attempt suicide in the absence of prominent depressive symptoms as a result of hallucinations, paranoia, disorganization, or other symptoms considered more primary to psychosis or other factors. Careful management of the illness as outlined above may reduce likelihood of suicide, as has been found in integrated first-episode treatment programs (Addington et al. 2004).

SUBSTANCE USE DISORDERS

Substance use and substance use disorders are common in first-episode patients (Green et al. 2004). Use of certain substances, particularly marijuana and psychostimulants, may be environmental factors that affect vulnerability to psychosis and impair recovery. Illicit substance use is also associated with poor adherence to treatment and thus is associated with increased relapse risk (Conus et al. 2010; Perkins et al. 2008). Thorough evaluation and targeted treatment of substance use is thus a critical component of first-episode treatment. The use of pharmacological strategies is not well researched, and clinicians often turn to strategies proven to be useful in substance-dependent patient populations.

SIDE-EFFECT MONITORING

During both the acute phase and the maintenance phase of treatment, close monitoring for medication side effects is necessary, as side effects impact subjective tolerability of medication, adherence, and overall health. Regular monitoring should be done for abnormal involuntary movements and parkinsonian symptoms, sexual side effects, weight gain, metabolic status (e.g., glucose, hemoglobin A1c [HgA1c], cholesterol, triglycerides), and sedation (Buchanan et al. 2010).

In first-episode patients, the emphasis is on prevention of adverse effects, especially weight gain. There is evidence that behavioral interventions may be effective, but only while patients are active participants in the program (Alvarez-Jiménez et al. 2008). Numerous clinical trials indicate that metformin (at dosages of 1,000–3,000 mg/day) may be particularly effective in prevention of weight gain and reversing lipid and glucose abnormalities (Bushe et al. 2009). Clinicians should consider early intervention in patients who are experiencing rapid weight gain. Strategies include switching to an antipsychotic with lower risk, and if switching is not a good option, then behavioral interventions should be offered. If weight gain continues, treatment with metformin or other pharmacological interventions (e.g., topiramate) should also be considered (Narula et al. 2010).

Prevention of movement disorders is also a priority in first-episode schizophrenia. Parkinsonian side effects should be considered unacceptable given their impact on function and the fact that their presence is a risk factor for future development of tardive dyskinesia. Early detection of tardive dyskinesia, together with early intervention (primarily switching to a medication with reduced risk, such as clozapine), may prevent or minimize the ultimate severity of involuntary movements.

MAINTENANCE PHASE TREATMENT

RELAPSE PREVENTION

Positive symptom remission or response is rarely sustained without maintenance antipsychotic treatment. Even a patient with a complete remission has a very high risk of relapse with antipsychotic discontinuation; about 75% experience positive symptom exacerbation within 1 year, and more than 90% relapse within 2 years of antipsychotic discontinuation (Gitlin et al. 2001; Wunderink et al. 2007). Relapse is associated with risk of clinical deterioration and neuroprogression, which limits eventual recovery (Lieberman 2007). Relapse prevention is thus the cornerstone of treatment of the first episode.

Relapse risk is greatly diminished by maintenance antipsychotic treatment (Alvarez-Jiménez et al. 2009). With each additional episode of psychosis, some proportion of patients will fail to recover, at least to the same degree as with their first episode. This process of psychotic relapse, treatment failure, and incomplete recovery leads many patients to a chronic course of illness. The deterioration process occurs predominantly in the early phases of the illness, especially during the first 5–10 years after the initial episode. Treatment guidelines for first-episode schizophrenia strongly recommend that clinicians consider long-term maintenance antipsychotic treatment in first-episode patients, even those with complete symptomatic and functional recovery.

Long-term adherence may be enhanced with psychotherapies based on motivational interviewing and cognitive-behavioral techniques (Gleeson et al. 2009). These therapies address attitudes and beliefs about illness and the benefits and risks associated with treatment, discover and address barriers to long-term adherence, and develop strategies to aid adherence (e.g., pill boxes, cell phone reminders). Long-acting injectable antipsychotics, individual and family therapeutic interventions, identification and treatment of comorbid substance use disorders, and assertive outreach to engage and maintain the patient in treatment may reduce risk of relapse (Alvarez-Jiménez et al. 2009; Smith et al. 2009).

FUNCTIONAL RECOVERY

First-episode patients treated in routine clinical settings typically have a deteriorating illness course despite good initial symptomatic response. For example, in a study of 349 patients followed up to 15 years after first onset of schizophrenia, 17% had no disability at follow-up, whereas 24% still had severe disability, and the remaining 59% had varying degrees of disability (Wiersma et al. 1998). Specialized first-episode treatment programs may improve functional outcomes, presumably by specifically addressing residual symptoms, promotion of long-term medication adherence, and provision of interventions targeted to social and vocational rehabilitation (Addington and Addington 2008; Henry et al. 2010; Petersen et al. 2008). Despite current best efforts, functional recovery is achieved by only a minority of patients; thus there is a huge need for research into treatments that foster sustained clinical and functional recovery.

Model First-Episode Programs

The best psychosocial interventions for first-episode patients remain unknown, although specialized first-episode treatment programs use a combination of strategies to promote symptomatic and functional recovery. In addition to optimal pharmacological therapy, model programs include family, individual, and group therapies. Many programs include an intense treatment model that is a modification of Assertive Community Treatment (ACT). The National Institute of Mental Health is sponsoring the RAISE (Recovery After an Initial Schizophrenia Episode) project, which includes a large-scale trial to evaluate the impact of integrated first-episode treatment on symptomatic and functional outcomes in first-episode schizophrenia in the United States (http://www.nimh.nih.gov/health/topics/schizophrenia/raise/index.shtml).

CONCLUSION

Early treatment of schizophrenia and related psychotic disorders is likely to minimize risk of the complications of untreated psychosis, including dangerous behaviors and functional impairments. Intervention soon after the onset of illness may increase the likelihood of recovery. Pharmacotherapy should be optimized, and family and individual psychotherapy should be considered to increase the likelihood of functional recovery. Once remission from the first episode is reached, the clinician and patient face the difficult issue of maintenance treatment duration. Despite remission, relapse risk is very high without antipsychotic treatment. Clinically useful predictors of the small minority who maintain remission without pharmacotherapy have not yet been identified, and thus long-term maintenance antipsychotic treatment is recommended. Prevention of recurrent relapse may reduce risk of clinical deterioration.

There is movement toward developing specialized programs to treat individuals in the early course of illness. The term *critical period* refers to the initial few years of illness, when attitudes and beliefs toward illness are developed and initial treatment occurs. Intense treatment, including family, group, and individual therapies, and assertive community outreach during this critical period may reduce the risk of suicide and relapse and may increase symptomatic and functional recovery.

REFERENCES

Addington J, Addington D: Outcome after discharge from an early psychosis program. Schizophr Res 106:363–366, 2008

Addington J, van Mastrigt S, Hutchinson J, et al: Pathways to care: help seeking behaviour in first episode psychosis. Acta Psychiatr Scand 106:358–364, 2002

Addington J, Williams J, Young J, et al: Suicidal behaviour in early psychosis. Acta Psychiatr Scand 109:116–120, 2004

Agid O, Remington G, Kapur S, et al: Early use of clozapine for poorly responding first-episode psychosis. J Clin Psychopharmacol 27:369–373, 2007

Alvarez-Jiménez M, Hetrick SE, González-Blanch C, et al: Non-pharmacological management of antipsychotic-induced weight gain: systematic review and meta-analysis of randomised controlled trials. Br J Psychiatry 193:101–107, 2008

Alvarez-Jiménez M, Parker AG, Hetrick SE, et al: Preventing the second episode: a systematic review and meta-analysis of psychosocial and pharmacological trials in first-episode psychosis. Schizophr Bull November 9, 2009 [Epub ahead of print]

Amminger GP, Schäfer MR, Papageorgiou K, et al: Long-chain omega-3 fatty acids for indicated prevention of psychotic disorders: a randomized, placebo-controlled trial. Arch Gen Psychiatry 67:146–154, 2010

an der Heiden W, Häfner H: The epidemiology of onset and course of schizophrenia. Eur Arch Psychiatry Clin Neurosci 250:292–303, 2000

Borgwardt SJ, Dickey C, Hulshoff Pol H, et al: Workshop on defining the significance of progressive brain change in schizophrenia: December 12, 2008 American College of Neuropsychopharmacology (ACNP) all-day satellite, Scottsdale, Arizona. The rapporteurs' report. Schizophr Res 112(1–3):32–45, 2009

Boter H, Peuskens J, Libiger J, et al: Effectiveness of antipsychotics in first-episode schizophrenia and schizophreniform disorder on response and remission: an open randomized clinical trial (EUFEST). Schizophr Res 115(2–3):97–103, 2009

Buchanan RW, Kreyenbuhl J, Kelly DL, et al: The 2009 schizophrenia PORT psychopharmacological treatment recommendations and summary statements. Schizophr Bull 36:71–93, 2010

Bushe CJ, Bradley AJ, Doshi S, et al: Changes in weight and metabolic parameters during treatment with antipsychotics and metformin: do the data inform as to potential guideline development? A systematic review of clinical studies. Int J Clin Pract 63:1743–1761, 2009

Cannon TD, Cadenhead K, Cornblatt B, et al: Prediction of psychosis in youth at high clinical risk: a multisite longitudinal study in North America. Arch Gen Psychiatry 65:28–37, 2008

Cassidy CM, Norman R, Manchanda R, et al: Testing definitions of symptom remission in first-episode psychosis for prediction of functional outcome at 2 years. Schizophr Bull 36:1001–1008, 2010

Conus P, Lambert M, Cotton S, et al: Rate and predictors of service disengagement in an epidemiological first-episode psychosis cohort. Schizophr Res 118:256–263, 2010

Corcoran CM, Kimhy D, Stanford A, et al: Temporal association of cannabis use with symptoms in individuals at clinical high risk for psychosis. Schizophr Res 106:286–293, 2008

Crossley NA, Constante M, McGuire P, et al: Efficacy of atypical v typical antipsychotics in the treatment of early psychosis: meta-analysis. Br J Psychiatry 196:434–439, 2010

Davidson M, Galderisi S, Weiser M, et al: Cognitive effects of antipsychotic drugs in first-episode schizophrenia and schizophreniform disorder: a randomized, open-label clinical trial (EUFEST). Am J Psychiatry 166:675–682, 2009

Derks EM, Fleischhacker WW, Boter H, et al: Antipsychotic drug treatment in first-episode psychosis: should patients be switched to a different antipsychotic drug after 2, 4, or 6 weeks of nonresponse? J Clin Psychopharmacol 30:176–180, 2010

Dixon LB, Perkins DO, Calmes C: Guideline watch (September 2009): Practice Guideline for the Treatment of Patients with Schizophrenia. Arlington, VA, American Psychiatric Association, 2009. Available at: http://www.psychiatryonline.com/content.aspx?aid=501001. Accessed December 10, 2010.

Dixon LB, Dickerson F, Bellack AS, et al: The 2009 schizophrenia PORT psychosocial treatment recommendations and summary statements. Schizophr Bull 36:48–70, 2010

Eack SM, Greenwald DP, Hogarty SS, et al: Cognitive enhancement therapy for early-course schizophrenia: effects of a two-year randomized controlled trial. Psychiatr Serv 60:1468–1476, 2009

Eack SM, Greenwald DP, Hogarty SS, et al: One-year durability of the effects of cognitive enhancement therapy on functional outcome in early schizophrenia. Schizophr Res 120:210–216, 2010a

Eack SM, Hogarty GE, Cho RY, et al: Neuroprotective effects of cognitive enhancement therapy against gray matter loss in early schizophrenia: results from a 2-year randomized controlled trial. Arch Gen Psychiatry 67:674–682, 2010b

Emsley R, Rabinowitz J, Medori R, et al: Remission in early psychosis: rates, predictors, and clinical and functional outcome correlates. Schizophr Res 89:129–139, 2007

Gitlin M, Nuechterlein K, Subotnik KL, et al: Clinical outcome following neuroleptic discontinuation in patients with remitted recent-onset schizophrenia. Am J Psychiatry 158:1835–1842, 2001

Gleeson JF, Cotton SM, Alvarez-Jiménez M, et al: A randomized controlled trial of relapse prevention therapy for first-episode psychosis patients. J Clin Psychiatry 70:477–486, 2009

Green AI, Tohen MF, Hamer RM, et al: First episode schizophrenia-related psychosis and substance use disorders: acute response to olanzapine and haloperidol. Schizophr Res 66:125–135, 2004

Häfner H, an der Heiden W: The course of schizophrenia in the light of modern follow-up studies: the ABC and WHO studies. Eur Arch Psychiatry Clin Neurosci
249 (suppl 4):14–26, 1999

Henry LP, Amminger GP, Harris MG, et al: The EPPIC follow-up study of first-
episode psychosis: longer-term clinical and functional outcome 7 years after index admission. J Clin Psychiatry 71:716–728, 2010

Huband N, Ferriter M, Nathan R, et al: Antiepileptics for aggression and associated
impulsivity. Cochrane Database Syst Rev 2:CD003499, 2010

Judge AM, Estroff SE, Perkins DO, et al: Recognizing and responding to early psychosis: a qualitative analysis of individual narratives. Psychiatr Serv 59:96–99,
2008

Keefe RS, Sweeney JA, Gu H, et al: Effects of olanzapine, quetiapine, and risperidone
on neurocognitive function in early psychosis: a randomized, double-blind 52-
week comparison. Am J Psychiatry 164:1061–1071, 2007

Lehman AF, Lieberman JA, Dixon LB, et al: Practice guideline for the treatment of
patients with schizophrenia (second edition). Am J Psychiatry 161 (2 suppl):1–
56, 2004

Lieberman JA: Neuroprotection: a new strategy in the treatment of schizophrenia:
neurobiological basis of neurodegeneration and neuroprotection. CNS Spectr
12(10, suppl 18):4–6, 2007

Lieberman JA, Phillips M, Gu H, et al: Atypical and conventional antipsychotic drugs
in treatment-naive first-episode schizophrenia: a 52-week randomized trial of
clozapine vs chlorpromazine. Neuropsychopharmacology 28:995–1003, 2003

Marx CE, Keefe RS, Buchanan RW, et al: Proof-of-concept trial with the neuroster-
oid pregnenolone targeting cognitive and negative symptoms in schizophrenia.
Neuropsychopharmacology 34:1885–1903, 2009

McEvoy JP, Lieberman JA, Perkins DO, et al: Efficacy and tolerability of olanzapine,
quetiapine, and risperidone in the treatment of early psychosis: a randomized,
double-blind 52-week comparison. Am J Psychiatry 164:1050–1060, 2007

McGorry PD, Yung AR, Phillips LJ, et al: Randomized controlled trial of interventions designed to reduce the risk of progression to first-episode psychosis in a
clinical sample with subthreshold symptoms. Arch Gen Psychiatry 59:921–928,
2002

McLaren JA, Silins E, Hutchinson D, et al: Assessing evidence for a causal link between
cannabis and psychosis: a review of cohort studies. Int J Drug Policy 21:10–19,
2010

Milev P, Ho BC, Arndt S, et al: Predictive values of neurocognition and negative
symptoms on functional outcome in schizophrenia: a longitudinal first-episode
study with 7-year follow-up. Am J Psychiatry 162:495–506, 2005

Morrison AP, French P, Walford L, et al: Cognitive therapy for the prevention of psychosis in people at ultra-high risk: randomised controlled trial. Br J Psychiatry
185:291–297, 2004

Morrison AP, French P, Parker S, et al: Three-year follow-up of a randomized controlled trial of cognitive therapy for the prevention of psychosis in people at ul-
trahigh risk. Schizophr Bull 33:682–687, 2007

Narula PK, Rehan HS, Unni KE, et al: Topiramate fro prevention of olanzapine associated weight gain and metabolic dysfunction in schizophrenia: a double-blind, placebo-controlled trial. Schizophr Res 118:218–223, 2010

Perkins DO, Leserman J, Jarskog LF, et al: Characterizing and dating the onset of symptoms in psychotic illness: the Symptom Onset in Schizophrenia (SOS) Inventory. Schizophr Res 44:1–10, 2000

Perkins DO, Gu H, Boteva K, et al: Relationship between duration of untreated psychosis and outcome in first-episode schizophrenia: a critical review and meta-analysis. Am J Psychiatry 162:1785–1804, 2005

Perkins DO, Gu H, Weiden PJ, et al: Predictors of treatment discontinuation and medication nonadherence in patients recovering from a first episode of schizophrenia, schizophreniform disorder, or schizoaffective disorder: a randomized, double-blind, flexible-dose, multicenter study. J Clin Psychiatry 69:106–113, 2008

Petersen L, Thorup A, Oghlenschlaeger J, et al Predictors of remission and recovery in a first-episode schizophrenia spectrum disorder sample: 2-year follow-up of the OPUS trial. Can J Psychiatry 53:660–670, 2008

Phillips LJ, McGorry PD, Yuen HP, et al: Medium term follow-up of a randomized controlled trial of interventions for young people at ultra high risk of psychosis. Schizophr Res 96:25–33, 2007

Smith TE, Weston CA, Lieberman JA: Schizophrenia (maintenance treatment). Clin Evid (Online) April 16, 2009

Tuominen HJ, Tiihonen J, Wahlbeck K, et al: Glutamatergic drugs for schizophrenia. Cochrane Database Syst Rev (2):CD003730, 2006

Verdoux H, Liraud F, Gonzales B, et al: Predictors and outcome characteristics associated with suicidal behaviour in early psychosis: a two-year follow-up of first-admitted subjects. Acta Psychiatr Scand 103:347–354, 2001

Whitehead C, Moss S, Cardno A, et al: Antidepressants for the treatment of depression in people with schizophrenia: a systematic review. Psychol Med 33:589–599, 2003

Wiersma D, Nienhuis FJ, Slooff CJ, et al: Natural course of schizophrenic disorders: a 15-year followup of a Dutch incidence cohort. Schizophr Bull 24:75–85, 1998

Woods SW, Breier A, Zipursky RB, et al: Randomized trial of olanzapine versus placebo in the symptomatic acute treatment of the schizophrenic prodrome. Biol Psychiatry 54:453–464, 2003

Woods SW, Addington J, Cadenhead KS, et al: Validity of the prodromal risk syndrome for first psychosis: findings from the North American Prodrome Longitudinal Study. Schizophr Bull 35:894–908, 2009

Wunderink L, Nienhuis FJ, Sytema S, et al: Guided discontinuation versus maintenance treatment in remitted first-episode psychosis: relapse rates and functional outcome. J Clin Psychiatry 68:654–661, 2007

Yung AR, Nelson B, Stanford C, et al: Validation of "prodromal" criteria to detect individuals at ultra high risk of psychosis: 2 year follow-up. Schizophr Res 105:10–17, 2008

NEUROCOGNITIVE IMPAIRMENTS

RICHARD S.E. KEEFE, PH.D.

CHARLES E. EESLEY, PH.D.

COGNITIVE IMPAIRMENT IN SCHIZOPHRENIA

COGNITION AS A CORE FEATURE OF SCHIZOPHRENIA

Cognitive impairment associated with schizophrenia is now viewed as a potential psychopharmacological target for treatment (Hyman and Fenton 2003). Although cognition is not a formal part of the current diagnostic criteria for schizophrenia, DSM-IV-TR (American Psychiatric Association 2000) includes seven references to cognitive dysfunction in the description of the disorder. Diagnostic and scientific experts increasingly have expressed the idea that neurocognitive impairment is a core feature of the illness and not simply the result of the symptoms or the current treatments of schizophrenia. It is likely that the fifth edition of DSM will include cognition as a domain that will need to be evaluated by clinicians in the course of a diagnostic assessment (Barch and Keefe 2010; Keefe and Fenton 2007).

PROFILE AND MAGNITUDE OF COGNITIVE IMPAIRMENT ASSOCIATED WITH SCHIZOPHRENIA

In several cognitive domains, the average cognitive impairment in schizophrenia can reach 2 standard deviations below the healthy control mean (Harvey and Keefe 1997; Heinrichs and Zakzanis 1998; Saykin et al. 1991). Although approximately 27% of patients with schizophrenia (and 85% of the general population) are not rated as "impaired" by clinical neuropsychological assessment (Palmer et al. 1997), these patients tend to have the highest levels of premorbid functioning (Kremen et al. 2000) and demonstrate cognitive functioning that is considerably below what would be expected of them based on their premorbid levels and the education level of their parents. Up to 98% of patients with schizophrenia perform more poorly on cognitive tests than would be predicted by their parents' education level (Keefe et al. 2005). In addition, comparisons of monozygotic twins discordant for schizophrenia suggest that almost all affected twins perform worse than their unaffected twin on cognitive tests (Goldberg et al. 1990). Therefore, it is likely that almost all patients with schizophrenia are functioning below the level that would be expected in the absence of the illness.

Neurocognitive tests often assess more than one domain of functioning, and many tests do not fit neatly into a single domain. Thus, descriptions of the profile of cognitive deficits in schizophrenia have varied across literature reviews. The opinion of a group of experts who served on the Neurocognition Subcommittee of the Measurement and Treatment Research to Improve Cognition in Schizophrenia (MATRICS) project (www.matrics.ucla.edu) is that the most important domains of cognitive deficit in schizophrenia are working memory, vigilance and attention, verbal learning and memory, visual learning and memory, reasoning and problem solving, speed of processing, and social cognition (Nuechterlein et al. 2004).

The most striking aspect of the profile of cognitive deficits in patients with schizophrenia is that so few cognitive functions remain similar to those in healthy control subjects (Harvey and Keefe 1997; Saykin et al. 1994). A review and meta-analysis of 204 studies shows a consistent and stable difference between patients with schizophrenia ($n=7,420$) and healthy control subjects ($n=5,865$) in a wide range of domains of cognitive functioning (Heinrichs and Zakzanis 1998). Examples of tests that measure the most important components of cognitive impairment in schizophrenia are reviewed briefly here.

Working Memory

Working memory is a core component of the cognitive impairment in schizophrenia (Goldman-Rakic 1994; Keefe 2001; Silver et al. 2003) and is related to functional outcomes such as employment status (McGurk and Meltzer 2000) and job tenure (Gold et al. 2002). Much of the clinical relevance of working memory deficits in schizophrenia comes from the strong correlations that working memory measures have with a variety of other cognitive domains impaired in schizophrenia, such as attention, planning, memory (reviewed in Keefe 2001), and intelligence (Baddeley 1992). Also, advanced understanding of the neuroanatomy of working memory functions in human and nonhuman primates suggests that neural circuitry that includes prefrontal cortical regions mediates aspects of working memory functions (Callicott et al. 1999; Goldman-Rakic 1987) and that this circuitry may be impaired in schizophrenia (Callicott et al. 1999).

Vigilance and Attention

Vigilance refers to the ability to maintain attention over time. Impairments in vigilance can result in difficulty following social conversations and an inability to follow important instructions; simple activities such as reading or watching television become labored or impossible. Vigilance deficits in patients with schizophrenia are related to various aspects of outcome, including social deficits, community functioning, and skills acquisition (Green 1996; Green et al. 2000).

Verbal Learning and Memory

The abilities involved in memory functioning include learning new information, retaining newly learned information over time, and recognizing previously presented material. In general, patients show larger deficits in learning than in retention. The tests used to measure learning typically involve the ability to learn lists of words or written passages. Much empirical evidence points to the connection between verbal memory impairment and social deficits in patients with schizophrenia (Green 1996).

Visual Learning and Memory

Because visual information is not as easily expressed as verbal information, fewer tests sensitive to the deficits of schizophrenia have been developed, and this area of cognitive function has generally been found not to be as impaired as verbal memory (Heinrichs and Zaksanis 1998).

Visual memory has been found to correlate modestly with employment status (Gold et al. 2003), job tenure (Gold et al. 2002), psychosocial rehabilitation success (Mueser et al. 1991), social functioning (Dickerson et al. 1999), quality of life ratings (Buchanan et al. 1994), and strongly with functional capacity (Twamley et al. 2003). Other studies have reported no significant correlations (Addington and Addington 2000; Addington et al. 1998; Ertugrul and Ulug 2002; Velligan et al. 2000).

Reasoning and Problem Solving

Although there are many tests of reasoning and problem solving, the most well known and most frequently used in schizophrenia research is the Wisconsin Card Sorting Test (WCST; Heaton 1981). The very poor performance of patients with schizophrenia on the WCST (Goldberg et al. 1987) and the reduced activity of the dorsolateral prefrontal cortex during performance of this test (Weinberger 1987) led to widespread pursuit of the hypothesis of frontal hypoactivation in schizophrenia. It is important to note, however, that the WCST measures a variety of cognitive functions and is not a pure measure of executive functions (Keefe 1995).

The rules of society and the workplace change regularly, and success in these arenas is often measured by one's ability to adapt to changes. Patients with schizophrenia who are impaired on measures of executive functions have difficulty adapting to the rapidly changing world around them.

Speed of Processing

Many neurocognitive tests require subjects to process information rapidly and can be compromised by impairments in processing speed. A standard example of this type of task is the Digit Symbol Test of the Wechsler Adult Intelligence Scale (Wechsler 1997). This nonspecific cognitive impairment has been found to correlate with a variety of clinically important features of schizophrenia, such as daily life activities (Evans et al. 2003), job tenure (Gold et al. 2002), and independent living status (Brekke et al. 1997).

Reduced processing speed can impair ability to keep in step with the task-oriented jobs that are frequently held by patients with schizophrenia. Increased response latency in social settings may hamper social relationships.

Social Cognition

Theory-of-mind skills and social perception have been the general focus of the literature on social cognition in schizophrenia. *Theory of mind* is the ability to infer another's intentions and/or to represent the mental states of others. Individuals with schizophrenia perform poorly on measures of theory-of-mind abilities (Corcoran et al. 1995; Drury et al. 1998; Sarfati et al. 1997). Facial affect recognition and social cue perception are the two general areas into which studies of social perception in schizophrenia can be broken down.

Reviews of the literature on facial affect recognition (Morrison et al. 1988; Penn et al. 1997) suggest that individuals with schizophrenia have stable deficits on tests of facial affect perception and that perception of negative emotions and fear may be particularly impaired (Addington and Addington 1998; Edwards et al. 2001; Gaebel and Wolwer 1992). Tests of social cue perception use more dynamic stimuli that require multiple sensory modalities, such as watching videotapes of persons interacting. Patients with schizophrenia show consistent impairments on these tasks (Bell et al. 1997; Corrigan et al. 1990). Social cognition is related to social impairments in schizophrenia, even after controlling for performance on neurocognitive tasks (Penn et al. 1996; Trumbetta and Mueser 2001).

SUMMARY

Experts in cognition and schizophrenia have come to a clear consensus that cognitive impairment is a core feature of the illness. The profile of deficits is broad and severe and is likely present in most, if not all, patients. Neurocognitive impairment has clear clinical relevance because cognitive impairment interferes with the everyday lives of patients in various important ways, from limiting social relationships to reducing the likelihood of employment.

NATURAL HISTORY OF NEUROCOGNITIVE IMPAIRMENT

The time course of the development of cognitive deficits in schizophrenia patients appears to follow a predictable pattern. Some deficits may be present in childhood, followed by a decline in cognitive function before the first episode. The severity of neurocognitive impairments increases once psychosis develops. The long-term stability of neurocognitive impairment over time is not clear, but evidence for progression in nonelderly patients is lacking.

DEFICITS IN CHILDREN AT RISK FOR SCHIZOPHRENIA

Individuals who are genetically vulnerable to schizophrenia have notable cognitive impairments (Cornblatt and Keilp 1994), whereas individuals who are examined with cognitive assessments before they develop schizophrenia are found to have impairments in a variety of areas (Davidson et al. 1999). High-risk studies of children with one or two biological parents with schizophrenia (Cornblatt et al. 1999) have suggested that attention deficits can predict which children will develop schizophrenia in the future.

Follow-Back Studies

In separate studies completed in the United Kingdom (Jones et al. 1994) and Sweden (David et al. 1997), children who went on to develop schizophrenia as adults differed significantly from the general population in a wide range of cognitive and behavioral domains. Similar findings were generated from a population-based study that investigated the risk of schizophrenia in the United States. Iowa Test scores from grades 4, 8, and 11 for 70 children who later developed schizophrenia were compared with those of children who did not develop schizophrenia. A significant drop in test scores was found between grades 8 and 11, corresponding with the onset of puberty (Fuller et al. 2002).

In Israel, a study of all adolescents ages 16–17 years suggested that cognitive functions are significantly impaired in those adolescents who are later hospitalized for schizophrenia. These cognitive deficits thus precede the onset of psychosis and, along with social isolation and impaired organizational ability, are a significant predictor of which young people will eventually develop a psychotic disorder (Davidson et al. 1999). In the young people who later experienced a first episode of schizophrenia, most of their cognitive impairments occurred prior to the first psychotic episode (Caspi et al. 2003).

Prodrome Studies

Cognitive deficits are also found in individuals who are identified as being at "ultra-high" risk (Yung and McGorry 1996) for schizophrenia by virtue of their family history of schizophrenia and/or the manifestation of mild signs and symptoms consistent with the prodromal symptoms of schizophrenia (Brewer et al. 2003; Hawkins et al. 2004). Preliminary data also suggest that olfactory identification deficits predict which individuals at ultra-high risk will develop schizophrenia (Brewer et al. 2003).

FIRST-EPISODE PSYCHOSIS STUDIES

Once psychosis develops, cognitive deficits are severe (Bilder et al. 2000; DeLisi et al. 1995; Hoff et al. 1999; Mohamed et al. 1999; Stirling et al. 2003). Patients with a first episode of schizophrenia who have never taken antipsychotic medication already exhibit cognitive impairment (Brickman et al. 2004; Mohamed et al. 1999; Saykin et al. 1994).

Cognitive Changes in Patients Recovering From Acute Exacerbation

Patients recovering from an acute exacerbation of illness do not appear to demonstrate substantial changes in the severity of their cognitive impairment despite clear improvements in symptoms with treatment (Gold 1999; Hughes et al. 2003; Nopoulos et al. 1994; Sweeney et al. 1991).

Longitudinal Change in Cognitive Function

The notion of neurodegeneration in schizophrenia has been controversial. Evidence has been presented suggesting that schizophrenia is a neurodegenerative process, and some have concluded that schizophrenia is progressive (Lieberman 1999). However, with a few notable exceptions (Bilder et al. 1992; Davidson et al. 1995; O'Donnell et al. 1995), cross-sectional studies generally have not found evidence of increased cognitive impairment in association with duration of illness, and older nonelderly patients do not manifest greater impairment than younger patients (Goldberg et al. 1993; Heaton and Drexler 1987; Hyde et al. 1994; Eyler Zorrilla et al. 2000).

Definitive answers to questions regarding possible progression of cognitive impairment in schizophrenia must come from longitudinal studies, and few have been completed. One longitudinal study traced 111 first-episode schizophrenia patients over 10–12 years and found that visuospatial function, although spared in the first episode, may deteriorate over time, whereas executive deficits do not (Stirling et al. 2003). Other longitudinal studies of neurocognitive impairment suggest that it is a stable, enduring feature of the illness, with very little change in patients with chronic schizophrenia between assessment periods of up to 5 years (Heaton et al. 2001; Rund 1998).

Summary

Neurocognitive impairment is present in a mild form before the onset of psychosis in young people destined to develop schizophrenia. Neurocognitive impairment is severe in patients who have experienced their first psychotic episode, even before antipsychotic treatment is initiated. Although some early-phase patients may demonstrate a slight improvement in neurocognitive impairment with treatment, many patients do not improve at all. Following this early phase, neurocognitive impairment appears to be remarkably consistent, even in the presence of symptom change, although few longitudinal studies have had follow-up periods of longer than 5 years.

RELATION OF NEUROCOGNITIVE IMPAIRMENT TO SCHIZOPHRENIA SYMPTOMS

If neurocognitive deficits were the result of the symptoms of the illness, then the deficits would disappear when the symptoms do. However, this is usually not the case in patients with schizophrenia. Unlike patients with psychotic bipolar illness, whose performance on cognitive tests may improve when their psychotic symptoms remit, patients with schizophrenia do not show any change in performance when psychosis remits (Harvey et al. 1990). The impact of antipsychotics on cognition is weak (Blyler and Gold 2000; Davidson et al. 2009; Keefe et al. 2007). The recalcitrance of neurocognitive impairment in the context of substantial symptom improvement is one of the most compelling lines of evidence of the independence of these symptom domains.

CROSS-SECTIONAL STUDIES OF THE RELATION TO SYMPTOMS OF SCHIZOPHRENIA

Positive Symptoms

Neurocognitive ability is not strongly correlated with severity of psychotic symptoms in patients with schizophrenia (Addington et al. 1991; Bilder et al. 1985; Strauss 1993). Although some exceptions exist, such as isolated reports of significant correlations of positive symptoms with working memory (Bressi et al. 1996; Carter et al. 1996), source monitoring (Keefe et al. 2002), and auditory distractibility (Walker and Lewine 1988), the overall trend is for general neurocognitive impairment not to be correlated with positive symptoms. This low correlation across various patient samples, including first-episode (Mohamed et al. 1999), chronic (Addington et al. 1991; Tamlyn et al. 1992), and elderly (Davidson et al. 1995) patients, confirmed in 1,331 patients assessed at entrance into the CATIE schizophrenia trial (Keefe et al. 2006), suggests that positive symptoms are clearly not the sole cause of the cognitive impairment found in patients with schizophrenia.

Negative Symptoms

Cognitive dysfunction is significantly correlated with various types of negative symptoms (Addington et al. 1991; Cuesta et al. 1995; Morris et al. 1995; Strauss 1993; Summerfelt et al. 1991; Tamlyn et al. 1992). The greater variance shared between neurocognition and negative symptoms may result from measurement overlap. For instance, the neurocognitive variable verbal fluency and the negative symptom variable poverty of speech both measure the speed at which a patient generates speech. A patient who generates speech at a slow rate will do so during a test of verbal fluency as well as in an interview during which he or she is being rated for poverty of speech.

Whether the negative symptom of reduced motivation underlies the poor performance of patients with schizophrenia on cognitive tests is controversial. Increases in pupil size are associated with increased cognitive processing demands (Granholm et al. 1996). Therefore, pupillary response can measure engagement in a task. If the cognitive deficits of patients with schizophrenia were caused by lack of interest or motivation, their pupillary response would be low throughout the period of cognitive assessment. Only during high-processing conditions do patients have abnormal pupillary responses, suggesting they put forth a normal amount of effort when being given cognitive tests, yet their decreased processing capacity leads them to be unable to engage in difficult tasks (Granholm et al. 1997).

On the contrary, cognitive deficits may cause reduced motivation. Individuals with cognitive deficits are less likely to be motivated to have goals and pursue them (reviewed by Deci and Flaste 1996). Patients with neurocognitive impairment are likely to be met with failure if they attempt to pursue employment, social, and even recreational avenues that require cognitive skill. Repeated failures are likely to cause discouragement and reduced motivation in people with schizophrenia.

Formal Thought Disorder

Deficits in semantic memory may lie at the heart of the cognition–thought disorder relation (Elvevag et al. 2002). Empirical data suggest that the difference between semantic fluency and phonological fluency, an indication of the severity of the impairment of the "semantic network" in patients with schizophrenia, predicts the severity of their formal thought disorder (Goldberg et al. 1998). Thus, a patient's ability to have verbal information available (referred to as "semantic priming") may be the most important cognitive factor in formal thought disorder.

Affective Symptoms

The distinction between depressive symptoms and negative symptoms is sometimes difficult for raters and clinicians to make (Goldman et al. 1992; McKenna et al. 1989), yet factor analyses suggest that they are separate dimensions of schizophrenia (Lindenmayer et al. 1995; Willem Van der Does et al. 1995). Higher depression scores were significantly correlated with worse verbal memory task performance, which remained even after controlling for psychomotor retardation and processing speed performance (Brebion et al. 2001). Thus, depression may influence the association between negative symptoms and cognitive impairments and also may have a direct deleterious effect on some aspects of neurocognitive impairment.

In conclusion, the cross-sectional correlations between neurocognitive impairment and symptoms are weaker than might be expected and vary depending on symptom domain. The consistency of this finding strongly supports the idea that neurocognitive impairment is not caused by psychosis.

Longitudinal Studies

The relative independence of neurocognitive impairment and symptoms in cross-sectional studies appears to be supported by longitudinal studies. When patients with schizophrenia are successfully treated with antipsychotics, the severity of their symptoms is substantially reduced (Kahn et al. 2008; Lieberman et al. 2003), yet antipsychotic treatment has only modest effects on cognition (Bilder et al. 2000; Davidson et al. 2009; Keefe et al. 2007). The stability of neurocognitive impairment occurs in the context of frequent variability of the symptoms of schizophrenia, especially the positive symptoms (Bilder et al. 2000; Harvey et al. 1996; Nopoulos et al. 1994). Studies that have calculated the correlation between change in neurocognitive impairment and symptom change have generally suggested that symptom change does not contribute substantially to cognitive change (Addington et al. 1991; Hoff et al. 1999).

Impact of Treatment on Cognition

Despite the centrality of cognition in schizophrenia, there are no proven pharmacological treatments for neurocognitive impairments currently available, and antipsychotics have minimal impact (Davidson et al. 2009; Keefe et al. 2007). Driven by the NIMH Measurement and Treatment Research to Improve Cognition in Schizophrenia (MATRICS) initiative, a pathway for FDA approval of compounds to improve cognition has been established. Included in the approved battery of tests is the MATRICS Consensus Cognitive Battery (MCCB), which includes 10 tests in the seven cognitive domains that were determined by the MATRICS Neurocognition Committee to be the most relevant cognitive treatment targets in schizophrenia (Nuechterlein et al. 2008).

SUMMARY

The literature on neurocognitive impairment demonstrates consistently that cognitive impairment is not caused by the symptoms of schizophrenia. Whereas other aspects of schizophrenia, such as negative symptoms, appear to correlate with neurocognitive impairment, there is as much or more evidence supporting the idea that neurocognitive impairment causes negative symptoms as there is evidence that negative symptoms cause neurocognitive impairment. Although there is limited evidence of a relationship between changes in neurocognitive impairment and changes in symptoms over time, there is no clear evidence that improvements in neurocognitive impairment are caused by improvements in symptoms. In fact, most data point to the relative independence of these two targets of treatment in schizophrenia.

CLINICAL IMPORTANCE OF NEUROCOGNITIVE IMPAIRMENT

CROSS-SECTIONAL CORRELATIONS WITH FUNCTION

Relation of Neurocognitive Impairment to Functioning

Cognition has been firmly established as a predictor of real-world community functioning and laboratory measures of functional capacity (Green 1996; Patterson et al. 2001). In a 1-year follow-up study of patients with first-episode psychosis, the size of the correlations between the number and quality of actual social relations and various cognitive measures were found to be in the 0.25–0.35 range (Malla et al. 2002). All of the key neurocognitive constructs have demonstrated significant relationships to functional outcome and effect sizes in the medium range (Green et al. 2000; Nuechterlein et al. 2004). Cognitive impairments are also correlated with deficits in the performance of specific skills critical for independent living (Evans et al. 2003; Patterson et al. 2001).

Unemployment

Ratings of work behavior/performance are related to baseline scores on cognitive tests in schizophrenia, and improvement in patient work performance in a 6-month work rehabilitation program was predicted by baseline performance on various cognitive tests (Bell and Bryson 2001; Lysaker and Bell 1995). Patients enrolled in school full-time or holding competitive employment show superior performance across measures of working memory, sustained attention, problem solving, and episodic memory when compared with unemployed patients (McGurk and Meltzer 2000; McGurk et al. 2003). Neurocognitive performance plays a more important role than clinical symptoms in the ability of patients with schizophrenia to work (McGurk et al. 2003).

Quality of Life

Reductions in quality of life are more strongly associated with cognitive deficits than other symptomatic features of the illness. Specifically, the relationship between subjective experience and social functioning has been shown to be mediated by executive functioning (Brekke et al. 2001). Fujii and Wylie (2003) studied the long-term effects of neurocognition on quality of life in patients with severe schizophrenia. They found that neurocognition does, in fact, have long-term predictive validity for quality of life and that therapeutics targeting neurocognition could improve quality of life in this population.

Relapse Prevention

Cognitive functions have been shown to be a strong predictor of patients' ability to manage medications (Jeste et al. 2003). Cognitive deficits contribute to patterns of medication mismanagement that are associated with poor adherence and risk of relapse (Fenton et al. 1997; Jarboe and Schwartz 1999). In one study, memory impairment was the best predictor of partial compliance (Donohoe et al. 2001). Patients performing poorly in medication management tests also had poor global scores on a dementia inventory (Patterson et al. 2002).

Medical Comorbidity

Neurocognitive impairment is also related to medical comorbidities in schizophrenia. Deficits in organization (executive skills) directly affect patients' ability to seek treatment for medical problems. In elderly patients with schizophrenia, cognitive and functional impairments predicted the later incidence of new-onset medical problems, whereas medical problems did not predict the subsequent worsening of cognitive and self-care deficits (Friedman et al. 2002). Inability of patients with schizophrenia to reduce damaging habits such as smoking has been correlated with deficits in memory and attention (Buchanan et al. 1994; George et al. 2000). Thus, cognitive impairments were shown directly to effect new-onset medical problems in older patients.

Costs

Cognitive impairment is also a major factor in the costs (direct and indirect) associated with schizophrenia (Sevy and Davidson 1995). Factors leading to the increased cost include loss of ability for self-care, level of inpatient and out-patient care needed, and loss of productivity (for both patient and caretaker).

CONCLUSION

A consensus has developed that cognitive impairment is a core feature of schizophrenia. The course of neurocognitive impairment follows a characteristic pattern and following the early phase is consistent even when positive and negative symptoms change. Consistent with the demonstration that cognitive impairments are not merely secondary to positive symptoms of schizophrenia, these two targets for treatment are largely independent. Functional status years later can be predicted with considerable accuracy from the extent of neurocognitive impairments. The relationship has been established between cognition and many other facets of schizophrenia, from social functioning to unemployment to relapse prevention. Current pharmacological treatment has little impact on cognitive function. Multiple efforts are under way to identify behavioral and pharmacological treatments that could improve cognition and the functional outcomes that it mediates.

REFERENCES

Addington J, Addington D: Facial affect recognition and information processing in schizophrenia and bipolar disorder. Schizophr Res 32:171–181, 1998

Addington J, Addington D: Neurocognitive and social functioning in schizophrenia: a 2.5 year follow-up study. Schizophr Res 44:47–56, 2000

Addington J, Addington D, Maticka-Tyndale E: Cognitive functioning and positive and negative symptoms in schizophrenia. Schizophr Res 5:123–134, 1991

Addington J, McCleary L, Munroe-Blum H: Relationship between cognitive and social dysfunction in schizophrenia. Schizophr Res 34:59–66, 1998

American Psychiatric Association: Diagnostic and Statistical Manual of Mental Disorders, 4th Edition, Text Revision. Washington, DC, American Psychiatric Association, 2000

Baddeley A: Working memory. Science 255:556–559, 1992

Barch DM, Keefe RS: Anticipating DSM-V: opportunities and challenges for cognition and psychosis. Schizophr Bull 36:43–47, 2010

Bell M, Bryson G: Work rehabilitation in schizophrenia: does cognitive impairment limit improvement? Schizophr Bull 27:269–279, 2001

Bell M, Bryson G, Lysaker P: Positive and negative affect recognition in schizophrenia: a comparison with substance abuse and normal control subjects. Psychiatry Res 73:73–82, 1997

Bilder RM, Mukherjee S, Rieder RO, et al: Symptomatic and neuropsychological components of defect states. Schizophr Bull 11:409–419, 1985

Bilder RM, Lipschutz-Broch L, Reiter G, et al: Intellectual deficits in first-episode schizophrenia: evidence for progressive deterioration. Schizophr Bull 18:437–448, 1992

Bilder RM, Goldman RS, Robinson D, et al: Neuropsychology of first-episode schizophrenia: initial characterization and clinical correlates. Am J Psychiatry 157:549–559, 2000

Blyer CR, Gold JM: Cognitive effects of conventional antipsychotics: another look, in Cognitive Functioning in Schizophrenia: Characteristics, Correlates, and Treatment. Edited by Sharma T, Harvey P. Oxford, England, Oxford University Press, 2000, pp 241–265

Brebion G, Gorman JM, Malaspina D, et al: Clinical and cognitive factors associated with verbal memory task performance in patients with schizophrenia. Am J Psychiatry 158:758–764, 2001

Brekke JS, Raine A, Ansel M, et al: Neuropsychological and psychophysiological correlates of psychosocial functioning in schizophrenia. Schizophr Bull 23:19–28, 1997

Brekke JS, Kohrt B, Green MF: Neuropsychological functioning as a moderator of the relationship between psychosocial functioning and the subjective experience of self and life in schizophrenia. Schizophr Bull 27:697–708, 2001

Bressi S, Miele L, Bressi C, et al: Deficit of central executive component of working memory in schizophrenia. New Trends in Experimental and Clinical Psychiatry 12:243–252, 1996

Brewer WJ, Wood SJ, McGorry PD, et al: Impairment of olfactory identification ability in individuals at ultra-high risk for psychosis who later develop schizophrenia. Am J Psychiatry 160:1790–1794, 2003

Brickman A, Buchsbaum M, Bloom R, et al: Neuropsychological functioning in first-break, never-medicated adolescents with psychosis. J Nerv Ment Dis 192:615–622, 2004

Buchanan RW, Holstein C, Breier A: The comparative efficacy and long-term effect of clozapine treatment on neuropsychological test performance. Biol Psychiatry 36:717–725, 1994

Callicott JH, Mattay VS, Bertolino A, et al: Physiological characteristics of capacity constraints in working memory as revealed by functional MRI. Cereb Cortex 9:20–26, 1999

Carter C, Robertson L, Nordahl T, et al: Spatial working memory deficits and their relationship to negative symptoms in unmedicated schizophrenia patients. Biol Psychiatry 40:930–932, 1996

Caspi A, Reichenberg A, Weiser M, et al: Cognitive performance in schizophrenia patients assessed before and following the first psychotic episode. Schizophr Res 65:87–94, 2003

Corcoran R, Mercer G, Frith CD: Schizophrenia, symptomatology and social influence: investigating "theory of mind" in people with schizophrenia. Schizophr Res 17:5–13, 1995

Cornblatt B, Keilp J: Impaired attention, genetics, and the pathophysiology of schizophrenia. Schizophr Bull 20:31–46, 1994

Cornblatt B, Obuchowski M, Roberts S, et al: Cognitive and behavioral precursors of schizophrenia. Dev Psychopathol 11:487–508, 1999

Corrigan PW, Davies-Farmer RM, Stolley MR: Social cue recognition in schizophrenia under variable levels of arousal. Cognit Ther Res 14:353–361, 1990

Cuesta MJ, Peralta V, Caro F, et al: Schizophrenic syndrome and Wisconsin Card Sorting Test dimensions. Psychiatry Res 58:45–51, 1995

David AS, Malmberg A, Brandt L, et al: IQ and risk for schizophrenia: a population-based cohort study. Psychol Med 27:1311–1323, 1997

Davidson M, Harvey PD, Powchik P, et al: Severity of symptoms in chronically institutionalized geriatric schizophrenic patients. Am J Psychiatry 152:197–207, 1995

Davidson M, Reichenberg A, Rabinowitz J, et al: Behavioral and intellectual markers for schizophrenia in apparently healthy male adolescents. Am J Psychiatry 156:1328–1335, 1999

Davidson M, Galderisi S, Weiser M, et al: Cognitive effects of antipsychotic drugs in first-episode schizophrenia and schizophreniform disorder: a randomized, open-label clinical trial (EUFEST). Am J Psychiatry 166:675–682, 2009

Deci EL, Flaste R: Why We Do What We Do: Understanding Self-Motivation. New York, Penguin, 1996

DeLisi LE, Tew W, Xie S, et al: A prospective follow-up study of brain morphology and cognition in first-episode schizophrenic patients: preliminary findings. Biol Psychiatry 38:349–360, 1995

Dickerson F, Boronow JJ, Ringel N, et al: Social functioning and neurocognitive deficits in outpatients with schizophrenia: a 2-year follow-up. Schizophr Res 37:13–20, 1999

Donohoe G, Owens N, O'Donnell C, et al: Predictors of compliance with neuroleptic medication among inpatients with schizophrenia: a discriminant function analysis. Eur Psychiatry 16:293–298, 2001

Drury VM, Robinson EJ, Birchwood M: "Theory of mind" skills during an acute episode of psychosis and following recovery. Psychol Med 28:1101–1112, 1998

Edwards J, Pattison PE, Jackson HJ, et al: Facial affect and affective prosody recognition in first-episode schizophrenia. Schizophr Res 48:235–253, 2001

Elvevag B, Weickert T, Wechsler M, et al: An investigation of the integrity of semantic boundaries in schizophrenia. Schizophr Res 53:187–198, 2002

Ertugrul A, Ulug B: The influence of neurocognitive deficits and symptoms on disability in schizophrenia. Acta Psychiatr Scand 105:196–201, 2002

Evans JD, Heaton RK, Paulsen JS, et al: The relationship of neuropsychological abilities to specific domains of functional capacity in older schizophrenic patients. Biol Psychiatry 53:422–430, 2003

Eyler Zorrilla LT, Heaton RK, McAdams LA, et al: Cross-sectional study of older outpatients with schizophrenia and healthy comparison subjects: no differences in age-related cognitive decline. Am J Psychiatry 157:1324–1326, 2000

Fenton WS, Blyler CR, Heinssen RK: Determinants of medication compliance in schizophrenia: empirical and clinical findings. Schizophr Bull 23:637–651, 1997

Friedman JI, Harvey PD, McGurk SR, et al: Correlates of change in functional status of institutionalized geriatric schizophrenic patients: focus on medical comorbidity. Am J Psychiatry 159:1388–1394, 2002

Fujii DE, Wylie AM: Neurocognition and community outcome in schizophrenia: long-term predictive validity. Schizophr Res 59:219–223, 2003

Fuller R, Nopoulos P, Arndt S, et al: Longitudinal assessment of premorbid cognitive functioning in patients with schizophrenia through examination of standardized scholastic test performance. Am J Psychiatry 159:1183–1189, 2002

Gaebel W, Wolwer W: Facial expression and emotional face recognition in schizophrenia and depression. Eur Arch Psychiatry Clin Neurosci 242:46–52, 1992

George TP, Ziedonis DM, Feingold A, et al: Nicotine transdermal patch and atypical antipsychotic medications for smoking cessation in schizophrenia. Am J Psychiatry 157:1835–1842, 2000

Gold JM, Goldberg RW, McNary SW, et al: Cognitive correlates of job tenure among patients with severe mental illness. Am J Psychiatry 159:1395–1402, 2002

Gold JM, Wilk CM, McMahon RP, et al: Working memory for visual features and conjunctions in schizophrenia. J Abnorm Psychol 112:61–71, 2003

Gold S: Longitudinal study of cognitive function in first-episode and recent-onset schizophrenia. Am J Psychiatry 156:1342–1348, 1999

Goldberg TE, Weinberger DR, Berman KF, et al: Further evidence for dementia of the prefrontal type in schizophrenia? A controlled study of teaching the Wisconsin Card Sorting Test. Arch Gen Psychiatry 44:1008–1014, 1987

Goldberg TE, Ragland JD, Torrey EF, et al: Neuropsychological assessment of monozygotic twins discordant for schizophrenia. Arch Gen Psychiatry 47:1066–1072, 1990

Goldberg TE, Hyde TM, Kleinman JE, et al: Course of schizophrenia: neuropsychological evidence for a static encephalopathy. Schizophr Bull 19:797–804, 1993

Goldberg TE, Aloia MS, Gourovitch ML, et al: Cognitive substrates of thought disorder; I: the semantic system. Am J Psychiatry 155:1671–1676, 1998

Goldman RS, Tandon R, Liberzon I, et al: Measurement of depression and negative symptoms in schizophrenia. Psychopathology 25:49–56, 1992

Goldman-Rakic PS: Circuitry of the frontal association cortex and its relevance to dementia. Arch Gerontol Geriatr 6:299–309, 1987

Goldman-Rakic PS: Working memory dysfunction in schizophrenia. J Neuropsychiatry Clin Neurosci 6:348–357, 1994

Granholm E, Asarnow RF, Sarkin AJ, et al: Pupillary responses index cognitive resource limitations. Psychophysiology 33:457–461, 1996

Granholm E, Morris SK, Sarkin AJ, et al: Pupillary responses index overload of working memory resources in schizophrenia. J Abnorm Psychol 106:458–467, 1997

Green MF: What are the functional consequences of neurocognitive deficits in schizophrenia? Am J Psychiatry 153:321–330, 1996

Green MF, Kern RS, Braff DL, et al: Neurocognitive deficits and functional outcome in schizophrenia: are we measuring the "right stuff"? Schizophr Bull 26:119–136, 2000

Harvey PD, Keefe RSE: Cognitive impairment in schizophrenia and implications of atypical neuroleptic treatment. CNS Spectr 2:1–11, 1997

Harvey PD, Keefe RS, Moskowitz J, et al: Attentional markers of vulnerability to schizophrenia: performance of medicated and unmedicated patients and normals. Psychiatry Res 33:179–188, 1990

Harvey PD, Lombardi J, Leibman M, et al: Cognitive impairment and negative symptoms in geriatric chronic schizophrenic patients: a follow-up study. Schizophr Res 22:223–231, 1996

Hawkins KA, Addington J, Keefe RS, et al: Neuropsychological status of subjects at high risk for a first episode of psychosis. Schizophr Res 67:115–122, 2004

Heaton RK: Wisconsin Card Sorting Test Manual. Odessa, FL, Psychological Assessment Resources, 1981

Heaton RK, Drexler M: Clinical neuropsychological findings in schizophrenia and aging, in Schizophrenia and Aging: Schizophrenia, Paranoia, and Schizophreniform Disorders in Later Life. Edited by Milner NE, Cohen GD. New York, Guilford, 1987, pp 145–161

Heaton RK, Gladsjo JA, Palmer BW, et al: Stability and course of neuropsychological deficits in schizophrenia. Arch Gen Psychiatry 58:24–32, 2001

Heinrichs RW, Zakzanis KK: Neurocognitive deficit in schizophrenia: a quantitative review of the evidence. Neuropsychology 12:426–444, 1998

Hoff AL, Sakuma M, Wieneke M, et al: Longitudinal neuropsychological follow-up study of patients with first-episode schizophrenia. Am J Psychiatry 156:1336–1341, 1999

Hughes C, Kumari V, Soni W, et al: Longitudinal study of symptoms and cognitive function in chronic schizophrenia. Schizophr Res 59:137–146, 2003

Hyde TM, Nawroz S, Goldberg TE, et al: Is there cognitive decline in schizophrenia? A cross-sectional study. Br J Psychiatry 164:494–500, 1994

Hyman SE, Fenton WS: What are the right targets for psychopharmacology? Science 299:350–351, 2003

Jarboe KS, Schwartz SK: The relationship between medication noncompliance and cognitive function in patients with schizophrenia. J Am Psychiatr Nurses Assoc 5:S2–S8, 1999

Jeste SD, Patterson TL, Palmer BW, et al: Cognitive predictors of medication adherence among middle-aged and older outpatients with schizophrenia. Schizophr Res 63:49–58, 2003

Jones P, Rodgers B, Murray R, et al: Child development risk factors for adult schizophrenia in the British 1946 birth cohort. Lancet 344:1398–1402, 1994

Kahn RS, Fleischhacker WW, Boter H, et al: Effectiveness of antipsychotic drugs in first-episode schizophrenia and schizophreniform disorder: an open randomized clinical trial. Lancet 371:1085–1097, 2008

Keefe RS: The contribution of neuropsychology to psychiatry. Am J Psychiatry 152:6–15, 1995

Keefe RS: Neurocognition, in Current Issues in the Psychopharmacology of Schizophrenia. Edited by Breier A, Tran PV, Herrera J, et al. Baltimore, MD, Lippincott Williams & Wilkins, 2001, pp 192–208

Keefe RS, Fenton WS: How should DSM-V criteria for schizophrenia include cognitive impairment? Schizophr Bull 33:912–920, 2007

Keefe RS, Arnold MC, Bayen UJ, et al: Source-monitoring deficits for self-generated stimuli in schizophrenia: multinomial modeling of data from three sources. Schizophr Res 57:51–67, 2002

Keefe RS, Eesley CE, Poe MP: Defining a cognitive function decrement in schizophrenia. Biol Psychiatry 57:688–691, 2005

Keefe RS, Bilder RM, Harvey PD, et al: Baseline neurocognitive deficits in the CATIE schizophrenia trial. Neuropsychopharmacology 31:2003–2046, 2006

Keefe RS, Sweeney JA, Gu H, et al: Effects of olanzapine, quetiapine, and risperidone on neurocognitive function in early psychosis: a randomized, double-blind 52 week comparison. Am J Psychiatry 164:1061–1071, 2007

Kremen WS, Seidman LJ, Faraone SV, et al: The paradox of normal neuropsychological function in schizophrenia. J Abnorm Psychol 109:743–752, 2000

Lieberman JA: Is schizophrenia a neurodegenerative disorder? A clinical and neurobiological perspective. Biol Psychiatry 46:729–739, 1999

Lieberman JA, Tollefson G, Tohen M, et al: Comparative efficacy and safety of atypical and conventional antipsychotic drugs in first-episode psychosis: a randomized, double-blind trial of olanzapine versus haloperidol. Am J Psychiatry 160:1396–1404, 2003

Lindenmayer JP, Grochowski S, Hyman RB: Five factor model of schizophrenia: replication across samples. Schizophr Res 14:229–234, 1995

Lysaker P, Bell M: Work rehabilitation and improvements in insight in schizophrenia. J Nerv Ment Dis 183:103–106, 1995

Malla AK, Norman RMG, Manchanda LT: Symptoms, cognition, treatment adherence and functional outcome in first-episode psychosis. Psychol Med 32:1109–1119, 2002

McGurk SR, Meltzer HY: The role of cognition in vocational functioning in schizophrenia. Schizophr Res 45:175–184, 2000

McGurk SR, Mueser KT, Harvey PD, et al: Cognitive and symptom predictors of work outcomes for clients with schizophrenia in supported employment. Psychiatr Serv 54:1129–1135, 2003

McKenna PJ, Lund CE, Mortimer AM: Negative symptoms: relationship to other schizophrenic symptom classes. Br J Psychiatry 7:104–107, 1989

Mohamed S, Paulsen JS, O'Leary D, et al: Generalized cognitive deficits in schizophrenia: a study of first-episode patients. Arch Gen Psychiatry 56:749–754, 1999

Morris RG, Rushe T, Woodruffe PW, et al: Problem solving in schizophrenia: a specific deficit in planning ability. Schizophr Res 14:235–246, 1995

Morrison RL, Bellack AS, Mueser KT: Deficits in facial-affect recognition and schizophrenia. Schizophr Bull 14:67–83, 1988

Mueser KT, Bellack AS, Douglas MS, et al: Prediction of social skill acquisition in schizophrenic and major affective disorder patients from memory and symptomatology. Psychiatry Res 37:281–296, 1991

Nopoulos P, Flashman L, Flaum M, et al: Stability of cognitive functioning early in the course of schizophrenia. Schizophr Res 14:29–37, 1994

Nuechterlein KH, Barch DM, Gold JM, et al: Identification of separable cognitive factors in schizophrenia. Schizophr Res 72:29–39, 2004

Nuechterlein KH, Green MF, Kern RS, et al: The MATRICS consensus cognitive battery, Part 1: test selection, reliability, and validity. Am J Psychiatry 165:203–213, 2008

O'Donnell BF, Faux SF, McCarley RW, et al: Increased rate of P300 latency prolongation with age in schizophrenia: electrophysiological evidence for a neurodegenerative process. Arch Gen Psychiatry 52:544–549, 1995

Palmer BW, Heaton RK, Paulsen JS, et al: Is it possible to be schizophrenic yet neuropsychologically normal? Neuropsychology 11:437–446, 1997

Patterson TL, Goldman S, McKibbin CL, et al: UCSD performance-based skills assessment: development of a new measure of everyday functioning for severely mentally ill adults. Schizophr Bull 27:235–245, 2001

Patterson TL, Lacro J, McKibbin CL, et al: Medication management ability assessment: results from a performance-based measure in older outpatients with schizophrenia. J Clin Psychopharmacol 22:11–19, 2002

Penn DL, Spaulding W, Reed D, et al: The relationship of social cognition to ward behavior in chronic schizophrenia. Schizophr Res 20:327–335, 1996

Penn DL, Corrigan PW, Bentall RP, et al: Social cognition in schizophrenia. Psychol Bull 121:114–132, 1997

Rund BR: A review of longitudinal studies of cognitive functions in schizophrenia patients. Schizophr Bull 24:425–435, 1998

Sarfati Y, Hardy-Bayle MC, Nadel J, et al: Attribution of mental states to others by schizophrenic patients. Cognitive Neuropsychiatry 2:1–17, 1997

Saykin AJ, Gur RC, Gur RE, et al: Neuropsychological function in schizophrenia: selective impairment in memory and learning. Arch Gen Psychiatry 48:618–624, 1991

Saykin AJ, Shtasel DL, Gur RE, et al: Neuropsychological deficits in neuroleptic naive patients with first-episode schizophrenia. Arch Gen Psychiatry 51:124–131, 1994

Sevy S, Davidson M: The cost of cognitive impairment in schizophrenia. Schizophr Res 17:1–3, 1995

Silver H, Feldman P, Bilker W, et al: Working memory deficit as a core neuropsychological dysfunction in schizophrenia. Am J Psychiatry 160:1809–1816, 2003

Stirling J, White C, Lewis S, et al: Neurocognitive function and outcome in first-episode schizophrenia: a 10-year follow-up of an epidemiological cohort. Schizophr Res 65:75–86, 2003

Strauss ME: Relations of symptoms to cognitive deficits in schizophrenia. Schizophr Bull 19:215–231, 1993

Summerfelt AT, Alphs LD, Funderburk FR, et al: Impaired Wisconsin Card Sort performance in schizophrenia may reflect motivational deficits. Arch Gen Psychiatry 48:282–283, 1991

Sweeney JA, Haas GL, Keilp JG, et al: Evaluation of the stability of neuropsychological functioning after acute episodes of schizophrenia: one-year follow-up study. Psychiatry Res 38:63–76, 1991

Tamlyn D, McKenna PJ, Mortimer AM, et al: Memory impairment in schizophrenia: its extent, affiliations and neuropsychological character. Psychol Med 22:101–115, 1992

Trumbetta SL, Mueser KT: Social functioning and its relationship to cognitive deficits over the course of schizophrenia, in Negative Symptom and Cognitive Deficit Treatment Response in Schizophrenia. Edited by Keefe RSE, McEvoy JP. Washington, DC, American Psychiatric Press, 2001, pp 33–67

Twamley EW, Doshi RR, Nayak GV, et al: Generalized cognitive impairments, ability to perform everyday tasks, and level of independence in community living situations of older patients with psychosis. Am J Psychiatry 159:2013–2020, 2003

Velligan DI, Bow-Thomas C, Mahurin RK, et al: Do specific neurocognitive deficits predict specific domains of community function in schizophrenia? J Nerv Ment Dis 188:518–524, 2000

Walker E, Lewine RJ: The positive/negative symptom distinction in schizophrenia: validity and etiological relevance. Schizophr Res 1:315–328, 1988

Wechsler D: Wechsler Adult Intelligence Scale—III. San Antonio, TX, Psychological Corporation, 1997

Weinberger DR: Implications of normal brain development for the pathogenesis of schizophrenia. Arch Gen Psychiatry 44:660–669, 1987

Willem Van der Does AJ, Dingemans PMAJ, Linszen DH, et al: Dimensions and subtypes of recent-onset schizophrenia: a longitudinal analysis. J Nerv Ment Dis 183:681–687, 1995

Yung AR, McGorry PD: The prodromal phase of first-episode psychosis: past and current conceptualizations. Schizophr Bull 22:353–370, 1996

SOCIAL AND FUNCTIONAL IMPAIRMENTS

AMY E. PINKHAM, PH.D.

KIM T. MUESER, PH.D.

DAVID L. PENN, PH.D.

SHIRLEY M. GLYNN, PH.D.

SUSAN R. MCGURK, PH.D.

JEAN ADDINGTON, PH.D.

SOCIAL FUNCTIONING

Problems with social relationships and role functioning, such as going to school or working, typically precede the onset of schizophrenia and continue throughout much of an affected person's life. In addition to psychotic symp-

93

toms that are hallmarks of schizophrenia, impaired social and vocational functioning are required for the diagnosis of schizophrenia according to both DSM-IV-TR (American Psychiatric Association 2000) and ICD-10 (World Health Organization 1992) classification systems. Thus, problems in social and vocational functioning are a critical feature of schizophrenia.

ONSET AND COURSE OF PSYCHOSOCIAL IMPAIRMENTS

Problems in social functioning in schizophrenia typically antedate the onset of prominent symptoms by many years. Although some people with schizophrenia have few social problems during childhood and adolescence before developing the early signs of schizophrenia, many others show one of two patterns of maladjustment (Baum and Walker 1995; Hans et al. 1992).

First, some individuals are shyer, are awkward when interacting with peers, have fewer friends, and are generally more anxious and withdrawn than others around them (Zigler and Glick 1986). These individuals may seem peculiar to others or are viewed as loners with reduced social drive. Their onset of schizophrenia is often very gradual, and the social impairments related to the illness appear to be mainly an exaggeration of problems in their premorbid social functioning.

Second, some individuals have impulse-control problems during childhood and adolescence with behavior marked by poor attention during school, fights, disregard for authority, and other problems commonly found in conduct disorder (Cannon et al. 1993; Robins 1966; Rutter 1997). These individuals' social problems stem more from their failure to recognize the rights and feelings of others than from their lack of understanding of basic social norms.

Although extensive research has documented problems in social functioning before the onset of schizophrenia, mounting evidence indicates that at least some of the pervasive social impairments observed in people who later develop schizophrenia may actually be early signs of the illness. Work by Häfner and his colleagues (Häfner 2000; Häfner et al. 2003) indicates that the first signs of schizophrenia include depression and mild negative symptoms, followed by cognitive impairment and difficulties in role functioning. Problems in these areas usually appear several years before the emergence of psychotic symptoms.

In addition to reporting that the first signs of schizophrenia include both mood and social problems that precede the onset of psychotic symptoms by several years, Häfner and colleagues (1993, 1999) found that the age at which these difficulties first emerge is related to the person's subsequent social functioning over the course of the illness. Specifically, the older an individual is when he or she develops the first signs and symptoms of schizophrenia, the more social roles that person has been able to fulfill and the better his or her social functioning will be over the course of the illness. The later age at onset of schizophrenia for women than for men accounts for women's better social functioning (Haas and Garratt 1998) and somewhat milder course of illness (Angermeyer et al. 1990), according to Häfner et al. (1993).

Over the long-term course of schizophrenia, psychosocial impairments tend to be relatively stable in the absence of concerted rehabilitation efforts. The consensus from long-term follow-up studies is that a significant proportion of patients has partial or full symptom remissions and improvements in social functioning (Häfner and an der Heiden 2003; Harding and Keller 1998). While some improvement is common, the extent of such gains has been the topic of much debate.

SOCIAL SKILLS AND SOCIAL FUNCTIONING

For many years, interventions for schizophrenia focused narrowly on relapse prevention and symptoms. However, the discovery of antipsychotic medications, followed by deinstitutionalization and the growth of community-based treatment, has shifted attention to helping patients with schizophrenia function competently in society. Improvement in the breadth of domains of functioning that most would consider integral to a successful life—work, intimacy, friendships, family, and avocations—is a major treatment priority. Psychiatric rehabilitation is a relatively new field that reflects this broader conceptualization of outcome (Corrigan et al. 2008).

In this chapter, the term *social functioning* refers to domains of behavior that involve interactions with others, including social relationships. Social functioning in schizophrenia has been operationalized at both the microcomponent and macrocomponent level. Many of the microcomponents of social functioning are subsumed under the rubric of *social skills*. These typically include the verbal, paralinguistic, and nonverbal components of interpersonal interactions, such as eye contact, facial expressions, and latency of speech utterances (Bellack et al. 2004). A related variable involves *social cognition*, a construct discussed in detail later in this chapter. Many of the core symptoms of schizophrenia, especially those pertaining to cognitive deficits and negative symptoms, are reflected in the poor social skills often shown by persons with the disorder.

At a more macro level, social functioning can be seen as analogous to social adjustment. Here, the primary issue is role functioning in domains such as work, school, and parenting. For adults, successful role functioning typically includes living independently, being financially self-sufficient through employment, having a strong social network of family and friends, and having satisfying avocations. In DSM-IV-TR, criterion B for schizophrenia reflects this impairment in role functioning.

Social Skills

Poor social skills have been understood as a core characteristic of schizophrenia from its first conceptualization as a disorder (Kraepelin 1919/1971). Among persons with schizophrenia, women tend to have better social skills (Mueser et al. 1990; Usall et al. 2002), as do those with less impaired cognitive functioning (Mueser et al. 2010) and less severe negative symptoms (Jackson et al. 1989; Patterson et al. 2001). Social skills are strongly related to the quality of social functioning and capacity for independent living (Bellack et al. 1990; Penn et al. 1995). When an individual is acutely psychotic, antipsychotic medications can lead to more appropriate social behavior, through both reducing the individual's attention to internal stimuli such as hallucinations and reducing the impact of delusions on what the person says and does. However, in the absence of an acute exacerbation of psychotic symptoms or concerted rehabilitation efforts, social skills tend to be quite stable over time in people with schizophrenia (Mueser et al. 1991).

Social skills training programs are the most common psychosocial interventions for schizophrenia. These programs involve the use of cognitive-behavioral techniques grounded in learning theory (e.g., coaching, prompting, modeling, chaining, positive reinforcement) to improve specific components of social skills (Bellack et al. 2004; Liberman et al. 1989). The generalization of social skills from training sessions to the natural environment is built into the program through strategies such as home practice assignments, in vivo trips to use skills in the community (Glynn et al. 2002), and involvement of natural supports such as family and friends to prompt skills as needed (Tauber et al. 2000). Sessions can be run individually or in a group and typically are offered in a time-limited fashion. Typical therapeutic goals might include improving conversational skills, making friends, resolving conflict, and enhancing community living skills (e.g., use of transportation, budgeting). Immediate outcome is usually assessed through role-plays or performance on mastery tests of the curriculum taught, while the primary longer-term goals are usually improving quality of relationships, role functioning, and independent living. The steps of social skills training are summarized in Table 5–1.

Recently, two meta-analyses of controlled research on social skills training have been published with remarkably similar conclusions regarding its effects (Kurtz and Mueser 2008; Pfammatter et al. 2006). Kurtz and Mueser (2008) hypothesized that the impact of social skills training would be strongest on outcomes that were most "proximal" or immediate to the training methods used, such as mastery tests of skills training content and perfor-

mance of role-play tests of social skill; moderate on outcomes related to social skill, such as social functioning and negative symptoms; and weakest on
outcomes more distally related to skills training, such as other symptoms and
relapses. Their hypotheses were largely supported, with significant effects
found on all of the domains listed above. Of greatest significance, social skills
training had a significant effect on improving social and community functioning, underscoring the importance of this method of psychiatric rehabilitation
for persons with schizophrenia.

Other Approaches to Improving Social Functioning

In addition to social skills training, a variety of other interventions are used
to improve social functioning in schizophrenia. Similar to its effects on social
skills, antipsychotic medications do not have a major impact on improving
social functioning, except to the extent of reducing or eliminating psychotic
symptoms that can have a deleterious effect on social and community adjustment. Therefore, the most effective treatments for improving social functioning tend to be psychosocial in nature.

Cognitive-behavioral therapy for psychosis is a psychotherapeutic approach to schizophrenia that involves systematically teaching individuals how
to examine, challenge, and (when inaccurate) change the thoughts, attributions, and beliefs underlying upsetting psychotic symptoms, poor self-esteem, and perceptions of interference with attaining functional goals (Beck
et al. 2009; Fowler et al. 1995; Kingdon and Turkington 2004; Morrison et
al. 2004). Cognitive-behavioral approaches also often teach coping skills for
dealing with persistent psychotic symptoms. Although cognitive-behavioral
therapy has been combined with social skills training (Granholm et al. 2005),
usually they are provided as separate interventions. The results of the most recent comprehensive meta-analysis provide support for the efficacy of cognitive-behavioral therapy for schizophrenia (Wykes et al. 2008); not only was
the intervention found to significantly reduce the severity of psychotic and
negative symptoms, but it was also found to improve social functioning.

Cognitive functioning is often impaired in schizophrenia (Heaton et al.
1994) and is strongly related to psychosocial functioning (Green et al. 2000).
Therefore, cognitive remediation aims at improving cognitive functioning in
areas such as attention, psychomotor speed, memory, and executive functions
with the intention of improving social and role functioning. A wide range of
cognitive training methods have been developed that often employ computer-
based cognitive exercises, and may also involve individual or group-based
practice of cognitive skills. Some of these programs are integrated or combined with other psychiatric rehabilitation methods, such as social skills or social cognition training (Hogarty et al. 2004; Roder et al. 2002; Silverstein et

---

TABLE 5–1.   Steps of social skills training

---

1. Establish rationale for the skill.

   - Elicit reasons for learning the skill from group participants.
   - Acknowledge all contributions.
   - Provide additional reasons not mentioned by group members.

2. Discuss the steps of the skill.

   - Break down the skill into three or four steps.
   - Write the steps on a board or poster.
   - Discuss the reason for each step.
   - Check for understanding of each step.

3. Model the skill in a role-play.

   - Explain that you will demonstrate the skill in a role-play.
   - Plan out the role-play.
   - Use two leaders to model the skill.
   - Keep the role-play simple.

4. Review the role-play with the participants.

   - Discuss whether each step of the skill was used in the role-play.
   - Ask group members to evaluate the effectiveness of the role model.
   - Keep the review brief and to the point.

5. Engage a patient in a role-play of the same situation.

   - Request the patient to try the skill in a role-play with one of the leaders.
   - Ask the patient questions to make sure he or she understands their goal.
   - Instruct members to observe the patient.
   - Start with a patient who is more skilled or is likely to be compliant.

6. Provide positive feedback.

   - Elicit positive feedback from group members about the patient's skills.
   - Encourage feedback that is specific.
   - Cut off any negative feedback.
   - Praise effort and provide hints to group members about good performance.

TABLE 5–1. Steps of social skills training *(continued)*

7. Provide corrective feedback.

- Elicit suggestions for how patient could do the skill better next time.
- Limit the feedback to one or two suggestions.
- Strive to communicate the suggestions in a positive, upbeat manner.

8. Engage the patient in another role-play of the same situation.

- Request that the patient change one behavior in the role-play.
- Check by asking questions to make sure the patient understands the suggestion.
- Try to work on behaviors that are salient and changeable.

9. Provide additional feedback.

- Focus first on the behavior that the patient was requested to change.
- Engage patient in two to four role-plays with feedback after each one.
- Use other behavior-shaping strategies to improve skills, such as coaching, prompting, supplemental modeling.
- Be generous but specific when providing positive feedback.

10. Assign homework.

- Give an assignment to practice the skill.
- Ask group members to identify situations in which they could use the skill.
- When possible, tailor the assignment to each patient's level of skill.

---

al. 2005). A recent meta-analysis of controlled trials of cognitive remediation for schizophrenia finds significant benefits on both cognitive functioning and psychosocial adjustment (McGurk et al. 2007b). Interestingly, although programs that provide another type of psychiatric rehabilitation in addition to cognitive remediation did not have stronger effects on cognitive functioning, the combination of both types of treatment is significantly more effective at improving psychosocial functioning than cognitive remediation alone.

Several other interventions may also improve social functioning in schizophrenia, with research providing less definitive support at this time. First, developing illness self-management skills (Mueser et al. 2002), such as developing a relapse prevention plan, managing stress, strategies to enhance medication adherence, and coping strategies for symptoms, may improve social functioning by reducing the interfering effects of symptoms and relapses on relationships and independent living (Hogarty et al. 1997a, 1997b; Levitt et al. 2009). Second, family psychoeducation that involves forming a partnership between the treatment team and the family (including the patient), teaching them about schizophrenia and its treatment, developing relapse prevention strategies, and reducing stress through more effective communication and problem solving strategies (Dixon et al. 2010) can improve social functioning by reducing relapses and fostering family support for the patient's goals (Barrowclough and Tarrier 1998). Third, environmental-based interventions may be useful in facilitating more independent living for patients with severe psychosocial impairments. For example, Velligan et al. (2000) find that implementing a set of compensatory strategies (e.g., color coding, checklists, audible prompts) tailored to the participants' impediments in motivation, impulse control, and executive functioning lead to significant improvements in functioning.

VOCATIONAL FUNCTIONING

Poor occupational functioning is common in patients with schizophrenia, with competitive employment rates typically in the range of 10%–20% (Brekke et al. 1993; Marwaha and Johnson 2004; Mueser et al. 2001). Long-term outcome studies report occupational decline from premorbid levels in a significant proportion of persons with schizophrenia (Johnstone et al. 1990; Marneros et al. 1992). Moreover, this decline is evident as early as 6–18 months after the first episode (Beiser et al. 1994; Ho et al. 1998).

The high rate of unemployment among persons with schizophrenia has important implications for the effect of the disorder on the individual, the family, and society. From an individual perspective, high costs are associated with unemployment in schizophrenia, such as living in poverty with an increased vulnerability to victimization (Goodman et al. 2001; Walsh et al. 2003). People with schizophrenia who are working tend to function better across a range of different domains, and the attainment of work in previously unemployed persons is associated with increases in self-esteem, decreases in depression and psychotic symptoms, improved satisfaction with finances, and better overall functioning (Arns and Linney 1993; Bond et al. 2001; Mueser et al. 1997), supporting the old adage that "work is good therapy" (Harding et al. 1987).

Low employment rates in schizophrenia also naturally lead to an increased dependence on the family for housing support and getting basic needs met, contributing to significant objective and subjective burden on relatives (Baronet 1999; Dyck et al. 1999).

In addition, unemployment, resulting in lost productivity and the need for supplemental income, is a primary source of the high cost of schizophrenia, estimated to exceed $6 billion per year (Rice 1999). Indeed, the loss of productivity over most of the adult lifetime is a major reason that the combined economic and social costs of schizophrenia place it among the world's top 10 causes of disability-adjusted life-years (Murray and Lopez 1996).

Finally, work is a critical component of how people in Western society define themselves, and the inability to work sets patients with schizophrenia apart from others and further contributes to their social marginalization (Crisp et al. 2000). Unfortunately, the stigma associated with schizophrenia may impede the ability of people with the illness to obtain jobs because of discrimination, which increases their stigmatization even more (Farina 1998; Wahl 1999). Increasing employment rates may decrease both stigmatizing public attitudes toward schizophrenia and self-stigmatizing beliefs among persons with the illness (Wahl 1997).

CORRELATES AND PREDICTORS OF WORK

A variety of sociodemographic, historical, and clinical correlates of work have been identified in schizophrenia. Schizophrenia is associated with a curtailed level of education (Kessler et al. 1995), and as in the general population, level of education is related to work in schizophrenia (Mueser et al. 2001). Some research suggests that social skills are related to work performance in persons with schizophrenia (Arns and Linney 1995; Bellack et al. 1990). However, an even greater wealth of evidence points to the importance of symptoms and cognitive functioning as contributing factors to impaired vocational functioning in schizophrenia. The severity of both psychotic and negative symptoms is correlated with, and predictive of, work in persons with schizophrenia (Glynn et al. 1992; McGurk and Mueser 2004; Racenstein et al. 2002).

Impaired cognitive functioning is the clinical feature of schizophrenia that is most strongly related to work (McGurk and Meltzer 2000), with multiple studies demonstrating the association. A review of correlates and predictors of work in schizophrenia and other severe mental illnesses concluded that although symptoms and cognitive functioning predict work in schizophrenia, the associations tend to be stronger in patients not receiving employment services than among patients receiving such services (McGurk and Mueser 2004). A possible implication of these findings is that vocational rehabilitation may serve to compensate for the effects of illness-related impairments, both symptom and cognitive, on work. Furthermore, there is some evidence from controlled trials that cognitive remediation may accentuate the effects of vocational rehabilitation programs on work outcomes (Bell et al. 2005, 2007; Lindenmayer et al. 2008; McGurk et al. 2005, 2007a, 2009; Vauth et al. 2005).

VOCATIONAL REHABILITATION

The high rates of unemployment in patients with schizophrenia underscore the importance of improving employment outcomes in these individuals. Furthermore, most persons with schizophrenia express a desire for competitive work (Mueser et al. 2001; Rogers et al. 1991). Various vocational rehabilitation models have been developed to address the poor work outcomes of persons with schizophrenia. Traditional approaches that use a "train-place" approach (i.e., where patients engage in extensive preparation before getting a competitive job, such as vocational counseling, skills training, or sheltered work) found few beneficial effects on competitive work outcomes (Bond 1992). In contrast, vocational rehabilitation models that emphasize rapid job search and attainment and include the provision of follow-along supports (most notably, supported employment) are empirically validated.

Supported Employment

Purpose and scope.   Supported employment focuses on helping patients find competitive jobs in integrated community settings and on providing ongoing supports to facilitate good job performance or to help in the transition to another job. The most widely studied approach to supported employment for severe mental illness is the Individual Placement and Support (IPS) model (Becker and Drake 2003). The IPS model of supported employment is defined by the principles outlined in Table 5–2.

Research on supported employment.   Over the past decade, a growing body of research has documented the effectiveness of supported employment for persons with schizophrenia and other severe mental illnesses. Most of the research has examined the IPS model (Becker and Drake 2003), although research also has evaluated other models of supported employment. Five quasi-experimental studies have examined the effects of closing day treatment programs and initiating supported employment programs in their place (Bailey et al. 1998; Becker et al. 2001; Drake et al. 1994, 1996a; M. Gold and Marrone 1998). Across the studies, the conversion to a supported employment program was associated with significant increases in work, without any untoward effects observed, such as increases in relapses or rehospitalizations.

In addition to these quasi-experimental studies, 16 randomized controlled trials have reported the superiority of supported employment to a variety of other vocational rehabilitation approaches across the United States and worldwide, as illustrated in Figure 5–1 (Bond et al. 2008). These studies have shown that IPS or other approaches to supported employment result in significantly higher levels of competitive employment over 1–2 years compared with a va-

TABLE 5–2.   Principles of the Individual Placement and Support (IPS) model of supported employment

1. Zero exclusion for participation in program
   - Eligibility to participate in supported employment program is determined solely by patient's desire to work.
   - No clinical stabilization criteria are imposed on patient's ability to participate in program.
2. Focus on competitive work
   - Emphasis is on competitive jobs paying competitive wages in integrated community settings.
   - Focus is on jobs "owned" by patient rather than rehabilitation agency.
   - Focus is on truly competitive jobs, rather than on protected or sheltered jobs for people with a disability.
3. Rapid job search
   - Uses brief rather than extensive assessment following enrollment in program.
   - Job search usually begins within month of patient joining program.
   - No prevocational skills training is required.
4. Follow-along supports
   - Time-unlimited supports are provided after individual obtains job.
   - A wide range of supports is possible, such as teaching job-related skills, teaching social skills related to the workplace, negotiating job accommodations with employer, teaching strategies to cope with cognitive difficulties or symptoms, problem solving work-related challenges, collaborating with natural supports (e.g., family).
5. Attention to patient preferences
   - Jobs are developed and sought based on patient's interests and preferences, rather than just availability.
   - Respect for patient preferences regarding whether to disclose his or her psychiatric disorder to a prospective or current employer.
6. Integration of vocational and clinical services
   - Vocational and clinical services are integrated at level of clinical treatment team.
   - When possible, vocational and clinical services are located together at same place.
   - At least weekly meetings between vocational service provider and clinical team are held.
7. Benefits counseling
   - All patients receive information about how work may affect their disability benefits.
   - Patients are informed about specific work incentive programs for persons with disabilities.

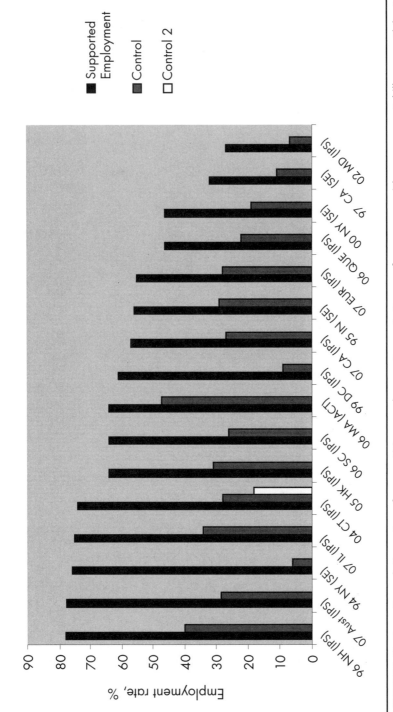

FIGURE 5–1. Cumulative rates of competitive employment over 1–2 years for persons with severe mental illness participating in 16 randomized controlled trials of supported employment programs.

ACT=Assertive Community Treatment; IPS=Individual Placement and Support model of supported employment; SE=other supported employment model. Specific vocational programs used in comparisons with IPS and SE included sheltered work, brokered vocational rehabilitation services, prevocational preparation and skills training, psychosocial rehabilitation programs, and diversified vocational placement (i.e., access to multiple types of programs). See text for details.

riety of other programs, including sheltered work in New York (Gervey and Bedell 1994); Washington, D.C. (Drake et al. 1999); and South Carolina (P.B. Gold et al. 2004); brokered vocational rehabilitation services in California (Chandler et al. 1997; Twamley et al. 2004), New York (McFarlane et al. 2000), and Connecticut (Mueser et al. 2004); prevocational preparation and skills training in Indiana (Bond et al. 1995) and New Hampshire (Drake et al. 1996b); psychosocial rehabilitation programs in Connecticut (Mueser et al. 2004) and Maryland (Lehman et al. 2002); certified psychosocial clubhouse vocational services in Massachusetts (Macias et al. 2006); diversified vocational placement (i.e., access to multiple types of programs) in Illinois (Bond et al. 2007); and traditional vocational services in Australia, Europe (Burns et al. 2007), Hong Kong (Wong et al. 2008), and Quebec (Latimer et al. 2005). Thus, significant research supports the effectiveness of supported employment for persons with severe mental illness.

SOCIAL COGNITION

To this point, we have discussed social and vocational impairment in schizophrenia, with a primary emphasis on remediation strategies that directly target these impairments. In the remainder of this chapter, we provide an overview of *social cognition*, a construct that has been firmly linked to functional outcome and that may provide additional insight into novel treatment strategies. Social cognition, which has been defined as "the human ability and capacity to perceive the intentions and dispositions of others" (Brothers 1990, p. 28), includes the cognitive processes involved in thoughts about the self, others, social situations, and social interactions (Penn et al. 1997). A related definition has been proposed by Adolphs (1999), who describes it as "the processes that subserve behavior in response to conspecifics, and, in particular, to those higher cognitive processes subserving the extreme, diverse, and flexible social behaviors that are seen in primates" (p. 469). These definitions characterize social cognition as being a key component of social behavior.

Unlike nonsocial cognition (or neurocognition), which has enjoyed a long history of investigation in schizophrenia, social cognition has only recently come to the forefront, motivated in part by several factors. First, individuals with schizophrenia show impairments in multiple domains of social cognition. Second, there is growing evidence that individuals with schizophrenia show abnormal functioning of a neural network—composed of the prefrontal cortex, fusiform gyrus, superior temporal sulcus, and amygdala—specialized for the processing of social information, and that these abnormalities may underlie social cognitive impairments (Phillips et al. 2003a, 2003b; Pinkham et al. 2003). Third, it is increasingly realized that social cognition is directly related to social functioning (Couture et al. 2006; Pinkham and Penn 2006) and may mediate the relationship between neurocognition and functional outcome (Addington et al. 2006b; Brekke et al. 2005; Nienow et al. 2006; Vaskinn et al. 2008). These findings identify social cognition as an important target for pharmacological and psychosocial treatments and indicate that improving social cognition may have a direct effect on real-world outcomes.

In the ensuing sections, we review three major domains of social cognition in schizophrenia (Figure 5–2): 1) theory of mind, 2) attributional style, and 3) facial affect perception, with particular emphasis on the salient issues relevant to each domain.

THEORY OF MIND IN SCHIZOPHRENIA

Theory of mind (ToM) refers to the ability to represent the mental states of others and/or to make inferences about another's intentions. Skills that fall under the rubric of ToM include understanding false beliefs, hints, intentions, deception, metaphor, irony, and faux pas. A common way to conceptualize ToM skills is to place them in a hierarchical ordering of complexity. For example, false beliefs are often referred to as being of either first- or second-order ToM. *First-order ToM* involves the ability to understand that someone can hold a false belief about the state of the world, whereas *second-order ToM* is the more complex ability to understand that someone can have a false belief about the belief of another character (Frith and Corcoran 1996). Accordingly, increasingly subtle ToM concepts such as hints, deception, metaphor, and irony are considered more difficult to understand than false beliefs.

In the following section, ToM is reviewed specifically as it relates to schizophrenia. ToM deficits that are evident in individuals with schizophrenia, as well as the relation of these deficits to general cognitive abilities, phases of illness, and social functioning, are discussed.

Mind Deficits

The finding that individuals with schizophrenia show impairments in ToM has been well established, with meta-analyses by Sprong et al. (2007) and Bora et al. (2009) reporting effect sizes of 1.255 and 1.10, respectively. Recent work also demonstrates that deficits may be present in first-episode (Bertrand et al. 2007; Kettle et al. 2008) and prodromal samples (Chung et al. 2008). Some debate remains, however, about whether certain symptom clusters are most related to this impairment. While some studies suggest greater impairment in individuals with predominantly negative symptoms (Corcoran et al. 1995; Pickup and Frith 2001), others have found that individuals with disorganiza-

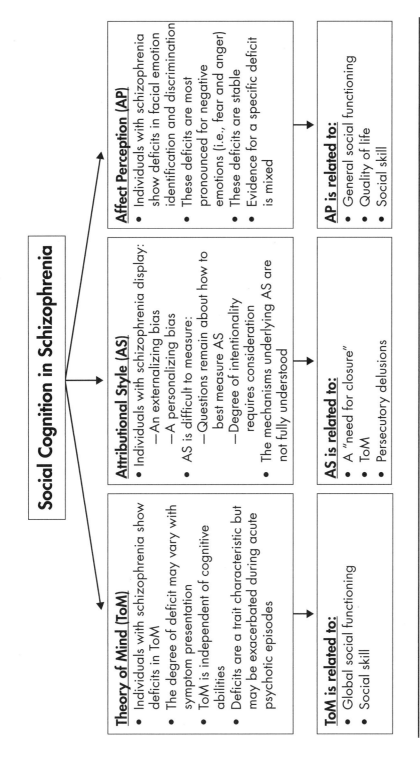

FIGURE 5–2.   Major domains of social cognition in schizophrenia.

tion have more difficulty (Pilowsky et al. 2000; Sarfati and Hardy-Bayle 1999; Sarfati et al. 1997, 1999). This latter finding has received support from the meta-analysis of Sprong and colleagues (2007), who found that disorganized subgroups performed worse than nondisorganized and paranoid subgroups. Of importance however, Sprong and colleagues qualified their results by noting inconsistencies across studies in patient subgrouping and by the use of hierarchical grouping procedures in which individuals in the disorganized subgroup may have also had the defining symptoms of other groups. Thus, it is possible that these results may be explained by greater symptom complexity in the disorganized group rather than reflect true differences between subgroups.

Cognitive Abilities

On the whole, it appears that ToM deficits are at least partially independent of cognitive functioning (for reviews, see Brune 2005a, 2005b; Harrington et al. 2005). Meta-analyses addressing this question have reported conflicting results, with Sprong et al. (2007) reporting no effect of IQ on effect size indices and Bora et al. (2009) reporting a significant influence of IQ impairment on ToM deficit. Individual studies also deserve consideration. For example, two studies that matched groups on IQ still found ToM impairments in individuals with schizophrenia compared with healthy and psychiatric control subjects (Frith and Corcoran 1996; Pickup and Frith 2001), and Brunet and colleagues (2003b) elegantly demonstrated that individuals with schizophrenia could successfully complete sequences of physical causality, both with and without social characters, but that they could not complete sequences involving the attribution of intentions or ToM. These results remained stable after controlling for verbal IQ.

In addition to these behavioral studies, neuroimaging research also supports the dissociation between ToM and cognitive abilities. Numerous neuroimaging studies of healthy individuals suggest that there are specific neural structures that subserve ToM (for review, see Pinkham et al. 2003). These structures, primarily the medial prefrontal cortex and, to some extent, the orbitofrontal cortex (Brodmann areas 8 and 9), are activated in healthy individuals during ToM tasks but not during comparable non-ToM cognitive tasks. As applied to schizophrenia, several studies have found reduced activation of the medial prefrontal cortex during tasks of mental state attribution and have suggested that these abnormalities may underlie ToM deficits (Brunet et al. 2003a; Pinkham et al. 2008; Russell et al. 2000). Thus, a strong case can be made that ToM is generally independent from general cognitive functioning and that impairments in ToM are not caused by deficits in general intellectual abilities.

A State or Trait Deficit?

An important question is whether ToM deficits are dependent on the individual's clinical state (i.e., stage of illness) or whether they are a trait characteristic. Several studies support the idea of a state-dependent relationship. One of the earliest studies to address this question found that individuals whose symptoms were in remission at the time of testing performed just as well as control subjects on a hinting ToM task (Corcoran et al. 1995)—a finding that has been replicated in multiple studies using a variety of ToM tasks, including first- and second-order false belief tasks (Frith and Corcoran 1996; Pickup and Frith 2001), metaphor and irony tasks (Drury et al. 1998), and the hinting task (Corcoran 2003). Despite these findings, evidence supporting a trait hypothesis is mounting. Perhaps most convincingly, both previously mentioned meta-analyses report that ToM deficits persist in patients whose symptoms are in remission (Bora et al. 2009; Sprong et al. 2007). Thus, at present, it appears that a combination of state and trait factors is likely involved such that deficits are exacerbated during acute episodes but remain even in asymptomatic individuals.

Social Functioning

Thus far, the majority of research on social functioning has focused on characterizing the nature of deficits in ToM; however, a growing number of studies has confirmed the presence of a strong relationship between ToM and social functioning and social outcome (Pinkham and Penn 2006; Pollice et al. 2002). For example, Brune (2005) found that ToM performance accounted for 24% of the variance in problem social behavior, and Roncone et al. (2002) reported that ToM accounted for 15% of the variance in social functioning. Thus, it appears that deficits in ToM have an association with social functioning, which provides support for targeting ToM in psychosocial treatment trials, as has been done in autism research (Hadwin et al. 1996, 1997; Ozonoff and Miller 1995; Swettenham 1996).

Overall, we may conclude that individuals with schizophrenia have impairments in ToM that appear to be somewhat independent from general cognitive abilities and that are likely present even in remitted states. Future work will likely be targeted toward further elucidating the relationship between specific symptoms and ToM deficits and developing ToM remediation programs that may ultimately result in improved functioning.

ATTRIBUTIONAL STYLE IN SCHIZOPHRENIA

Attributions refer to how one explains the causes for positive and negative outcomes. Much of the work on attributions, as applied to clinical populations, grew out of the groundbreaking research by Seligman and colleagues, who reported that individuals with depression make internal, stable, and global attributions for negative events (Abramson et al. 1978). Thus, a depressed individual who fails an exam will think that he or she is stupid (an internal attribution), that he or she will always fail exams (a stable attribution), and that he or she is a failure at everything (a global attribution).

In this section, we discuss attributional style and schizophrenia. The bulk of the research in this area has focused on attributional style in individuals with paranoia or persecutory delusions; thus, this will be the focus of our review. We begin by providing an overview of the two most common attributional biases observed in individuals with persecutory delusions: a self-serving attributional style and a personalizing bias. We conclude this section with a discussion of unanswered questions in this area.

Self-Serving and Personalizing Biases

Attributional style in schizophrenia has received much attention over the past 15 years, and unlike depression, the internal dimension has fostered the greatest interest in schizophrenia research.

Richard Bentall, the pioneer in this area, and colleagues observed that individuals with paranoia or persecutory delusions (the former referring to diagnostic subtypes, the latter to symptom severity) tended to show a self-serving bias (i.e., taking credit for successful outcomes and denying responsibility for negative outcomes) that was, they argued, an exaggeration of the bias seen in nonclinical control subjects (and opposite to what is typically observed in depressed individuals) (Bentall et al. 1994, 2001; Blackwood et al. 2001; Kaney and Bentall 1989).

However, as pointed out in a number of excellent reviews (Bentall et al. 2001; Garety and Freeman 1999), direct replication of the self-serving bias has been limited (Candido and Romney 1990), with studies either finding no evidence of a self-serving bias (Martin and Penn 2002) or providing only partial support in the form of only an external attribution for negative outcomes (rather than the additional positive attribution for positive outcomes) (Fear et al. 1996; Garety and Freeman 1999; Kinderman and Bentall 1997; Krstev et al. 1999; Lyon et al. 1994; Sharp et al. 1997). Perhaps as a result, several more recent studies have utilized the broader term "externalizing bias," rather than the more specific self-serving bias, when reporting on attributional style in schizophrenia (Janssen et al. 2006; Langdon et al. 2006, 2010).

The investigation of the tendency of individuals with persecutory delusions to attribute negative outcomes to external factors can be refined by distinguishing between external "personal" attributions (i.e., causes that are attributed to other people) and external "situational" attributions (i.e., causes that are attributed to situational factors) (Kinderman and Bentall 1996a, 1996b). This distinction is in accord with the clinical experience of individuals with persecutory delusions, who often explain negative outcomes (e.g., someone not returning a phone call right away) as being due to malevolent intentions (e.g., that person is angry at them) rather than to a situational context (e.g., the person is out of town). Kinderman and Bentall (1996b) described this style of attributing negative outcomes to others, rather than to situations, as a "personalizing bias."

There is growing evidence in support of a personalizing bias for individuals with persecutory delusions (reviewed in Bentall et al. 2001; Garety and Freeman 1999; see also Aarke et al. 2009; Langdon et al. 2010). Specifically, a tendency toward a personalizing bias has been observed in people with persecutory delusions relative to individuals with depression (Kinderman and Bentall 1997), nonparanoid individuals with schizophrenia (Aarke et al. 2009), and nonclinical control subjects (Kinderman and Bentall 1997; Martin and Penn 2002) and may be most pronounced in individuals with acute, rather than remitted, symptoms (Aarke et al. 2009; Randall et al. 2003). This tendency to blame others likely increases negative affect, defensiveness, avoidance, and possibly aggressive behaviors (Waldheter et al. 2005).

Unanswered Questions

The study of attributional style has demonstrated that attributions may be best understood within symptom rather than diagnostic category models and that people with persecutory delusions have a tendency to blame others, rather than situations, for negative outcomes. There remain, however, a number of unanswered questions that plague this area of research. First and foremost is how to measure attributions in this clinical population. Current measures of attributional style have been criticized as having poor psychometric properties (e.g., ASQ) or, because of being composed of hypothetical scenarios, as having questionable external validity (e.g., IPSAQ) (Bentall et al. 2001; Garety and Freeman 1999).

In addition, the most widely used measures of attributional style in schizophrenia research do not make a distinction among negative outcomes that vary in degree of intentionality. For example, most people would agree that the following scenario involves a negative outcome in which the intent is clear: "A person jumps ahead of you on a grocery line and says, 'I'm in a rush.'" However, what would be the intent in the following situation? "You walk past a group of teenagers, and as you pass by you hear them laugh." One could argue that it is the latter type of situation, in which the intent is ambiguous, that is particularly problematic for individuals with persecutory delusions. Of note, however, a new measure, the Ambiguous Intentions Hostility

Questionnaire (AIHQ; Combs et al. 2007b), has been developed to address this possibility, and initial results show a strong relationship between a hostile social cognitive bias and paranoia (Combs et al. 2007b).

Perhaps the most pressing unanswered question in this area is the mechanism by which persecutory beliefs lead to attributional biases or vice versa. As reviewed by Penn et al. (2008), current models posit a beneficial role for attributional biases, as the tendency to blame others for negative outcomes may protect the individual with persecutory delusions from low self-esteem. One trade-off, however, is that continually blaming others for negative outcomes can lead to increasingly negative views of others—views that are not corrected over time even in the face of exonerating evidence.

Bentall and colleagues (2001) hypothesize that two factors may prevent people with persecutory delusions from correcting for situational information. First, individuals with persecutory beliefs may have a greater need for "closure" (i.e., a desire to get a specific answer on a topic or issue, rather than dealing with ambiguity)—a hypothesis with some preliminary support in samples with both nonclinical (Colbert and Peters 2002) and clinical (Bentall and Swarbrick 2003) levels of delusional ideation. Second, individuals with persecutory delusions may be ignoring not only social context but also the "mental" context of others; in other words, impairments in theory of mind may contribute to personalizing biases. Recent evidence from nonclinical (Kinderman et al. 1998; Taylor and Kinderman 2002) and clinical (Randall et al. 2003) samples supports the association between deficits in theory of mind and the tendency to make external-personal attributions.

While promising, this model may be somewhat incomplete, as other social cognitive biases, such as the tendency to "jump to conclusions" or to display a confirmation bias (i.e., giving more weight to information that supports an already held belief than information that does not support it), have also been linked to paranoid ideation (for a review, see Freeman 2007; see also Merrin et al. 2007). In fact, an impressive and recent transdiagnostic study of paranoid ideation found that the best predictive model of paranoid thinking included a combination of pessimistic thinking style (low self-esteem, a tendency to make global and stable attributions, and negative emotion) and impaired cognitive performance (executive function, jumping to conclusions, and ToM) (Bentall et al. 2009). Unfortunately, externalizing bias could not be included in the analysis because of inadequate reliability, raising the possibility that even this advanced model may be incomplete. It is therefore clear that further examination of these relationships is needed to form a comprehensive model of the mechanisms underlying attributional style and persecutory delusions.

FACIAL AFFECT RECOGNITION

One important component of social cognition that has been widely studied in schizophrenia is the ability to recognize affect in the faces of others. It has been relatively well established that individuals with schizophrenia generally show deficits in both identification and discrimination of facial affect, and a recent meta-analysis reported a large overall effect size ($d=-0.91$; Kohler et al. 2010). The many studies in this area have been reviewed previously (Edwards et al. 2002; Mandal et al. 1998; Pinkham et al. 2003, 2007a). However, several questions have arisen that include the specificity of the deficit in terms of schizophrenia, the emotional valence of the deficit, the stability of the deficit, and the nature of the deficit, namely, whether the impairment is specific to emotions or due to generalized poor performance. Further, the relationship of facial affect recognition with both social and cognitive functioning requires consideration.

Is the Deficit Specific to Schizophrenia?

Studies have shown that individuals with schizophrenia perform more poorly than nonpatient and psychiatric control subjects on tests of facial affect recognition (Mandal 1986; Morrison et al. 1988; Muzekari and Bates 1977; Walker et al. 1980). However, variability is evident depending on the type of psychiatric comparison group. Specifically, several studies demonstrate an advantage for individuals with depression compared with those with schizophrenia (e.g., Gaebel and Wolwer 1992; Gessler et al. 1989; Weniger et al. 2004; see Schneider et al. 1995 for an exception), but, as compared with bipolar disorder, findings have been less consistent. Addington and Addington (1998) reported that individuals with schizophrenia performed significantly worse on facial affect recognition tasks than individuals with bipolar disorder, and this finding was replicated with a first-episode sample (Edwards et al. 2001). In contrast, however, Bellack and colleagues (1996) did not find any differences between subjects with schizophrenia and subjects with bipolar disorder. Finally, Bolte and Poustka (2003) found that individuals with schizophrenia performed better than individuals with autism on a facial recognition test; however, Sasson et al. (2007) reported no difference between individuals with autism and individuals with schizophrenia in emotion recognition performance despite differences in visual orienting to faces. Overall, these findings suggest that although individuals with schizophrenia are impaired in facial affect recognition relative to nonclinical control subjects, performance deficits compared with clinical control subjects are less consistently shown.

Does the Deficit Occur With All Emotions?

Further research suggests that difficulties in affect recognition are a function of the specific emotions being identified. Individuals with schizophrenia appear to have more difficulty when tasks involve identification or discrimination of negative emotions (e.g., fear, anger) compared with more positive emotions (i.e., happiness; Bigelow et al. 2006; Borod et al. 1993; Edwards et al. 2001) , and recognition deficits may be most pronounced for fear (Kohler et al. 2003). Further, individuals with schizophrenia may tend to misattribute neutral features as negative (Kohler et al. 2003; Pinkham et al. 2011).

Is the Deficit Stable Over Time?

A number of cross-sectional studies have demonstrated a decrease in affect recognition deficits during remission (Gaebel and Wolwer 1992; Gessler et al. 1989). Penn and colleagues (2000) found that acutely ill individuals with schizophrenia perform worse than chronically ill yet stable inpatients on emotion perception tasks. The few longitudinal studies examining the stability of these deficits, however, suggest that such deficits tend to remain. In Addington and Addington's (1998) study, despite a highly significant improvement in positive and negative symptoms from the time of hospitalization to 3-month follow-up, patients showed no improvement in facial affect recognition, suggesting that deficits are stable and do not improve with symptom remission. This finding supports and improves on the results of Gaebel and Wolwer (1992) and Streit and colleagues (1997), whose follow-up periods were only 4 weeks. In a more recent study, the longitudinal stability (1 year) of deficits in facial affect recognition has been supported (Kee et al. 2003).

Is the Deficit a Result of a Specific or Generalized Impairment?

One question that arises is whether these deficits in affect recognition are the result of a specific impairment in facial affect recognition or whether they are related to general cognitive or face processing impairments.

Several studies argue for a differential deficit (Heimberg et al. 1992; Kosmidis et al. 2007; Penn et al. 2000; Schneider et al. 2006; Silver et al. 2009; Walker et al. 1984); however, others have shown that although schizophrenia subjects perform more poorly than control subjects on facial affect recognition tasks, they also perform more poorly on a control task, usually a facial recognition task (Addington and Addington 1998; Feinberg et al. 1986; Gessler et al. 1989; Kerr and Neale 1993; Martin et al. 2005; Mueser et al. 1996; Novic et al. 1984; Sachs et al. 2004; Salem et al. 1996).

While these findings suggest that facial affect impairment is more likely to be a generalized impairment than a specific impairment, Penn and colleagues (1997) highlight an important consideration—namely, the nature of the "control" task, which typically is a face perception test. Although this type of task controls for the affective quality of the stimulus, it is also a social stimulus and therefore limits the conclusions that can be made about a specific versus generalized deficit in social cognition proper. Work that uses a differential deficit design, which must include both social and nonsocial perception tasks, is clearly warranted to further our understanding of the deficit's specificity.

Relationship Among Facial Affect Recognition, Neurocognition, and Social Functioning

Several studies have demonstrated that facial affect recognition is significantly related to various aspects of social functioning, such as social skill, general social functioning, and quality of life (Hooker and Park 2002; Ihnen et al. 1998; Kee et al. 2003; Mueser et al. 1996; Penn et al. 1996; Pinkham and Penn 2006; for a review, see Couture et al. 2006). This finding suggests that social cognition has *functional* significance for individuals with schizophrenia. Perhaps more importantly, a few more recent studies have demonstrated that the relationship between neurocognition and functional outcome may depend on affect recognition, either as a moderator (Nienow et al. 2006) or as a mediator (Addington et al. 2006a; Horton and Silverstein 2008). Thus, this preliminary evidence suggests that facial affect recognition, although related to cognitive and social functioning, may be a distinct construct that is independently related to social functioning.

Unanswered Questions

A number of unanswered questions remain. First, given the heterogeneity of schizophrenia, it is important to determine whether specific symptoms relate, or contribute, to facial recognition deficits. For example, there is some evidence that individuals with persecutory delusions or paranoia perform better on facial recognition tasks relative to nonparanoid individuals with schizophrenia (Davis and Gibson 2000; Kline et al. 1992; Lewis and Garver 1995; for an exception, see Pinkham et al. 2011). Conversely, negative symptoms or the deficit syndrome may impair emotion perception (Bryson et al. 1998; Gur et al. 2006; Mueser et al. 1996; for exceptions, see Silver and Shlomo 2001; Streit et al. 1997). This finding suggests that a finer-grained analysis of facial affect recognition in schizophrenia may be obtained by forming symptom subgroups of individuals. Second, it is still unclear exactly when affect recognition deficits emerge. Recent work suggests that impairments are present during the first-episode (Edwards et al. 2001), as well as early in the course of the illness (Kucharska-Pietura et al. 2005; Pinkham et al. 2007a), and perhaps even in individuals who are at risk of developing psychosis (Addington et al. 2008). Clarifying the period of onset will likely provide important information about potential vulnerability markers for psychosis and may shed light on a potential mechanism for social decline. Third, we are still learning about the mechanisms underlying performance deficits in this social cognitive area. While numerous investigations have linked abnormal functioning of a neural circuit centered on the amygdala to emotion processing deficits (for reviews, see Li et al. 2010; Pinkham et al. 2007b), abnormal visual scanning of faces and social scenes may also be particularly relevant. Several studies have highlighted aberrant patterns of visual attention in schizophrenia (Loughland et al. 2002; Sasson et al. 2007; Streit et al. 1997), and these may be most pronounced for individuals with persecutory delusions (Phillips and David 1998; Phillips et al. 2000). Investigation of potential interactions between visual scanning and neural activation (Dalton et al. 2005) may provide unique insight into why individuals with schizophrenia have difficulty perceiving the emotions of others.

CONCLUSION

Impairments in social and vocational functioning are a defining characteristic of schizophrenia and include poor quality of social relationships and difficulty with role functioning in areas such as school, work, and parenting. Problems in social functioning appear to be at least partly related to symptoms of the illness, including psychotic, negative, and cognitive symptoms, but are not fully explained by those symptoms. Economic constraints and environmental factors such as stigma and discrimination also play a role in limiting social functioning.

Although impairments in functioning tend to be relatively stable and long term in schizophrenia, significant advances have been made in the development of interventions for improving functioning. Most notable among those interventions are social skills training, cognitive-behavioral therapy for psychosis, and cognitive remediation to improve social functioning, and supported employment to improve vocational outcomes.

The study of social cognition also provides a promising avenue for intervention. As reviewed here, individuals with schizophrenia display impairments in multiple domains of social cognition, and such deficits are related to social functioning. These findings, however, are just a start, and there is still a great deal of work that is needed before a more complete understanding of the role of social cognition in schizophrenia can be gained. Likely targets for future efforts include remediation strategies and refined measures. Newly developed social cognitive remediation programs show promise for ameliorative change (Combs et al. 2007a; Horan et al. 2009; Roberts and Penn 2009); however, additional work is needed to fully establish the efficacy of these interventions and to investigate the impact of these programs on social functioning. Likewise, despite the considerable advancements reviewed here, the measurement of social cognitive abilities remains difficult, as the majority of currently used measures have only limited psychometric development. Before social cognition can be a truly meaningful treatment target, reliable and valid measures are necessary. Improved measurement may also help answer many of the questions raised here and, as such, should be a priority for future investigations.

REFERENCES

Aarke JM, Seghers JP, St.-Hilaire A, et al: Attributional style in delusional patients: a comparison of remitted paranoid, remitted nonparanoid, and current paranoid patients with nonpsychiatric controls. Schizophr Bull 35:994–1002, 2009

Abramson LY, Seligman MEP, Teasdale JD: Learned helplessness in humans: critique and reformulation. J Abnorm Psychol 78:40–74, 1978

Addington J, Addington D: Facial emotion recognition and information processing in schizophrenia and bipolar disorder. Schizophr Res 32:171–181, 1998

Addington J, Saeedi H, Addington D: Facial affect recognition: a mediator between cognitive and social functioning in psychosis? Schizophr Res 85:142–150, 2006a

Addington J, Saeedi H, Addington D: Influence of social perception and social knowledge on cognitive and social functioning in early psychosis. Br J Psychiatry 189:373–378, 2006b

Addington J, Penn D, Woods SW, et al: Facial affect recognition in individuals at clinical high risk for psychosis. Br J Psychiatry 192:67–68, 2008

Adolphs R: Social cognition and the human brain. Trends Cogn Sci 3:469–479, 1999

American Psychiatric Association: Diagnostic and Statistical Manual of Mental Disorders, 4th Edition, Text Revision. Washington, DC, American Psychiatric Association, 2000

Angermeyer MC, Kuhn L, Goldstein JM: Gender and the course of schizophrenia: differences in treated outcome. Schizophr Bull 16:293–307, 1990

Arns PG, Linney JA: Work, self, and life satisfaction for persons with severe and persistent mental disorders. Psychosocial Rehabilitation Journal 17:63–79, 1993

Arns PG, Linney JA: Relating functional skills of severely mentally ill clients to subjective and societal benefits. Psychiatr Serv 46:260–265, 1995

Bailey EL, Ricketts SK, Becker DR, et al: Do long-term day treatment clients benefit from supported employment? Psychiatr Rehabil J 22:24–29, 1998

Baronet A-M: Factors associated with caregiver burden in mental illness: a critical review of the research literature. Clin Psychol Rev 19:819–841, 1999

Barrowclough C, Tarrier N: Social functioning and family interventions, in Handbook of Social Functioning in Schizophrenia. Edited by Mueser KT, Tarrier N. Boston, MA, Allyn & Bacon, 1998, pp 327–341

Baum KM, Walker EF: Childhood behavioral precursors of adult symptom dimensions in schizophrenia. Schizophr Res 16:111–120, 1995

Beck AT, Rector NA, Stolar N, et al: Schizophrenia: Cognitive Theory, Research, and Therapy. New York, Guilford, 2009

Becker DR, Drake RE: A Working Life for People With Severe Mental Illness. New York, Oxford University Press, 2003

Becker DR, Bond GR, McCarthy D, et al: Converting day treatment centers to supported employment programs in Rhode Island. Psychiatr Serv 52:351–357, 2001

Beiser M, Bean G, Erickson D, et al: Biological and psychosocial predictors of job performance following a first episode of psychosis. Am J Psychiatry 151:857–863, 1994

Bell MD, Bryson GJ, Greig TC, et al : Neurocognitive enhancement therapy with work therapy: productivity outcomes at 6- and 12-month follow-ups. J Rehabil Res Dev 42:829–838, 2005

Bell MD, Fiszdon J, Greig T, et al: Neurocognitive enhancement therapy with work therapy in schizophrenia: 6-month followup of neuropsychological performance. J Rehabil Res Dev 44:761–770, 2007

Bellack AS, Morrison RL, Wixted JT, et al: An analysis of social competence in schizophrenia. Br J Psychiatry 156:809–818, 1990

Bellack AS, Blanchard JJ, Muser KT: Cue availability and affect perception in schizophrenia. Schizophr Bull 22:535–544, 1996

Bellack AS, Mueser KT, Gingerich S, et al: Social Skills Training for Schizophrenia: A Step-By-Step Guide, 2nd Edition. New York, Guilford, 2004

Bentall RP, Swarbrick R: The best laid schemas of paranoid patients: autonomy, sociotropy, and need for closure. Psychol Psychother 76:163–171, 2003

Bentall RP, Kinderman P, Kaney S: The self, attributional processes and abnormal beliefs: towards a model of persecutory delusions. Behav Res Ther 32:331–341, 1994

Bentall RP, Corcoran R, Howard R, et al: Persecutory delusions: a review and theoretical integration. Clin Psychol Rev 21:1143–1192, 2001

Bentall RP, Rowse G, Shryane N, et al: The cognitive and affective structure of paranoid delusions. Arch Gen Psychiatry 66:236–247, 2009

Bertrand MC, Sutton H, Achim AM, et al: Social cognitive impairments in first-episode psychosis. Schizophr Res 95:124–133, 2007

Bigelow NO, Paradiso S, Adolphs R, et al: Perception of socially relevant stimuli in schizophrenia. Schizophr Res 83:257–267, 2006

Blackwood NJ, Howard RJ, Bentall RP, et al: Cognitive neuropsychiatric models of persecutory delusions. Am J Psychiatry 158:527–539, 2001

Bolte S, Poustka F: The recognition of facial affect in autistic and schizophrenic subjects and their first-degree relatives. Psychol Med 33:907–915, 2003

Bond GR: Vocational rehabilitation, in Handbook of Psychiatric Rehabilitation. Edited by Liberman RP. New York, MacMillan, 1992, pp 244–275

Bond G, Dietzen L, McGrew J, et al: Accelerating entry into supported employment for persons with severe psychiatric disabilities. Rehabil Psychol 40:91–111, 1995

Bond GR, Resnick SG, Drake RE, et al: Does competitive employment improve nonvocational outcomes for people with severe mental illness? J Consult Clin Psychol 69:489–501, 2001

Bond GR, Salyers MP, Dincin J, et al: A randomized controlled trial comparing two vocational models for persons with severe mental illness. J Consult Clin Psychol 75:968–982, 2007

Bond GR, Drake RE, Becker DR: An update on randomized controlled trials of evidence-based supported employment. Psychiatr Rehabil J 31:280–290, 2008

Bora E, Yucel M, Pantelis C: Theory of mind impairment in schizophrenia: meta-analysis. Schizophr Res 109:1–9, 2009

Borod JC, Martin CC, Alpert M, et al: Perception of facial emotion in schizophrenic and right brain-damaged patients. J Nerv Ment Dis 181:494–501, 1993

Brekke JS, Levin S, Wolkon GH, et al: Psychosocial functioning and subjective experience in schizophrenia. Schizophr Bull 19:600–608, 1993

Brekke J, Kay DD, Lee KS, et al: Biosocial pathways to functional outcome in schizophrenia. Schizophr Res 80:213–225, 2005

Brothers L: The social brain: a project for integrating primate behavior and neurophysiology in a new domain. Concepts in Neuroscience 1:27–51, 1990

Brune M: Emotion recognition, "theory of mind," and social behavior in schizophrenia. Psychiatry Res 133:135–147, 2005a

Brune M: Theory of mind in schizophrenia: a review of the literature. Schizophr Bull 31:21–42, 2005b

Brunet E, Sarfati Y, Hardy-Bayle MC, et al: Abnormalities of brain function during a nonverbal theory of mind task in schizophrenia. Neuropsychologia 41:1574–1582, 2003a

Brunet E, Sarfati Y, Hardy-Bayle MC: Reasoning about physical causality and other's intentions in schizophrenia. Cogn Neuropsychiatry 8:129–139, 2003b

Bryson G, Bell M, Kaplan E, et al: Affect recognition in deficit syndrome schizophrenia. Psychiatry Res 77:113–120, 1998

Burns T, Catty J, Becker T, et al: The effectiveness of supported employment for people with severe mental illness: a randomized controlled trial. Lancet 370:1146–1152, 2007

Candido CL, Romney DM: Attributional style in paranoid versus depressed patients. Br J Med Psychol 63:355–363, 1990

Cannon TD, Mednick SA, Parnas J, et al: Developmental brain abnormalities in the offspring of schizophrenic mothers. Arch Gen Psychiatry 50:551–564, 1993

Chandler D, Meisel J, Hu T, et al: A capitated model for a cross-section of severely mentally ill clients: employment outcomes. Community Ment Health J 33:501–516, 1997

Chung YS, Kang DH, Shin NY, et al: Deficit of theory of mind in individuals at ultra-high-risk for schizophrenia. Schizophr Res 99:111–118, 2008

Colbert SM, Peters ER: Need for closure and jumping-to-conclusions in delusion-prone individuals. J Nerv Ment Dis 190:27–31, 2002

Combs DR, Adams SD, Penn DL, et al: Social Cognition and Interaction Training (SCIT) for inpatients with schizophrenia spectrum disorders: preliminary findings. Schizophr Res 91:112–116, 2007a

Combs DR, Penn DL, Wicher M, et al: The Ambiguous Intentions Hostility Questionnaire (AIHQ): a new measure for evaluating hostile social-cognitive biases in paranoia. Cogn Neuropsychiatry 12:128–143, 2007b

Corcoran R: Inductive reasoning and the understanding of intention in schizophrenia. Cogn Neuropsychiatry 8:223–235, 2003

Corcoran R, Mercer G, Frith CD: Schizophrenia, symptomatology and social inference: investigating "theory of mind" in people with schizophrenia. Schizophr Res 17:5–13, 1995

Corrigan PW, Mueser KT, Bond GR, et al: The Principles and Practice of Psychiatric Rehabilitation: An Empirical Approach. New York, Guilford, 2008

Couture SM, Penn DL, Roberts DL: The functional significance of social cognition in schizophrenia: a review. Schizophr Bull 32 (suppl 1):S44–S63, 2006

Crisp AH, Gelder MG, Rix S, et al: Stigmatization of people with mental illnesses. Br J Psychiatry 177:4–7, 2000

Dalton KM, Nacewicz BM, Johnstone T, et al: Gaze fixation and the neural circuitry of face processing in autism. Nature Neurosci 8:519–526, 2005

Davis PJ, Gibson MG: Recognition of posed and genuine facial expressions of emotion in paranoid and non-paranoid schizophrenia. J Abnorm Psychol 109:445–450, 2000

Dixon LB, Dickerson F, Bellack AS, et al: The 2009 PORT psychosocial treatment recommendations and summary statements. Schizophr Bull 36:48–70, 2010

Drake RE, Becker DR, Biesanz JC, et al: Rehabilitative day treatment vs supported employment, I: vocational outcomes. Community Ment Health J 30:519–532, 1994

Drake RE, Becker DR, Biesanz BA, et al: Day treatment versus supported employment for persons with severe mental illness: a replication study. Psychiatr Serv 47:1125–1127, 1996a

Drake RE, McHugo GJ, Becker DR, et al: The New Hampshire Study of Supported Employment for people with severe mental illness: vocational outcomes. J Consult Clin Psychol 64:391–399, 1996b

Drake RE, McHugo GJ, Bebout RR, et al: A randomized clinical trial of supported employment for inner-city patients with severe mental illness. Arch Gen Psychiatry 56:627–633, 1999

Drury VW, Robinson EJ, Birchwood M: "Theory of mind" skills during an acute episode of psychosis and following recovery. Psychol Med 28:1101–1112, 1998

Dyck DG, Short R, Vitaliano PP: Predictors of burden and infectious illness in schizophrenia caregivers. Psychosom Med 61:411–419, 1999

Edwards J, Jackson HJ, Pattison PE, et al: Facial affect and affective prosody recognition in first-episode schizophrenia. Schizophr Res 48:235–253, 2001

Edwards J, Jackson HJ, Pattitson PE: Emotion recognition via facial expression and affective prosody in schizophrenia: a methodological review. Clin Psychol Rev 22:789–832, 2002

Farina A: Stigma, in Handbook of Social Functioning in Schizophrenia. Edited by Mueser KT, Tarrier N. Boston, MA, Allyn & Bacon, 1998, pp 247–279

Fear CF, Sharp H, Healy D: Cognitive processes in delusional disorders. Br J Psychiatry 168:1–8, 1996

Feinberg TE, Rifkin A, Schaffer C, et al: Facial discrimination and emotional recognition in schizophrenia and affective disorders. Arch Gen Psychiatry 43:276–279, 1986

Fowler D, Garety P, Kuipers E: Cognitive Behaviour Therapy for Psychosis: Theory and Practice. Chichester, West Sussex, UK, Wiley, 1995

Freeman D: Suspicious minds: the psychology of persecutory delusions. Clin Psychol Rev 27:425–457, 2007

Frith CD, Corcoran R: Exploring "theory of mind" in people with schizophrenia. Psychol Med 26:521–530, 1996

Gaebel W, Wolwer W: Facial expression and emotional face recognition in schizophrenia and depression. Eur Arch Psychiatry Clin Neurosci 242:46–52, 1992

Garety PA, Freeman D: Cognitive approaches to delusions: a critical review of theories and evidence. Br J Clin Psychol 38:113–154, 1999

Gervey R, Bedell JR: Supported employment in vocational rehabilitation, in Psychological Assessment and Treatment of Persons With Severe Mental Disorders. Edited by Bedell JR. Washington, DC, Taylor & Francis, 1994, pp 139–163

Gessler S, Cutting J, Frith CD, et al: Schizophrenic inability to judge facial emotion: a controlled study. Br J Clin Psychol 28:19–29, 1989

Glynn SM, Randolph ET, Eth S, et al: Schizophrenic symptoms, work adjustment, and behavioral family therapy. Rehabil Psychol 37:323–328, 1992

Glynn SM, Marder SR, Liberman RP, et al: Supplementing clinic-based skills training with manual-based community support sessions: effects on social adjustment of patients with schizophrenia. Am J Psychiatry 159:829–837, 2002

Gold M, Marrone J: Mass Bay Employment Services (a service of Bay Cove Human Services, Inc.): a story of leadership and vision resulting in employment for people with mental illness. Roses and Thorns From the Grassroots: A Series Highlighting Organizational Change in Massachusetts, Vol 1, Spring 1998

Gold PB, Meisler N, Santos AB, et al: Randomized trial of supported employment integrated with Assertive Community Treatment in the rural south: employment outcomes for persons with severe mental illness. Schizophr Bull 32:378–395, 2004

Goodman LA, Salyers MP, Mueser KT, et al: Recent victimization in women and men with severe mental illness: prevalence and correlates. J Trauma Stress 14:615–632, 2001

Granholm E, McQuaid JR, McClure FS, et al: A randomized, controlled trial of cognitive behavioral social skills training for middle-aged and older outpatients with chronic schizophrenia. Am J Psychiatry 162:520–529, 2005

Green MF, Kern RS, Braff DL, et al: Neurocognitive deficits and functional outcome in schizophrenia: are we measuring the "right stuff"? Schizophr Bull 26:119–136, 2000

Gur RE, Kohler CG, Ragland JD, et al: Flat affect in schizophrenia: relation to emotion processing and neurocognitive measures. Schizophr Bull 32:279–287, 2006

Haas GL, Garratt LS: Gender differences in social functioning, in Handbook of Social Functioning in Schizophrenia. Edited by Mueser KT, Tarrier N. Boston, MA, Allyn & Bacon, 1998, pp 149–180

Hadwin J, Baron-Cohen S, Howlin P, et al: Can we teach children with autism to understand emotions, belief, or pretense? Dev Psychopathol 8:345–365, 1996

Hadwin J, Baron-Cohen S, Howlin P, et al: Does teaching theory of mind have an effect on the ability to develop conversation in children? J Autism Dev Disord 27:519–535, 1997

Häfner H: Onset and early course as determinants of the further course of schizophrenia. Acta Psychiatr Scand 102 (suppl 407):44–48, 2000

Häfner H, an der Heiden W: Course and outcome of schizophrenia, in Schizophrenia, 2nd Edition. Edited by Hirsch SR, Weinberger DR. Oxford, England, Blackwell Scientific, 2003, pp 101–141

Häfner H, Maurer K, Löffler W, et al: The influence of age and sex on the onset and early course of schizophrenia. Br J Psychiatry 162:80–86, 1993

Häfner H, Löffler W, Maurer K, et al: Depression, negative symptoms, social stagnation and social decline in the early course of schizophrenia. Acta Psychiatr Scand 100:105–118, 1999

Häfner H, Maurer K, Löffler W, et al: Modeling the early course of schizophrenia. Schizophr Bull 29:325–340, 2003

Hans SL, Marcus J, Henson L, et al: Interpersonal behavior of children at risk for schizophrenia. Psychiatry 55:314–335, 1992

Harding CM, Keller AB: Long-term outcome of social functioning, in Handbook of Social Functioning in Schizophrenia. Edited by Mueser KT, Tarrier N. Boston, MA, Allyn & Bacon, 1998, pp 134–148

Harding C, Strauss J, Hafez H, et al: Work and mental illness, I: toward an integration of the rehabilitation process. J Nerv Ment Dis 175:317–326, 1987

Harrington L, Siegert RJ, McClure J: Theory of mind in schizophrenia: a critical review. CognNeuropsychiatry 10:249–286, 2005

Heaton R, Paulsen JS, McAdams LA, et al: Neuropsychological deficits in schizophrenics: relationship to age, chronicity, and dementia. Arch Gen Psychiatry 51:469–476, 1994

Heimberg C, Gur RE, Erwin RJ, et al: Facial emotion discrimination, III: behavioral findings in schizophrenia. Psychiatry Res 42:253–265, 1992

Higgins ET: Self-discrepancy: a theory relating self and affect. Psychol Rev 94:319–340, 1987

Ho BC, Nopoulos PM, Flaum M, et al: Two-year outcome in first-episode schizophrenia: predictive value of symptoms for quality of life. Am J Psychiatry 155:1196–1201, 1998

Hogarty GE, Greenwald D, Ulrich RF, et al: Three-year trials of personal therapy among schizophrenic patients living with or independent of family, II: effects of adjustment on patients. Am J Psychiatry 154:1514–1524, 1997a

Hogarty GE, Kornblith SJ, Greenwald D, et al: Three-year trials of personal therapy among schizophrenic patients living with or independent of family, I: description of study and effects on relapse rates. Am J Psychiatry 154:1504–1513, 1997b

Hogarty GE, Flesher S, Ulrich R, et al: Cognitive enhancement therapy for schizophrenia: effects of a 2-year randomized trial on cognition and behavior. Arch Gen Psychiatry 61:866–876, 2004

Hooker C, Park S: Emotion processing and its relationship to social functioning in schizophrenia patients. Psychiatry Res 112:41–50, 2002

Horan WP, Kern RS, Shokat-Fadai K, et al: Social cognitive skills training in schizophrenia: an initial efficacy study of stabilized outpatients. Schizophr Res 107:47–54, 2009

Horton HK, Silverstein SM: Social cognition as a mediator of cognition and outcome among deaf and hearing people with schizophrenia. Schizophr Res 105:125–137, 2008

Ihnen GH, Penn DL, Corrigan PW, et al: Social perception and social skill in schizophrenia. Psychiatry Res 80:275–286, 1998

Jackson HJ, Minas IH, Burgess PM, et al: Negative symptoms and social skills performance in schizophrenia. Schizophr Res 2:457–463, 1989

Janssen I, Versmissen D, Campo JA, et al: Attributional style and psychosis: evidence for an externalizing bias in patients but not in individuals at high risk. Psychol Med 36:771–778, 2006

Johnstone EC, Macmillan JF, Frith CD, et al: Further investigation of the predictors of outcome following first schizophrenic episodes. Br J Psychiatry 157:182–189, 1990

Kaney S, Bentall RP: Persecutory delusions and attributional style. Br J Med Psychol 62:191–198, 1989

Kee KS, Green MF, Mintz J, et al: Is emotion processing a predictor of functional outcome in schizophrenia? Schizophr Bull 29:487–497, 2003

Kerr SL, Neale JM: Emotional perception in schizophrenia: specific deficit or further evidence of generalized poor performance? J Abnorm Psychol 102:312–318, 1993

Kessler RC, Foster CL, Saunders WB, et al: Social consequences of psychiatric disorders, I: educational attainment. Am J Psychiatry 152:1026–1032, 1995

Kettle JWL, O'Brien-Simpson L, Allen NB: Impaired theory of mind in first-episode schizophrenia: comparison with community, university, and depressed controls. Schizophr Res 99:96–102, 2008

Kinderman P, Bentall RP: A new measure of causal locus: the Internal, Personal, and Situational Attributions Questionnaire. Pers Individ Dif 20:261–264, 1996a

Kinderman P, Bentall RP: Self-discrepancies and persecutory delusions: evidence for a model of paranoid ideation. J Abnorm Psychol 105:106–113, 1996b

Kinderman P, Bentall RP: Causal attributions in paranoia and depression: internal, personal, and situational attributions for negative events. J Abnorm Psychol 106:341–345, 1997

Kinderman P, Dunbar R, Bentall RP: Theory of mind deficits and causal attributions. Br J Psychol 89:191–204, 1998

Kingdon DG, Turkington D: Cognitive Therapy of Schizophrenia. New York, Guilford, 2004

Kline JS, Smith JE, Ellis HC: Paranoid and nonparanoid schizophrenic processing of facially displayed affect. J Psychiatr Res 26:169–182, 1992

Kohler CG, Turner TH, Bilker WB, et al: Facial emotion recognition in schizophrenia: intensity effects and error patterns. Am J Psychiatry 160:1768–1774, 2003

Kohler CG, Walker JB, Martin EA, et al: Facial emotion perception in schizophrenia: a meta-analytic review. Schizophr Bull 36:1009–1019, 2010

Kosmidis MH, Bozikas VP, Giannakou M, et al: Impaired emotion perception in schizophrenia: a differential deficit. Psychiatry Res 149:279–284, 2007

Kraepelin E: Dementia Praecox and Paraphrenia (1919). Translated by Barclay RM. New York, Krieger, 1971

Krstev H, Jackson H, Maude D: An investigation of attributional style in first-episode psychosis. Br J Clin Psychol 38:181–194, 1999

Kucharska-Pietura K, David AS, Masiak M, et al: Perception of facial and vocal affect by people with schizophrenia in early and late stages of illness. Br J Psychiatry 187:523–528, 2005

Kurtz MM, Mueser KT: A meta-analysis of controlled research on social skills training for schizophrenia. J Consult Clin Psychol 76:491–504, 2008

Langdon R, Corner T, McLaren J, et al: Externalizing and personalizing biases in persecutory delusions: The relationship with poor insight and theory-of-mind. Behav Res Ther 44:699–713, 2006

Langdon R, Ward PB, Coltheart M: Reasoning anomalies associated with delusions in schizophrenia. Schizophr Bull 36:321–330, 2010

Latimer E, Lecomte T, Becker DR, et al: Generalizability of the IPS model of supported employment for people with severe mental illness: results and economic implications of a randomized trial in Montreal, Canada. J Ment Health Policy Econ 8 (suppl 1):S29, 2005

Lehman AF, Goldberg R, Dixon LB, et al: Improving employment outcomes for persons with severe mental illnesses. Arch Gen Psychiatry 59:165–172, 2002

Levitt A, Mueser KT, DeGenova J, et al: A randomized controlled trial of illness management and recovery in multi-unit supported housing. Psychiatr Serv 60:1629–1636, 2009

Lewis SF, Garver DL: Treatment and diagnostic subtype in facial affect recognition in schizophrenia. J Psychiatr Res 29:5–11, 1995

Li H, Chan RCK, McAlonan GM, et al: Facial emotion processing in schizophrenia: a meta-analysis of functional neuroimaging data. Schizophr Bull 36:1029–1039, 2010

Liberman RP, DeRisi WJ, Mueser KT: Social Skills Training for Psychiatric Patients. Needham Heights, MA, Allyn & Bacon, 1989

Lindenmayer JP, McGurk SR, Mueser KT, et al: Cognitive remediation in persistently mentally ill inpatients: a randomized controlled trial. Psychiatr Serv 59:241–247, 2008

Loughland CM, Williams LM, Gordon E: Visual scanpaths to positive and negative facial emotions in an outpatient schizophrenia sample. Schizophr Res 55:159–170, 2002

Lyon HM, Kaney S, Bentall RP: The defensive function of persecutory delusions: evidence from attributional tasks. Br J Psychiatry 164:637–646, 1994

Macias C, Rodican CF, Hargreaves WA, et al: Supported employment outcomes of a randomized controlled trial of ACT and clubhouse models. Psychiatr Serv 57:1406–1415, 2006

Mandal MK: Judgment of facial affect among depressive and schizophrenics. Br J Clin Psychol 25:87–92, 1986

Mandal MK, Pandey R, Prasad AB: Facial expression of emotions and schizophrenia: a review. Schizophr Bull 24:399–412, 1998

Marneros A, Deister A, Rohde A: Comparison of long-term outcome of schizophrenic, affective and schizoaffective disorders [published erratum appears in Br J Psychiatry 161:868, 1992]. Br J Psychiatry Suppl (18):44–51, 1992

Martin J, Penn DL: Attributional style among outpatients with schizophrenia with and without persecutory delusions. Schizophr Bull 28:131–141, 2002

Martin F, Baudouin JY, Tiberghien G, et al: Processing emotional expression and facial identity in schizophrenia. Psychiatry Res 134:43–53, 2005

Marwaha S, Johnson S: Schizophrenia and employment: a review. Soc Psychiatry Psychiatr Epidemiol 39:337–349, 2004

McFarlane WR, Dushay RA, Deakins SM, et al: Employment outcomes in family aided assertive community treatment. Am J Orthopsychiatry 70:203–214, 2000

McGurk SR, Meltzer HY: The role of cognition in vocational functioning in schizophrenia. Schizophr Res 45:175–184, 2000

McGurk SR, Mueser KT: Cognitive functioning, symptoms, and work in supported employment: a review and heuristic model. Schizophr Res 70:147–174, 2004

McGurk SR, Mueser KT, Pascaris A: Cognitive training and supported employment for persons with severe mental illness: one year results from a randomized controlled trial. Schizophr Bull 31:898-909, 2005

McGurk SR, Mueser KT, Feldman K, et al: Cognitive training for supported employment: 2–3 year outcomes of a randomized controlled trial. Am J Psychiatry 164:437–441, 2007a

McGurk SR, Twamley EW, Sitzer DI, et al: A meta-analysis of cognitive remediation in schizophrenia. Am J Psychiatry 164:1791–1802, 2007b

McGurk SR, Mueser KT, DeRosa T, et al: Work, recovery, and comorbidity in schizophrenia: a randomized controlled trial of cognitive remediation. Schizophr Bull 35:319–335, 2009

Merrin J, Kinderman P, Bentall RP: "Jumping to conclusions" and attributional style in persecutory delusions. Cognitive Therapy Research 31:741–758, 2007

Morrison AP, Renton JC, Dunn H, et al: Cognitive Therapy for Psychosis: A Formulation-Based Approach. New York, Brunner-Routledge, 2004

Morrison RL, Bellack AS, Bashore TR: Perception of emotion among schizophrenic patients. Journal of Psychopathology and Behavioral Assessment 10:319–332, 1988

Mueser KT, Bellack AS, Morrison RL, et al: Gender, social competence, and symptomatology in schizophrenia: a longitudinal analysis. J Abnorm Psychol 99:138–147, 1990

Mueser KT, Bellack AS, Douglas MS, et al: Prevalence and stability of social skill deficits in schizophrenia. Schizophr Res 5:167–176, 1991

Mueser KT, Doonan R, Penn DL, et al: Emotional recognition and social competence in chronic schizophrenia. J Abnorm Psychol 105:271–275, 1996

Mueser KT, Becker DR, Torrey WC, et al: Work and nonvocational domains of functioning in persons with severe mental illness: a longitudinal analysis. J Nerv Ment Dis 185:419–426, 1997

Mueser KT, Salyers MP, Mueser PR: A prospective analysis of work in schizophrenia. Schizophr Bull 27:281–296, 2001

Mueser KT, Corrigan PW, Hilton D, et al: Illness management and recovery for severe mental illness: a review of the research. Psychiatr Serv 53:1272-1284, 2002

Mueser KT, Clark RE, Haines M, et al: The Hartford study of supported employment for severe mental illness. J Consult Clin Psychol 72:479–490, 2004

Mueser KT, Pratt SI, Bartels SJ, et al: Neurocognition and social skill in older persons with schizophrenia and major mood disorders: an analysis of gender and diagnosis effects. J Neurolinguistics 23:297–317, 2010

Murray CJL, Lopez AD (eds): The Global Burden of Disease and Injury Series, Vol 1: A Comprehensive Assessment of Mortality and Disability From Diseases, Injuries, and Risk Factors in 1990 and Projected to 2020. Cambridge, MA, Harvard School of Public Health on behalf of the World Health Organization and the World Bank, Harvard University Press, 1996

Muzekari LH, Bates ME: Judgment of emotion among chronic schizophrenics. J Clin Psychol 33:662–666, 1977

Nienow TM, Docherty NM, Cohen AS, et al: Attentional dysfunction, social perception, and social competence: what is the nature of the relationship? J Abnorm Psychol 115:408–417, 2006

Novic J, Luchins DJ, Perline R: Facial affect recognition in schizophrenia: is there a differential deficit? Br J Psychiatry 144:533–537, 1984

Ozonoff S, Miller JN: Teaching theory of minds: a new approach to social skills training for individuals with autism. J Autism Dev Disord 25:415–433, 1995

Patterson TL, Moscona S, McKibbin CL, et al: Social skills performance assessment among older patients with schizophrenia. Schizophr Res 30:351–360, 2001

Penn DL, Mueser KT, Spaulding W, et al: Information processing and social competence in chronic schizophrenia. Schizophr Bull 21:269–281, 1995

Penn DL, Spaulding W, Reed D, et al: The relationship of social cognition to ward behavior in chronic schizophrenia. Schizophr Res 20:327–335, 1996

Penn DL, Corrigan PW, Bentall RP, et al: Social cognition in schizophrenia. Psychol Bull 121:114–132, 1997

Penn DL, Combs DR, Ritchie M, et al: Emotion recognition in schizophrenia: further investigations of generalized versus specific deficit models. J Abnorm Psychol 109:512–516, 2000

Penn DL, Sanna LJ, Roberts DL: Social cognition in schizophrenia: an overview. Schizophr Bull 34:408–411, 2008

Pfammatter M, Junghan UM, Brenner HD: Efficacy of psychological therapy in schizophrenia: conclusions from meta-analyses. Schizophr Bull 32 (suppl 1):S64–S68, 2006

Phillips ML, David AS: Abnormal visual scan paths: a psychophysiological marker of delusions in schizophrenia. Schizophr Res 29:235–245, 1998

Phillips ML, Senior C, David AS: Perception of threat in schizophrenics with persecutory delusions: an investigation using visual scan paths. Psychol Med 30:157–167, 2000

Phillips ML, Drevets WC, Rauch SL, et al: Neurobiology of emotion perception, I: the neural basis of normal emotion perception. Biol Psychiatry 54:504–514, 2003a

Phillips ML, Drevets WC, Rauch SL, et al: Neurobiology of emotion perception, II: implications for major psychiatric disorders. Biol Psychiatry 54:515–528, 2003b

Pickup GJ, Frith CD: Theory of mind impairments in schizophrenia: symptomatology, severity, and specificity. Psychol Med 31:207–220, 2001

Pilowsky T, Yirmiya N, Arbelle S, et al: Theory of mind abilities of children with schizophrenia, children with autism, and normally developing children. Schizophr Res 42:145–155, 2000

Pinkham AE, Penn DL: Neurocognitive and social cognitive predictors of interpersonal skill in schizophrenia. Psychiatry Res 143:167–178, 2006

Pinkham AE, Penn DL, Perkins DO, et al: Implications for the neural basis of social cognition for the study of schizophrenia. Am J Psychiatry 160:815–824, 2003

Pinkham AE, Gur RE, Gur RC: Affect recognition deficits in schizophrenia: neural substrates and psychopharmacological implications. Expert Review of Neurotherapeutics 7:807–816, 2007a

Pinkham AE, Penn DL, Perkins DO, et al: Emotion perception and social skill over the course of psychosis: a comparison of individuals "at-risk" for psychosis and individuals with early and chronic schizophrenia spectrum illness. Cogn Neuropsychiatry 12:198–212, 2007b

Pinkham AE, Hopfinger JB, Ruparel K, et al: An investigation of the relationship between activation of a social cognitive neural network and social functioning. Schizophr Bull 34:688–697, 2008

Pinkham AE, Brensinger C, Kohler C, et al: Actively paranoid patients with schizophrenia over attribute anger to neutral faces. Schizophr Res 125:174–178, 2011

Pollice R, Roncone R, Falloon IRH, et al: Is theory of mind in schizophrenia more strongly associated with clinical and social functioning than with neurocognitive deficits? Psychopathology 35:280–288, 2002

Racenstein JM, Harrow M, Reed R, et al: The relationship between positive symptoms and instrumental work functioning in schizophrenia: a 10-year follow-up study. Schizophr Res 56:95–103, 2002

Randall F, Corcoran R, Day JC, et al: Attention, theory of mind, and causal attributions in people with persecutory delusions: a preliminary investigation. Cogn Neuropsychiatry 8:287–294, 2003

Rice DP: Economic burden of mental disorders in the United States. Economics of Neuroscience 1:40–44, 1999

Roberts DL, Penn DL: Social Cognition and Interaction Training (SCIT) for outpatients with schizophrenia: a preliminary study. Psychiatry Res 166:141–147, 2009

Robins LN: Deviant Children Grown Up. Huntington, NY, Robert E Krieger Publishing, 1966

Roder V, Brenner HD, Muller D, et al: Development of specific social skills training programmes for schizophrenia patients: results of multicentre study. Acta Psychiatr Scand 105:363–371, 2002

Rogers ES, Walsh D, Masotta L, et al: Massachusetts Survey of Client Preferences for Community Support Services (Final Report). Boston, MA, Center for Psychiatric Rehabilitation, 1991

Roncone R, Falloon IRH, Mazza M, et al: Is theory of mind in schizophrenia more strongly associated with clinical and social functioning than with neurocognitive deficits? Psychopathology 35:280–288, 2002

Russell TA, Rubia K, Bullmore ET, et al: Exploring the social brain in schizophrenia: left prefrontal underactivation during mental state attribution. Am J Psychiatry 157:2040–2042, 2000

Rutter ML: Nature-nurture integration: the example of antisocial behavior. Am Psychol 52:390–398, 1997

Sachs G, Steger-Wuchese D, Krypsin-Exner I, et al: Facial recognition deficits and cognition in schizophrenia. Schizophr Res 68:27–35, 2004

Salem JE, Kring AM, Kerr SL: More evidence for generalized poor performance in facial emotion perception in schizophrenia. J Abnorm Psychol 105:480–483, 1996

Sarfati Y, Hardy-Bayle M: How do people with schizophrenia explain the behaviour of others? A study of theory of mind and its relationship to thought and speech disorganization in schizophrenia. Psychol Med 29:613–620, 1999

Sarfati Y, Hardy-Bayle M, Nadel J, et al: Attribution of mental states to others by schizophrenic patients. Cogn Neuropsychiatry 2:1–17, 1997

Sarfati Y, Hardy-Bayle M, Brunet E, et al: Investigating theory of mind in schizophrenia: influence of verbalization in disorganized and non-disorganized patients. Schizophr Res 37:183–190, 1999

Sasson N, Tsuchiya N, Hurley R, et al: Orienting to social stimuli differentiates social cognitive impairment in autism and schizophrenia. Neuropsychologia 45:2580–2588, 2007

Schneider F, Gur RC, Gur RF, et al: Emotional processing in schizophrenia: neurobehavioral probes in relation to psychopathology. Schizophr Res 17:67–75, 1995

Schneider F, Gur RC, Koch K, et al: Impairment in the specificity of emotion processing in schizophrenia. Am J Psychiatry 163:442–447, 2006

Sharp HM, Fear CF, Healy D: Attributional style and delusions: an investigation based on delusional content. Eur Psychiatry 12:1–7, 1997

Silver H, Bilker W, Goodman C: Impaired recognition of happy, sad and neutral expressions in schizophrenia is emotion, but not valence, specific and context dependent. Psychiatry Res 169:101–106, 2009

Silverstein SM, Hatashita-Wong M, Solak BA, et al: Effectiveness of a two-phase cognitive rehabilitation intervention for severely impaired schizophrenia patients. Psychol Med 35:829–837, 2005

Sprong M, Schothorst P, Vos E, et al: Theory of mind in schizophrenia. Br J Psychiatry 191:5–13, 2007

Streit M, Wolwer W, Gaebel W: Facial affect recognition and visual scanning behaviour in the course of schizophrenia. Schizophr Res 24:311–317, 1997

Swettenham J: Can children with autism be taught to understand false belief using computers? J Child Psychol Psychiatry 37:157–165, 1996

Tauber R, Wallace CJ, Lecomte T: Enlisting indigenous community supporters in skills training programs for persons with severe mental illness. Psychiatr Serv 51:1428–1432, 2000

Taylor JL, Kinderman P: An analogue study of attributional complexity, theory of mind deficits and paranoia. Br J Psychol 93:137–140, 2002

Twamley EW, Bartels SJ, Becker D, et al: Individual placement and support for middle-aged and older clients with schizophrenia. Paper presented at the International Association of Psychosocial Services, San Diego, CA, May 2004

Usall J, Haro JM, Ochoa S, et al: Influence of gender on social outcome in schizophrenia. Acta Psychiatr Scand 106:337–342, 2002

Vaskinn A, Sundet K, Friis S, et al: Emotion perception and learning potential: mediators between neurocognition and social problem-solving in schizophrenia? J Int Neuropsychol Soc 14:279–288, 2008

Vauth R, Corrigan PW, Clauss M, et al: Cognitive strategies versus self-management skills as adjunct to vocational rehabilitation. Schizophr Bull 31:55–66, 2005

Velligan DI, Bow-Thomas CC, Huntzinger C, et al: Randomized controlled trial of the use of compensatory strategies to enhance adaptive functioning in outpatients with schizophrenia. Am J Psychiatry 157:1317–1323, 2000

Wahl O: Consumer Experience of Stigma. Fairfax, VA, George Mason University, Department of Psychology, 1997

Wahl OF: Telling Is Risky Business: Mental Health Consumers Confront Stigma. New Brunswick, NJ, Rutgers University Press, 1999

Waldheter EJ, Jones NT, Johnson ER, et al: Utility of social cognition and insight in the prediction of inpatient violence among individuals with a severe mental illness. J Nerv Ment Dis 9:609–618, 2005

Walker E, Marwit S, Emory E: A cross-sectional study of emotion recognition in schizophrenics. J Abnorm Psychol 89:428–436, 1980

Walker E, McGuire M, Bettes B: Recognition and identification of facial stimuli by schizophrenics and patients with affective disorders. Br J Clin Psychol 23:37–44, 1984

Walsh E, Moran P, Scott C, et al: Prevalence of violent victimisation in severe mental illness. Br J Psychiatry 183:233–238, 2003

Weniger G, Lange C, Ruther E, et al: Differential impairments of facial affect recognition in schizophrenia subtypes and major depression. Psychiatry Res 30:135–146, 2004

Wong KK, Chiu R, Tang B, et al: A randomized controlled trial of a supported employment program for persons with long-term mental illness in Hong Kong. Psychiatr Serv 59:84–90, 2008

World Health Organization: The ICD-10 Classification of Mental and Behavioural Disorders: Clinical Descriptions and Diagnostic Guidelines. Geneva, World Health Organization, 1992

Wykes T, Steel C, Everitt B, et al: Cognitive behavior therapy (CBTp) for schizophrenia: effect sizes, clinical models and methodological rigor. Schizophr Bull 34:523–537, 2008

Zigler E, Glick M: A Developmental Approach to Adult Psychopathology. New York, Wiley, 1986

CO-OCCURRING SUBSTANCE USE AND OTHER PSYCHIATRIC DISORDERS

MARY F. BRUNETTE, M.D.

DOUGLAS L. NOORDSY, M.D.

ALAN I. GREEN, M.D.

More than half of all patients with schizophrenia experience at least one co-occurring (i.e., comorbid) psychiatric disorder (Bermanzohn et al. 2000; Bland et al. 1987; Cassano et al. 1998) (Table 6–1). Detection and effective treatment of co-occurring disorders are essential if patient outcomes are to be optimized.

Some co-occurring conditions may have a genetic link to schizophrenia, and research aimed at establishing whether patients with schizophrenia are at increased risk for certain disorders may expand our understanding of the causes of schizophrenia.

TABLE 6–1. Co-occurring substance use and other psychiatric disorders in schizophrenia

Co-occurring disorder	Estimated lifetime prevalence (%)	Recommended treatments
Substance use disorders	47–59	Integrated treatments for mental illness and substance use disorders; medications for substance use disorders; clozapine may be better than other antipsychotics
Depressive disorders	Up to 81	Antipsychotics are the primary treatment modality; addition of antidepressant medication; psychosocial treatments for depression
Panic disorder	6–30	Case reports suggest addition of antipanic medications and cognitive-behavioral therapy
Social phobia	15–40	Case reports suggest addition of antidepressants and cognitive-behavioral therapy
Posttraumatic stress disorder	14–43	Treatments effective in general population (antidepressant medications and cognitive-behavioral therapy) should be considered
Obsessive-compulsive disorder	4–24	Case reports suggest addition of serotonin reuptake inhibitors and cognitive-behavioral therapy

Co-occurring disorders also may provide clues about the neurobiology of schizophrenia. For example, Green and colleagues (1999) proposed a neurobiological hypothesis to explain the high rates of substance use disorders observed in patients with schizophrenia. This hypothesis suggests that dysfunctional mesocorticolimbic brain reward pathways may underlie the symptoms of schizophrenia and the high vulnerability to substance abuse.

Although medications and psychosocial interventions are effective for the treatment of symptoms of schizophrenia and its associated cognitive deficits, identifying and treating co-occurring conditions remain major clinical challenges. In this chapter, we address co-occurring substance use disorder, depressive disorder, suicide, panic, social phobia, trauma and posttraumatic stress disorder (PTSD), and obsessive-compulsive disorder (OCD).

SUBSTANCE USE DISORDERS

PREVALENCE AND ETIOLOGY

The lifetime prevalence of *substance use disorders* in patients with schizophrenia is surprisingly high. The Epidemiologic Catchment Area study reported a lifetime prevalence of 47% in people with schizophrenia as compared with 16% of the general population (Regier et al. 1990). Alcohol is the most commonly abused substance in patients with schizophrenia, followed by cannabis (Drake and Mueser 1996; Kendler et al. 1996; Mueser et al. 1990; Selzer and Lieberman 1993). In addition, most people with schizophrenia are dependent on nicotine (58%–90%) (Dalack et al. 1998; Hughes et al. 1986).

Substance use disorders complicate the course of illness and treatment of patients with schizophrenia. Substance use is associated with treatment non-adherence; suicidality; hospitalization; homelessness; victimization; violence; increased risk for HIV, hepatitis B, and hepatitis C infection; and lower functioning in general (Brady et al. 1990; Drake and Mueser 1996; Drake et al. 1989; Hurlburt et al. 1996; Lysaker et al. 1994; Neria et al. 2002; Owen et al. 1996; Rosenberg et al. 2001a). Substance use disorders in first-episode patients may complicate assessment of the psychosis and delay treatment (Addington and Addington 2001; Green et al. 2004).

DETECTION AND MANAGEMENT

Co-occurring substance use disorders are often underdetected and under-treated in mental health settings (Ananth et al. 1989; Ridgely et al. 1990). Screening and assessment can be assisted through the use of standardized measures, especially instruments specifically developed for patients with mental illness (e.g., Dartmouth Assessment of Lifestyle Instrument [Rosenberg et al. 1998], Alcohol Use Scale [Mueser et al. 1995], and Drug Use Scale [Mueser et al. 1995]). Clinicians should supplement their observation of behaviors consistent with substance use (e.g., frequent missed appointments and financial or legal problems) with collateral information from family members, case managers, and significant others. A functional analysis of substance use incorporates the patient's view of both the positive and the negative aspects of substance use and actively involves the patient in the assessment process while simultaneously providing the foundation for cognitive-behavioral

TABLE 6–2. Principles of integrated dual-disorder treatment for patients with schizophrenia

Integration of mental health and substance use disorder treatments

Stagewise treatment that is tailored to the patient's motivation for change

Comprehensive services that include medication management, psychosocial rehabilitation, skills training, and residential and vocational services

Long-term perspective

substance abuse counseling. A nonjudgmental attitude reinforces honest communication about substance use and improves detection and treatment (Miller and Rollnick 2002).

In a review of 26 controlled studies of outpatient and residential programs, Drake and colleagues (2004) emphasized that integrating the treatment of the psychotic and the substance use disorders, thereby allowing for the coordination of pharmacotherapy, psychosocial treatments, and substance abuse counseling into one comprehensible package, results in improved patient outcomes (Barrowclough et al. 2001; Blankertz and Cnaan 1994; Drake et al. 1998). Important components of the effective integrated treatment of dual disorders include 1) integration of mental health and substance use disorder treatments; 2) staged interventions that are tailored to the patient's motivation for change (e.g., assertive outreach and motivational interviewing); 3) comprehensive services (e.g., medication management, rehabilitation, and social support interventions); and 4) a long-term perspective (Drake et al. 2004) (see Table 6–2). One such treatment program, Integrated Dual Disorder Treatment (Brunette et al. 2002; Mueser et al. 2003a), recommends that multidisciplinary teams provide the components of integrated care via case management, individual counseling, treatment groups, and family interventions.

Research on the optimal pharmacotherapy for dual-diagnosis patients has not yet established a standardized treatment approach (Green et al. 2008; Krystal et al. 1999; Noordsy and Green 2003; Wilkins 1997). While it is clear that antipsychotic agents decrease symptoms of psychosis in patients with co-occurring substance abuse disorder, many of these patients continue to use substances and experience poor outcomes despite such treatment (Drake et al. 1989; Salyers and Mueser 2001). Six preliminary studies, however, have suggested that clozapine may be helpful in treating substance use disorders (Brunette et al. 2006; Buckley et al. 1999; Drake et al. 2000; Green et al. 2003; Lee 1998; Zimmet et al. 2000).

Research findings on the effect of risperidone (Albanese 2001; Green et al. 2003; Smelson et al. 2002), olanzapine (Littrell et al. 2001; Longo 2002; Noordsy et al. 2001; Tsuang et al. 2002), quetiapine (Brown et al. 2002; Brunette et al. 2009; Potvin et al. 2006), and aripiprazole (Beresford et al. 2005; Brown et al. 2005; Warsi et al. 2005) at present appear less promising. Clozapine may be uniquely effective for patients with schizophrenia and substance use disorders because it potently blocks α_2-noradrenergic receptors, increases norepinephrine levels, and weakly blocks dopamine$_2$ (D_2) receptors, which may allow it to normalize the signal detection capability of dysfunctional mesocorticolimbic brain reward circuits (Green et al. 1999). Clearly, more studies are required to assess the effects of antipsychotics in this population.

Other medications demonstrated to be effective for the treatment of substance abuse in the general population show some promise for patients with schizophrenia. The following have evidence for efficacy: bupropion (Evins et al. 2001, 2005; George et al. 2002; Weiner et al. 2001) and varenicline for smoking cessation (Nino-Gomez et al. 2010); desipramine and imipramine for cocaine use disorder (Siris et al. 1993; Ziedonis et al. 1992); and disulfiram (Kofoed et al. 1986; Mueser et al. 2003b), and naltrexone (Dougherty 1997; Maxwell and Shinderman 1997, 2000; Petrakis et al. 2004, 2005) for alcohol disorders. Prescription benzodiazepine use is common for people with dual disorders (Clark et al. 2004), but these medications do not appear to improve outcomes and are associated with the development of benzodiazepine use disorders (Brunette et al. 2003).

A shared decision-making approach to prescribing medications is useful (Noordsy et al. 2000). Clinicians should encourage patients to take appropriate psychotropic medication, despite ongoing substance use, to stabilize the mental illness and to facilitate participation in substance abuse counseling. Comprehensive, integrated psychosocial and psychopharmacological treatments of both the psychotic and the substance use disorders delivered by multidisciplinary teams are recommended (Drake et al. 2001; Mueser et al. 2003a).

DEPRESSIVE DISORDERS

PREVALENCE AND OUTCOME

Although schizophrenia is viewed primarily as a psychotic disorder, patients with schizophrenia experience a variety of depressive states, ranging from dysphoria to major depression. The National Comorbidity Study (Kendler et al. 1996), as well as other studies (Bland et al. 1987; Hafner et al. 1999; Koreen et al. 1993; Martin et al. 1985), reported a lifetime risk of depression in patients with schizophrenia of up to 81%, with the point prevalence of major depression ranging from 10% to 30% (Baynes et al. 2000; Delahanty et al. 2001; Hafner et al. 1999; Herbener and Harrow 2002; Jin et al. 2001; Messias et al. 2001). Depression can be a symptom of the prodromal period prior to onset of psychotic symptoms (Hafner et al. 1999). It can also be an integral component of an acute episode of schizophrenia (McGlashan and Carpenter 1976; Sax et al. 1996), resolving as the psychosis remits (J. Addington et al. 2003; Hafner et al. 1999; Koreen et al. 1993; Oosthuizen et al. 2002; Tollefson et al. 1999).

Depression is associated with a risk of relapse of psychosis (Mandel et al. 1982), readmission (Shepherd et al. 1989), worse functioning (Jin et al. 2001), lower quality of life (Delahanty et al. 2001), and suicide (Drake et al. 1986), and relatives report more distress over this symptom cluster than over others (Boye et al. 2001).

DETECTION AND MANAGEMENT

Symptoms of depression are common during exacerbations of psychosis (Baynes et al. 2000; Hafner et al. 1999; Jin et al. 2001; Oosthuizen et al. 2002) and usually improve as the psychosis remits (Birchwood et al. 2000; Hafner et al. 1999; Koreen et al. 1993; Tollefson et al. 1999). Postpsychotic depression classically emerges after the resolution of psychotic symptoms and is most common after the first episode of schizophrenia (Birchwood et al. 2000; Koreen et al. 1993). In patients with schizoaffective disorder, depressed type, symptoms of depression are present concurrently with psychosis for a substantial proportion of the total duration of the psychotic illness.

Other clinically significant depressive phenomena, such as dysphoria and demoralization, occur frequently in patients with schizophrenia (Iqbal et al. 2000; Siris 2000a), although classic vegetative symptoms of depression may not be present in such patients (Bartels and Drake 1988). Some patients develop a sense of hopelessness, helplessness, and external locus of control, phenomena that Hoffman and colleagues (2000) found to be more powerful predictors of poor outcome in rehabilitation than depressive symptoms per se.

Symptoms of depression in patients with schizophrenia can be mistaken for negative symptoms, including affective flattening, alogia, avolition, apathy, anhedonia, and asociality (Birchwood et al. 2000; Sax et al. 1996; Siris 2000a), or for medication side effects, such as sedation, akinesia, and parkinsonism (Norman et al. 1998; Siris 1987). Key features of depression that distinguish it from negative symptoms include the presence of depressed mood, nondelusional guilt, and neurovegetative symptoms. By contrast, flat affect and anhedonic indifference without mood changes are more characteristic of negative symptoms than depression (Herbener and Harrow 2002; Mc-Glashan and Carpenter 1976). Cognitive impairment, another relatively independent aspect of schizophrenia (Tamminga et al. 1998), has been shown to correlate with depressive symptoms and syndromes (Brebion et al. 1997, 2000; Holthausen et al. 1999).

Although some clinical trials suggest that second-generation antipsychotics may be more effective than first-generation agents in treating acutely psychotic patients with schizophrenia and depression symptoms (Azorin 1995; Banov et al. 1994; Emsley et al. 2003; Marder et al. 1997; Tollefson et al. 1998), several studies found that risperidone treatment does not improve symptoms of depression more than haloperidol (Ceskova and Cvesta 1993; Moller et al. 1995; Peuskens 1995).

The results of controlled studies of the adjunctive use of antidepressant medications with antipsychotics have been mixed: 9 of 17 studies reported improvement compared with placebo or a comparison medication (D. Addington et al. 2002; Becker 1983; Dufresne et al. 1988; Hogarty et al. 1995; Johnson 1981; Kirli and Caliskan 1998; Kramer et al. 1989; Kurland and Nagaraju 1981; Mulholland et al. 2003; Muller-Siecheneder et al. 1998; Prusoff et al. 1979; Singh et al. 1978; Siris et al. 1987, 1989a, 1992; Vlokh et al. 2000; Waehrens and Gerlach 1980); however, many of these studies were limited by small sample size.

Psychosocial interventions that may be helpful for the treatment of depression include problem-solving training, coping skills training, cognitive therapy, exercise, family therapy, and support (Siris 1990, 2000b). For people who are demoralized, interventions geared toward meaningful activities can be helpful (Provencher et al. 2002).

Management of depressive symptoms in patients with schizophrenia depends on when such symptoms appear during the disorder as well as on their severity and their persistence. Because depressive symptoms may herald psychotic relapse, the patient should be monitored carefully for the emergence or exacerbation of psychosis. If the depression is part of a psychotic exacerbation, antipsychotic medication treatment should be optimized. If depressive symptoms persist or worsen in the absence of a psychotic exacerbation, use of an antidepressant medication or ECT can be considered.

SUICIDE

PREVALENCE AND RISK FACTORS

Suicide is the leading cause of premature death in people with schizophrenia (Black et al. 1985; Osby et al. 2000). Nearly 50% of patients with schizophrenia attempt suicide, and their lifetime risk of death by suicide is 5%–10% (Inskip et al. 1998; Palmer et al. 2005; Tsuang et al. 1999), a rate at least 10-fold higher than in the general population (Baxter and Appleby 1999; Dutta et al. 2010). Suicide in patients with schizophrenia has been associated with depression, anxiety, hopelessness, and a sense of failure (Bartels et al. 1992; Drake and Cotton 1986; Drake et al. 1985; Funahashi et al. 2000; Heila et al. 1997; Saarinen et al. 1999; Westermeyer et al. 1991). Drake and Cotton (1986) found that patients with schizophrenia who succeeded in a suicide attempt had been more depressed and isolated than were those who did not succeed. Moreover, suicide can be a "nonpsychotic reaction to a severe illness" (Drake et al. 1985), a notion that is supported by data showing a relation between higher levels of awareness and increased suicide risk in these patients (Amador et al. 1996).

Predictors of suicide in people with schizophrenia include a history of previous suicide attempts, earlier age at onset, and poor functioning (Alleback et al. 1987; Burgess et al. 2000; Nordentoft et al. 2002; Rossau and Mortensen 1997; Roy 1982). Men are at higher risk (Rossau and Mortensen 1997), and patients who attempt or commit suicide score higher on impulsivity scales (Dervaux et al. 2001). Risk of suicide is elevated 3 months after discharge from a psychiatric hospitalization (Heila et al. 1999; Rossau and Mortensen 1997; Roy 1982).

The early and active phases of the illness (Baxter and Appleby 1999; Heila et al. 1997; Osby et al. 2000; Westermeyer et al. 1991) are times of increased risk. Patients with prominent negative symptoms may have a somewhat reduced risk for suicide as compared with patients with mostly positive symptoms (Fenton et al. 1997). Although substance abuse is an established risk factor for suicide in the general population (Weiss and Hufford 1999), the evidence is mixed as to whether it is a risk factor among patients with schizophrenia (Alleback et al. 1987; Drake and Cotton 1986; Gupta et al. 1998; Meltzer 2002).

DETECTION AND MANAGEMENT

The detection of suicidal ideation and prevention of suicide in patients with schizophrenia can be difficult, as many suicide attempts are impulsive (Alleback et al. 1987; Gut-Fayand et al. 2001), and because patients may use highly lethal methods (Breier and Astrachan 1984; Heila et al. 1997) and give no advance disclosure (Earle et al. 1994).

Harkavy-Friedman and Nelson (1997) suggested that psychosocial and biological issues should be addressed. Listening and responding to the patient's reports of distress is crucial (Cohen et al. 1990). Burgess and colleagues (2000) pointed out that increasing the level of supervision and support, and ensuring continuity of care across systems, are essential for suicide prevention. Hospitalization can maintain safety as well as provide an opportunity for review and adjustment of psychopharmacological treatments. When the patient is discharged, engagement into treatment should be assured; intensive outreach may be required to engage patients with schizophrenia (Burgess et al. 2000).

Adequate psychopharmacological treatment of psychosis is essential. In a study of 88 patients with schizophrenia who died by suicide, Heila et al. (1999) found that more than half either had been prescribed inadequate doses of antipsychotic medication or had not been compliant with treatment; and an additional 23% had been judged nonresponsive to medication treatment. Psychoeducation and close monitoring may increase compliance with pharmacological treatment. Studies suggest that clozapine may decrease suicidal ideation, suicide attempts, and suicide completion in persons with schizophrenia more effectively than first-generation antipsychotic medications (Meltzer and Okayli 1995; Reid et al. 1998; Walker et al. 1997). Moreover, Meltzer and colleagues (2003) found that clozapine was more effective in decreasing suicidality than olanzapine in a large international trial of high-risk patients.

Optimal treatment for patients with schizophrenia who are at risk for suicide includes careful assessment of risk factors for suicide, the use of active outreach to engage patients in treatment and reduce isolation, psychosocial rehabilitation and skills training to improve coping skills, and effective pharmacotherapy.

ANXIETY SYMPTOMS AND DISORDERS

Anxiety symptoms and disorders are common in patients with schizophrenia. In diagnosing a co-occurring anxiety disorder, anxiety symptoms occurring during psychotic episodes must be differentiated from paranoia, reactions to delusions, and agitation related to psychosis. For example, Bayle and colleagues (2001) noted that panic attacks can be related to paranoid ideas. Additionally, anxiety must be differentiated from antipsychotic medication–induced side effects, such as akathisia, as well as other comorbid syndromes, such as substance-induced symptoms (e.g., cocaine intoxication or alcohol withdrawal) and depressive disorders (Zisook et al. 1999).

PANIC ATTACKS AND PANIC DISORDER

Prevalence and Outcome

Up to 45% of patients with schizophrenia experience panic attacks (Argyle 1990; Bayle et al. 2001; Bermanzohn et al. 2000; Bland et al. 1987; Craig et al. 2002; Goodwin et al. 2002; Labbate et al. 1999; Moorey and Soni 1994; Tibbo et al. 2003). Full panic disorder, with recurring spontaneous panic attacks and associated disability, occurs in 6%–33% (Argyle 1990; Bermanzohn et al. 2000; Cosoff and Hafner 1998; Kendler et al. 1996; Labbate et al. 1999; Pallanti et al. 2004; Stratkowsky et al. 1993; Tibbo et al. 2003). The National Comorbidity Study found that 26% of patients with schizophrenia had panic disorder (Kendler et al. 1996).

Patients with schizophrenia and panic attacks are more likely to be female, Caucasian, and married as well as to have less education (Goodwin et al. 2002).

The effect of panic on the course of schizophrenia and its relation to positive symptoms of psychosis remain poorly understood. Panic has been associated with comorbid depression and suicidal ideation in patients with schizophrenia (Bermanzohn et al. 2000; Cutler and Siris 1991; Goodwin et al. 2002).

Detection and Management

Patients with schizophrenia and panic experience the full spectrum of classic panic symptoms (Goodwin et al. 2002). Goodwin and colleagues (2002) reported that trembling, feelings of unreality, and fear of dying are particularly prominent symptoms. Although patients with schizophrenia and panic are more likely to seek mental health and medical treatment than are patients with schizophrenia who do not have panic symptoms (Goodwin et al. 2002), panic is dramatically underrecognized in these patients (Craig et al. 2002).

In a small, uncontrolled study of cognitive-behavioral therapy (CBT) for panic in patients with schizophrenia, Arlow and colleagues (1997) attempted a 16-week CBT program, including psychoeducation, cognitive restructuring, and in vivo exposure. They found that 73% of the patients were able to complete treatment; of those who completed the treatment, 75% experienced symptom improvement.

Although antipsychotic medications generally reduce anxiety (Marder et al. 1997), no studies have assessed the effect of antipsychotic medications on panic per se. No controlled studies have assessed the effectiveness of antidepressants or benzodiazepines for panic disorder in patients with schizophrenia. A report of two patients showed that panic symptoms that had not responded to antipsychotic medication did respond to imipramine augmentation of fluphenazine (Siris et al. 1989b). In addition, two studies showed that benzodiazepines reduced panic attacks in 10 patients with schizophrenia (Argyle 1990; Kahn et al. 1988) and that psychotic symptoms improved as the panic improved.

SOCIAL PHOBIA

Prevalence and Outcome

Many patients with schizophrenia have social anxiety and resulting social dysfunction (Morrison and Bellack 1987). A full social phobia syndrome was found in 15%–36% of small groups of patients with schizophrenia and schizoaffective disorders (Argyle 1990; Cosoff and Hafner 1998; Pallanti et al. 2004; Tibbo et al. 2003) and in 40% of the patients with schizophrenia in the National Comorbidity Study (Kendler et al. 1996).

Detection and Management

Patients with schizophrenia and social anxiety show levels of social fear (Penn et al. 1994) and social phobia (Pallanti et al. 2004) similar to those in persons with primary social phobia. However, social anxiety and fear of social situations must be carefully delineated from paranoia, withdrawal, and apathy (Pallanti et al. 2004; Penn et al. 1994). The key identifying features of social phobia are *fear of social situations* in which the individual might be scrutinized by others and *avoidance* of those situations or *endurance* of them only with intense anxiety. Evidence of embarrassment regarding scrutiny, rather than fear of persecution, will help identify patients with schizophrenia and social fear.

One controlled study of cognitive-behavioral group treatment for schizophrenia patients with social phobia found that social anxiety and depression improved in the treatment group as compared with the control group (Halperin et al. 2000). Social skills training and other rehabilitation efforts should incorporate education and gradual exposure to feared social situations (Heinssen and Glass 1990; Penn et al. 1994).

Antipsychotic medications alone may not always be helpful. Pallanti and colleagues (1999) described 12 patients taking clozapine whose social phobia symptoms became clinically detectable when their psychosis remitted during clozapine treatment. Further studies are needed to systematically test behavioral and pharmacological treatments.

TRAUMA AND POSTTRAUMATIC STRESS DISORDER

Prevalence and Outcome

Lifetime trauma is very common, reported by 85%–98% of patients with schizophrenia (Gearon et al. 2003; Goodman et al. 1995, 2001; Hutchings and Dutton 1993; Jacobson and Richardson 1987; Mueser et al. 1998). Approximately half (34%–65%) of patients with schizophrenia report childhood physical or sexual abuse (Darves-Bornoz et al. 1995; Goodman et al. 2001; Greenfield et al. 1994; Ross et al. 1994).

Studies of patients with schizophrenia report high rates of PTSD, ranging between 14% and 43% (Craine et al. 1988; Fenton 2001; Frame and Morrison 2001; Kendler et al. 1996; Mueser et al. 1998, 2004; Neria et al. 2002). Among patients with schizophrenia with a history of trauma, 27%–66% develop PTSD (Craine et al. 1988; Gearon et al. 2003; Mueser et al. 1998; Neria et al. 2002). More trauma experiences and childhood sexual abuse are significant predictors of the development of PTSD in this group (Gearon et al. 2003; Mueser et al. 1998; Neria et al. 2002).

Like people in the general population, patients with schizophrenia who have experienced trauma report more symptoms of anxiety, depression, suicidality, and dissociation than do those who have not experienced trauma (Goodman and Dutton 1996; Goodman et al. 1997; Priebe et al. 1998; Read and Argyle 1999; Schwartz and Cohen 2001). A history of trauma and PTSD is associated with worse role function (Lysaker et al. 2001), substance abuse (Goodman et al. 2001; Neria et al. 2002), homelessness (Goodman et al. 2001), lower quality of life, and less employment (Priebe et al. 1998).

Detection and Management

Because trauma and PTSD are so common in patients with schizophrenia and are associated with a variety of negative outcomes, clinicians should assess for the presence of PTSD symptoms and address the symptoms and functional correlates of trauma and PTSD. People who have been traumatized benefit from additional services, including education about trauma and its sequelae, training and support to enhance their current safety, and assistance to secure safe housing (Harris 2003). Clinicians should take care to be respectful and to assume a supportive stance when discussing trauma with patients.

CBT is helpful for people with primary PTSD in the general population (Harvey et al. 2003) and is being adapted for patients with schizophrenia (Rosenberg et al. 2001b) but has not yet been systematically studied. One study found CBT to be effective for patients with severe mental illness (15% schizophrenia) and PTSD (Mueser et al. 2008). Although antidepressants reduce PTSD symptoms (Albucher and Liberzon 2002), these drugs have not been studied in patients with schizophrenia and co-occurring PTSD. Further research is necessary to clarify how trauma and PTSD affect the course and treatment of schizophrenia and to assess interventions to reduce PTSD symptoms and prevent or reduce the negative sequelae of trauma in patients with schizophrenia.

OBSESSIVE-COMPULSIVE SYMPTOMS AND
OBSESSIVE-COMPULSIVE DISORDER

Prevalence and Outcome

Most contemporary studies report obsessive-compulsive symptoms in 10%–
26% of patients with schizophrenia (Berman et al. 1995a; Cassano et al. 1998;
Craig et al. 2002; Fabisch et al. 2001; Nechmad et al. 2003), and full OCD
with obsessions and compulsions not related to delusions has been documented
in 4%–24% of inpatients and outpatients with schizophrenia (Cosoff and
Hafner 1998; Craig et al. 2002; Eisen et al. 1997; Ohta et al. 2003; Pallanti et
al. 2004; Poyurovsky et al. 2001).

Although obsessions and compulsions in patients with schizophrenia are
similar to those in patients without psychosis (e.g., contamination/washing,
harm/checking) (Eisen et al. 1997; Fenton and McGlashan 1986; Ohta et al.
2003; Poyurovsky et al. 2001), distinguishing between delusions, preoccupations, and obsessions can be difficult in patients with thought disorders
(Eisen et al. 1997). Classically, *delusions* are described as fixed, false beliefs that
are ego-syntonic and actively embraced by the patient, whereas *obsessions* are
ego-dystonic and recognized as pathological intrusions (Hwang and Opler
2000). However, this distinction does not always hold true in clinical inter-
views of patients with primary OCD or in patients with psychosis. About 15%
of the patients with primary OCD have poor insight (Attiullah et al. 2000;
Marazziti et al. 2002); moreover, there appears to be a continuum of insight in
patients with schizophrenia, and for some patients, obsessions and delusions
may be overlapping (Bermanzohn et al. 1997).

Patients with obsessive-compulsive symptoms tend to be more socially isolated, to be less treatment responsive, and to have longer hospitalizations (Berman et al. 1995a; Fenton and McGlashan 1986; Hwang et al. 2000). Moreover,
research suggests an association between obsessive-compulsive symptoms and
poorer neurocognitive function in schizophrenia (Berman et al. 1998; Hwang
and Opler 2000; Lysaker et al. 2000; Schmidtke et al. 1998). Three studies
found that patients with schizophrenia and obsessive-compulsive symptoms
have higher levels of psychotic symptoms (Hwang et al. 2000; Lysaker et al.
2000; Nechmad et al. 2003), whereas five studies found no difference (Berman
et al. 1998; Craig et al. 2002; Ohta et al. 2003; Poyurovsky et al. 1999a, 2001).

Obsessive-compulsive symptoms in persons with schizophrenia may
have heterogeneous causes. Some authors have suggested that a supersensi-
tivity of serotonin receptors may occur during antipsychotic treatment, causing transient obsessive-compulsive symptoms (Baker et al. 1992; Kopala and
Honer 1994; Morrison et al. 1998; Poyurovsky et al. 1996, 1998), although
this was not evident in a controlled trial (Baker et al. 1996). Furthermore, several

studies found that obsessive-compulsive symptoms predated psychotic symptoms in more than half of the patients with co-occurring obsessive-compulsive symptoms and schizophrenia (Craig et al. 2002; Hwang and Opler 2000; Ohta et al. 2003).

Detection and Management

The types of obsessions and compulsions experienced by patients with schizophrenia are similar to those found in classic OCD. Most contemporary studies have reliably used the Yale-Brown Obsessive Compulsive Scale (Goodman et al. 1989) to detect obsessive-compulsive symptoms in these patients.

Antipsychotic medications used alone appear to be ineffective in the treatment of obsessive-compulsive symptoms in patients with schizophrenia (Poyurovsky et al. 2000). Although one report suggested that risperidone may enhance treatment response (McDougle et al. 2000), other reports suggested that clozapine may occasionally increase obsessive-compulsive symptoms (Patel et al. 1997; Strous et al. 1999). However, serotonin reuptake inhibitors used in combination with antipsychotics have been reported to reduce obsessive-compulsive symptoms in patients with schizophrenia (Berman et al. 1995b; Patel et al. 1997; Poyurovsky et al. 2003; Strous et al. 1999). A review (Chang and Berman 1999) of trials using clomipramine, imipramine, or fluoxetine reported that 67% of the patients showed improvement in obsessive-compulsive symptoms with no worsening of psychosis, whereas 19% showed worsening of psychosis. Similar results were found in a 12-week case series of 10 patients who received fluvoxamine augmentation (Poyurovsky et al. 1999b).

CBT has not been systematically studied in patients with schizophrenia and co-occurring obsessive-compulsive symptoms. The potential value of CBT may be influenced by the level of cognitive function and insight (Goff 1999).

CONCLUSION

Co-occurring disorders, such as substance abuse, major depression, and anxiety disorders, are common in patients with schizophrenia and are associated with a more difficult course of illness. These co-occurring disorders can be reliably identified, if clinicians look for them. Treatment protocols for some co-occurring disorders have been established, while for others further study will be required to define best practices guidelines. As a general rule, however, identification of these co-occurring disorders and integration of specific pharmacological and psychosocial interventions for them within schizophrenia treatment programs will be essential if clinical outcomes for patients with schizophrenia are to be improved.

REFERENCES

Addington D, Addington J, Patten S, et al: Double-blind, placebo-controlled comparison of the efficacy of sertraline as treatment for a major depressive episode in patients with remitted schizophrenia. J Clin Psychopharmacol 22:20–25, 2002

Addington J, Addington D: Impact of an early psychosis program on substance use. Psychiatr Rehabil J 25(1):60–67, 2001

Addington J, Leriger E, Addington D: Symptom outcome 1 year after admission to an early psychosis program. Can J Psychiatry 48:204–207, 2003

Albanese MJ: Safety and efficacy of risperidone in substance abusers with psychosis. Am J Addict 10:190–191, 2001

Albucher RC, Liberzon I: Psychopharmacological treatment in PTSD: a critical review. J Psychiatr Res 36:355–367, 2002

Alleback P, Varla A, Kristjansson E, et al: Risk factors for suicide among patients with schizophrenia. Acta Psychiatr Scand 76:414–419, 1987

Amador XF, Friedman JH, Kasapis C, et al: Suicidal behavior in schizophrenia and its relationship to awareness of illness. Am J Psychiatry 153:1185–1188, 1996

Ananth J, Vandewater S, Kamal M, et al: Missed diagnosis of substance abuse in psychiatric patients. Hosp Community Psychiatry 40:297–299, 1989

Argyle N: Panic attacks in chronic schizophrenia. Br J Psychiatry 157:430–433, 1990

Arlow PB, Moran ME, Bermanzohn PC, et al: Cognitive-behavioral treatment of panic attacks in chronic schizophrenia. J Psychother Pract Res 6:145–150, 1997

Attiullah N, Eisen JL, Rasmussen SA: Clinical features of obsessive-compulsive disorder. Psychiatr Clin North Am 23(3):469–491, 2000

Azorin JM: Long term treatment of mood disorders in schizophrenia. Acta Psychiatr Scand 91 (suppl):20–23, 1995

Baker RW, Chengappa KN, Baird JW, et al: Emergence of obsessive compulsive symptoms during treatment with clozapine. J Clin Psychiatry 53:439–442, 1992

Baker RW, Ames D, Umbricht DS, et al: Obsessive-compulsive symptoms in schizophrenia: a comparison of olanzapine and placebo. Psychopharmacol Bull 32:89–93, 1996

Banov MD, Zarate CA, Tohen M, et al: Clozapine therapy in refractory affective disorders: polarity predicts response in long-term follow-up. J Clin Psychiatry 55:295–300, 1994

Barrowclough C, Haddock G, Tarrier N, et al: Randomized controlled trial of motivational interviewing, cognitive behavior therapy, and family intervention for patients with comorbid schizophrenia and substance use disorders. Am J Psychiatry 158:1706–1713, 2001

Bartels SJ, Drake RE: Depressive symptoms in schizophrenia: comprehensive differential diagnosis. Compr Psychiatry 29:467–483, 1988

Bartels SJ, Drake RE, McHugo GJ: Alcohol abuse, depression, and suicidal behavior in schizophrenia. Am J Psychiatry 149:394–395, 1992

Baxter D, Appleby L: Case register study of suicide risk in mental disorders. Br J Psychiatry 175:322–326, 1999

Bayle F, Krebs M, Epelbaum C, et al: Clinical features of panic attacks in schizophrenia. Eur Psychiatry 16:349–353, 2001

Baynes D, Mulholland C, Cooper SJ, et al: Depressive symptoms in stable chronic schizophrenia: prevalence and relationship to psychopathology and treatment. Schizophr Res 45:47–56, 2000

Becker RE: Implications of the efficacy of thiothixene and a chlorpromazine-imipramine combination for depression in schizophrenia. Am J Psychiatry 140:208–211, 1983

Beresford TP, Clapp L, Martin B, et al: Aripiprazole in schizophrenia with cocaine dependence: a pilot study. J Clin Psychopharmacol 25:363–366, 2005

Berman I, Kalinowski A, Berman SM, et al: Obsessive and compulsive symptoms in chronic schizophrenia. Compr Psychiatry 36:6–10, 1995a

Berman I, Sapers BL, Chang HH, et al: Treatment of obsessive-compulsive symptoms in schizophrenic patients with clomipramine. J Clin Psychopharmacol 15:206–210, 1995b

Berman I, Merson A, Viegner B, et al: Obsessions and compulsions as a distinct cluster of symptoms: schizophrenia: a neuropsychological study. J Nerv Ment Dis 186:150–156, 1998

Bermanzohn PC, Porto L, Arlow PB, et al: Obsessions and delusions: separate and distinct or overlapping? CNS Spectrums 2:58–61, 1997

Bermanzohn PC, Porto L, Arlow PB, et al: Hierarchical diagnosis in chronic schizophrenia: a clinical study of co-occurring syndromes. Schizophr Bull 26:517–525, 2000

Birchwood M, Iqbal Z, Chadwick P, et al: Cognitive approach to depression and suicidal thinking in psychosis, 1: ontogeny of post-psychotic depression. Br J Psychiatry 177:516–521, 2000

Black DW, Warrack G, Winokur G: The Iowa record-linkage study, I: suicides and accidental deaths among psychiatric patients. Arch Gen Psychiatry 42:71–75, 1985

Bland RC, Newman SC, Orn H: Schizophrenia: lifetime co-morbidity in a community sample. Acta Psychiatr Scand 75:383–391, 1987

Blankertz LE, Cnaan RA: Assessing the impact of two residential programs for dually diagnosed homeless individuals. Soc Serv Rev 68:536–560, 1994

Boye B, Bentsen H, Ulstein I, et al: Relatives' distress and patients' symptoms and behaviours: a prospective study of patients with schizophrenia and their relatives. Acta Psychiatr Scand 104:42–50, 2001

Brady K, Anton R, Ballenger JC, et al: Cocaine abuse among schizophrenic patients. Am J Psychiatry 147:1164–1167, 1990

Brebion G, Smith M, Amador XF, et al: Clinical correlates of memory in schizophrenia: differential links between depression, positive and negative symptoms, and two types of memory impairment. Am J Psychiatry 154:1538–1543, 1997

Brebion G, Amador XF, Smith M, et al: Depression, psychomotor retardation, negative symptoms, and memory in schizophrenia. Neuropsychiatry Neuropsychol Behav Neurol 13:177–183, 2000

Breier A, Astrachan BM: Characterization of schizophrenic patients who commit suicide. Am J Psychiatry 141:206–209, 1984

Brown ES, Nejtek VA, Perantie DC, et al: Quetiapine in bipolar disorder and cocaine dependence. Bipolar Disord 4:406–411, 2002

Brown ES, Jeffress J, Liggin JD, et al: Switching outpatients with bipolar or schizoaffective disorders and substance abuse from their current antipsychotic to aripiprazole. J Clin Psychiatry 66:756–760, 2005

Brunette MF, Drake RE, Lynde D, et al: Toolkit for Integrated Dual Disorders Treatment. Rockville, MD, Substance Abuse and Mental Health Services Administration, 2002

Brunette M, Noordsy DL, Xie H, et al: Benzodiazepine use and abuse among patients with severe mental illness and co-occurring substance use disorders. Psychiatr Serv 54:1395–1401, 2003

Brunette MF, Drake RE, Xie H, et al: Clozapine use and relapses of substance use disorder among patients with co-occurring schizophrenia and substance use disorders. Schizophr Bull 32:637–643, 2006

Brunette MF, O'Keefe C, Dawson R, et al: An open label study of quetiapine in patients with schizophrenia and alcohol disorders. Mental Health and Substance Use: Dual Diagnosis 2:203–211, 2009

Buckley P, McCarthy M, Chapman P, et al: Clozapine treatment of comorbid substance abuse in patients with schizophrenia (abstract). Schizophr Res 36:272, 1999

Burgess P, Pirkis J, Morton J, et al: Lessons from a comprehensive clinical audit of users of psychiatric services who committed suicide. Psychiatr Serv 51:1555–1560, 2000

Cassano GB, Pini S, Saettoni M, et al: Occurrence and clinical correlates of psychiatric comorbidity in patients with psychotic disorders. J Clin Psychiatry 59:60–68, 1998

Ceskova E, Cvesta J: Double-blind comparison of risperidone and haloperidol in schizophrenia and schizoaffective psychosis. Psychopharmacopsychiatry 26:121–124, 1993

Chang HH, Berman I: Treatment issues for patients with schizophrenia who have obsessive-compulsive symptoms. Psychiatr Ann 29:529–535, 1999

Clark RE, Xie H, Brunette MF: Benzodiazepine prescription practices and substance abuse in persons with severe mental illness. J Clin Psychiatry 65:151–155, 2004

Cohen LJ, Test MA, Brown RL: Suicide and schizophrenia: data from a prospective community treatment study [published erratum appears in Am J Psychiatry 147:1110]. Am J Psychiatry 147:602–607, 1990

Cosoff S, Hafner RJ: The prevalence of comorbid anxiety in schizophrenia, schizoaffective disorder and bipolar disorder. Aust N Z J Psychiatry 32:67–72, 1998

Craig T, Hwang MY, Bromet EJ: Obsessive-compulsive and panic symptoms in patients with first-admission psychosis. Am J Psychiatry 159:592–598, 2002

Craine L, Henson C, Colliver J, et al: Prevalence of a history of sexual abuse among female psychiatric patients in a state hospital system. Hosp Community Psychiatry 39:300–304, 1988

Cutler JL, Siris SG: "Panic-like" symptomatology in schizophrenic and schizoaffective patients with postpsychotic depression: observations and implications. Compr Psychiatry 32:465–473, 1991

Dalack GW, Healy DJ, Meador-Woodruff JH: Nicotine dependence in schizophrenia: clinical phenomena and laboratory findings. Am J Psychiatry 155:1490–1501, 1998

Darves-Bornoz J, Lemperiere T, Degiovanni A, et al: Sexual victimization in women with schizophrenia and bipolar disorder. Soc Psychiatry Psychiatr Epidemiol 30:78–84, 1995

Delahanty J, Ram R, Postrado L, et al: Differences in rates of depression in schizophrenia by race. Schizophr Bull 27:29–38, 2001

Dervaux A, Bayle F, Laqueille X, et al: Is substance abuse in schizophrenia related to impulsivity, sensation seeking, or anhedonia? Am J Psychiatry 158:492–494, 2001

Dougherty RJ: Naltrexone in the treatment of alcohol dependent dual diagnosed patients (abstract). J Addict Dis 16:107, 1997

Drake RE, Cotton PG: Depression, hopelessness and suicide in chronic schizophrenia. Br J Psychiatry 148:554–559, 1986

Drake RE, Mueser KT: Alcohol-use disorder and severe mental illness. Alcohol Health Res World 20:87–93, 1996

Drake RE, Gates C, Whitaker A, et al: Suicide among schizophrenics: a review. Compr Psychiatry 26:90–100, 1985

Drake RE, Gates C, Cotton PG: Suicide among schizophrenics: a comparison of attempters and completed suicides. Br J Psychiatry 149:784–787, 1986

Drake RE, Osher FC, Wallach MA: Alcohol use and abuse in schizophrenia: a prospective community study. J Nerv Ment Dis 177:408–414, 1989

Drake RE, McHugo GJ, Clark RE, et al: Assertive community treatment for patients with co-occurring severe mental illness and substance use disorder: a clinical trial. Am J Orthopsychiatry 68:201–215, 1998

Drake RE, Xie H, McHugo GJ, et al: The effects of clozapine on alcohol and drug use disorders among schizophrenic patients. Schizophr Bull 26:441–449, 2000

Drake RE, Essock SM, Shaner A, et al: Implementing dual diagnosis services for clients with severe mental illness. Psychiatr Serv 52:469–472, 2001

Drake RE, Mueser KT, Brunette MF, et al: A review of treatments for people with severe mental illnesses and co-occurring substance use disorders. Psychiatr Rehabil J 27:360–374, 2004

Dufresne RL, Kass DJ, Becker RE: Bupropion and thiothixene versus placebo and thiothixene in the treatment of depression in schizophrenia. Drug Dev Res 12:259–266, 1988

Dutta R, Murray RM, Hotopf M, et al: Reassessing the long-term risk of suicide after a first episode of psychosis. Arch Gen Psychiatry 67:1230–1237, 2010

Earle KA, Forquer SL, Volo AM, et al: Characteristics of outpatient suicides. Hosp Community Psychiatry 45:123–126, 1994

Eisen JL, Beer DA, Pato MT, et al: Obsessive-compulsive disorder in patients with schizophrenia or schizoaffective disorder. Am J Psychiatry 154:271–273, 1997

Emsley R, Buckley P, Jones AM, et al: Differential effect of quetiapine on depressive symptoms in patients with partially responsive schizophrenia. J Psychopharmacol (Oxf) 17:210–215, 2003

Evins AE, Mays VK, Rigotti NA, et al: A pilot trial of bupropion added to cognitive behavioral therapy for smoking cessation in schizophrenia. Nicotine Tob Res 3:397–403, 2001

Evins AE, Cather C, Deckersbach T, et al: A double-blind placebo-controlled trial of bupropion sustained-release for smoking cessation in schizophrenia. J Clin Psychopharmacol 25:218–225, 2005

Fabisch K, Fabisch H, Langs G, et al: Incidence of obsessive-compulsive phenomena in the course of acute schizophrenia and schizoaffective disorder. Eur Psychiatry 16:336–341, 2001

Fenton WS: Comorbid conditions in schizophrenia. Curr Opin Psychiatry 14:17–23, 2001

Fenton WS, McGlashan TH: The prognostic significance of obsessive-compulsive symptoms in schizophrenia. Am J Psychiatry 143:437–441, 1986

Fenton WS, McGlashan TH, Victor BJ, et al: Symptoms, subtype, and suicidality in patients with schizophrenia spectrum disorders. Am J Psychiatry 154:199–204, 1997

Frame L, Morrison AP: Causes of posttraumatic stress disorder in psychotic patients. Arch Gen Psychiatry 58:305–306, 2001

Funahashi TM, Ibuki YM, Domon YM, et al: A clinical study on suicide among schizophrenics. Psychiatry Clin Neurosci 54:173–179, 2000

Gearon JS, Kaltman SI, Brown C, et al: Traumatic life events and PTSD among women with substance use disorders and schizophrenia. Psychiatr Serv 54:523–528, 2003

George TP, Vessicchio JC, Termine A, et al: A placebo controlled trial of bupropion for smoking cessation in schizophrenia. Biol Psychiatry 52:53–61, 2002

Goff DC: The comorbidity of obsessive-compulsive disorder and schizophrenia. Psychiatr Ann 29:533–536, 1999

Goodman LA, Dutton MA: The relationship between victimization and cognitive schemata among episodically homeless, seriously mentally ill women. Violence Vict 11:159–174, 1996

Goodman WK, Price LH, Rasmussen SA, et al: The Yale-Brown Obsessive Compulsive Scale: development, use, and reliability. Arch Gen Psychiatry 46:1006–1011, 1989

Goodman LA, Dutton MA, Harris M: Episodically homeless women with serious mental illness: prevalence of physical and sexual assault. Am J Orthopsychiatry 65:468–478, 1995

Goodman LA, Dutton MA, Harris M: The relationship between violence dimensions and symptom severity among homeless, mentally ill women. J Trauma Stress 10:51–70, 1997

Goodman LA, Salyers MP, Mueser KT, et al: Recent victimization in women and men with severe mental illness: prevalence and correlates. J Trauma Stress 14:615–632, 2001

Goodwin R, Lyons J, McNally R: Panic attacks in schizophrenia. Schizophr Res 58:213–220, 2002

Green AI, Zimmet SV, Strous RD, et al: Clozapine for comorbid substance use disorder and schizophrenia: do patients with schizophrenia have a reward-deficiency syndrome that can be ameliorated by clozapine? Harv Rev Psychiatry 6:287–296, 1999

Green AI, Burgess ES, Zimmet SV, et al: Alcohol and cannabis use in schizophrenia: effects of clozapine and risperidone. Schizophr Res 60:81–85, 2003

Green AI, Tohen M, Hamer RM, et al: First episode schizophrenia-related psychosis and substance use disorders: acute response to olanzapine and haloperidol. Schizophr Res 66:125–135, 2004

Green AI, Noordsy DL, Brunette MF, et al: Substance abuse and schizophrenia: pharmacotherapeutic intervention. J Subst Abuse Treat 34:61–71, 2008

Greenfield SF, Strakowski SM, Tohen M, et al: Childhood abuse in first-episode psychosis. Br J Psychiatry 164:831–834, 1994

Gupta S, Black DW, Arndt S, et al: Factors associated with suicide attempts among patients with schizophrenia. Psychiatr Serv 49:1353–1355, 1998

Gut-Fayand A, Dervaux A, Olie J, et al: Substance abuse and suicidality in schizophrenia: a common risk factor linked to impulsivity. Psychiatry Res 102:65–72, 2001

Hafner H, Loffler W, Maurer K, et al: Depression, negative symptoms, social stagnation and social decline in the early course of schizophrenia. Acta Psychiatr Scand 100:105–118, 1999

Halperin S, Nathan P, Drummond P, et al: A cognitive-behavioural, group-based intervention for social anxiety in schizophrenia. Aust N Z J Psychiatry 34:809–813, 2000

Harkavy-Friedman JM, Nelson E: Management of the suicidal patient with schizophrenia. Psychiatr Clin North Am 20:625–640, 1997

Harris M: Modifications in service delivery and clinical treatment for women diagnosed with severe mental illness who are also the survivors of sexual abuse trauma. J Ment Health Adm 21:397–406, 2003

Harvey AG, Bryant RA, Tarrier N: Cognitive behaviour therapy for posttraumatic stress disorder. Clin Psychol Rev 23:501–522, 2003

Heila H, Isometsa ET, Henriksson MM, et al: Suicide and schizophrenia: a nationwide psychological autopsy study on age- and sex-specific clinical characteristics of 92 suicide victims with schizophrenia. Am J Psychiatry 154:1235–1242, 1997

Heila H, Isometsa ET, Henriksson MM, et al: Suicide victims with schizophrenia in different treatment phases and adequacy of antipsychotic medication. J Clin Psychiatry 60:200–208, 1999

Heinssen RKJ, Glass CR: Social skills, social anxiety, and cognitive factors in schizophrenia, in Handbook of Social and Evaluation Anxiety. Edited by Leitenberg H. New York, Plenum, 1990, pp 325–355

Herbener ES, Harrow M: The course of anhedonia during 10 years of schizophrenic illness. J Abnorm Psychol 111:237–248, 2002

Hoffmann H, Kupper Z, Kunz B: Hopelessness and its impact on rehabilitation outcome in schizophrenia: an exploratory study. Schizophr Res 43:147–158, 2000

Hogarty GE, McEvoy JP, Ulrich RF, et al: Pharmacotherapy of impaired affect in recovering schizophrenic patients. Arch Gen Psychiatry 52:29–41, 1995

Holthausen E, Wiersma D, Knegtering R, et al: Psychopathology and cognition in schizophrenia spectrum disorders: the role of depressive symptoms. Schizophr Res 39:65–71, 1999

Hughes JR, Hatsukami DK, Mitchell JE, et al: Prevalence of smoking among schizophrenic outpatients. Am J Psychiatry 143:993–997, 1986

Hurlburt MS, Hough RL, Wood PA: Effects of substance abuse on housing stability of homeless mentally ill persons in supported housing. Psychiatr Serv 47:731–736, 1996

Hutchings PS, Dutton MA: Sexual assault history in a community mental health center clinical population. Community Ment Health J 29:59–63, 1993

Hwang MY, Opler LA: Management of schizophrenia with obsessive-compulsive disorder. Psychiatr Ann 30:23–28, 2000

Hwang MY, Morgan JE, Losconzey MF: Clinical and neuropsychological profiles of obsessive-compulsive schizophrenia: a pilot study. J Neuropsychiatry Clin Neurosci 12:91–94, 2000

Inskip HM, Harris EC, Barraclough B: Lifetime risk of suicide for affective disorder, alcoholism and schizophrenia. Br J Psychiatry 172:35–37, 1998

Iqbal Z, Birchwood M, Chadwick P, et al: Cognitive approach to depression and suicidal thinking in psychosis, 2: testing the validity of a social ranking model. Br J Psychiatry 177:522–528, 2000

Jacobson A, Richardson B: Assault experiences of 100 psychiatric inpatients: evidence of the need for routine inquiry. Am J Psychiatry 144:508–513, 1987

Jin H, Zisook S, Palmer BW, et al: Association of depressive symptoms with worse functioning in schizophrenia: a study in older outpatients. J Clin Psychiatry 62:797–803, 2001

Johnson DA: Depressions in schizophrenia: some observations on prevalence, etiology, and treatment. Acta Psychiatr Scand Suppl 291:137–144, 1981

Kahn JP, Puertollano MA, Schane MD, et al: Adjunctive alprazolam for schizophrenia with panic anxiety: clinical observation and pathogenetic implications. Am J Psychiatry 145:742–744, 1988

Kendler KS, Gallagher TJ, Abelson JM, et al: Lifetime prevalence, demographic risk factors, and diagnostic validity of nonaffective psychosis as assessed in a US community sample: the national comorbidity survey. Arch Gen Psychiatry 53:1022–1031, 1996

Kirli S, Caliskan M: A comparative study of sertraline versus imipramine in postpsychotic depressive disorder of schizophrenia. Schizophr Res 33:103–111, 1998

Kofoed LL, Kania J, Walsh T, et al: Outpatient treatment of patients with substance abuse and coexisting psychiatric disorders. Am J Psychiatry 143:867–872, 1986

Kopala L, Honer WG: Risperidone, serotonergic mechanisms, and obsessive-compulsive symptoms in schizophrenia. Am J Psychiatry 151:1714–1715, 1994

Koreen AR, Siris SG, Chakos M, et al: Depression in first-episode schizophrenia. Am J Psychiatry 150:1643–1648, 1993

Kramer MS, Vogel WH, DiJohnson C: Antidepressants in "depressed" schizophrenic inpatients: a controlled trial. Arch Gen Psychiatry 46:922–928, 1989

Krystal JH, D'Souza DC, Madonick S, et al: Toward a rational pharmacotherapy of comorbid substance abuse in schizophrenic patients. Schizophr Res 35:35–49, 1999

Kurland AA, Nagaraju A: Viloxazine and the depressed schizophrenic: methodological issues. J Clin Pharmacol 21:37–41, 1981

Labbate LA, Young PC, Arana GW: Panic disorder in schizophrenia. Can J Psychiatry 44:488–490, 1999

Lee ML: Clozapine and substance abuse in patients with schizophrenia. Can J Psychiatry 45:855–856, 1998

Littrell KH, Petty RG, Hilligoss NM, et al: Olanzapine treatment for patients with schizophrenia and substance abuse. J Subst Abuse Treat 21:217–221, 2001

Longo LP: Olanzapine for cocaine craving and relapse prevention in 2 patients. J Clin Psychiatry 63(7):595–596, 2002

Lysaker PH, Bell MD, Beam-Goulet J, et al: Relationship of positive and negative symptoms to cocaine abuse in schizophrenia. J Nerv Ment Dis 182:109–112, 1994

Lysaker PH, Marks KA, Picone JB, et al: Obsessive and compulsive symptoms in schizophrenia: clinical and neurocognitive correlates. J Nerv Ment Dis 188:78–83, 2000

Lysaker PH, Meyer PS, Evans JD, et al: Childhood sexual trauma and psychosocial functioning in adults with schizophrenia. Psychiatr Serv 52:1485–1488, 2001

Mandel MR, Severe JB, Schooler NR, et al: Development and prediction of postpsychotic depression in neuroleptic-treated schizophrenics. Arch Gen Psychiatry 39:197–203, 1982

Marder SR, Davis JM, Chouinard G: The effects of risperidone on the five dimensions of schizophrenia derived by factor analysis: combined results of the North American trials. J Clin Psychiatry 58:538–546, 1997

Marazziti D, Dell'Osso L, Di Nasso E, et al: Insight in obsessive-compulsive disorder: a study of an Italian sample. Eur Psychiatry 17:407–410, 2002

Martin RL, Cloninger CR, Guze SB, et al: Frequency and differential diagnosis of depressive syndromes in schizophrenia. J Clin Psychiatry 46:9–13, 1985

Maxwell S, Shinderman MS: Naltrexone in the treatment of dually diagnosed patients (abstract). J Addict Dis 16:125, 1997

Maxwell S, Shinderman MS: Use of naltrexone in the treatment of alcohol use disorders in patients with concomitant major mental illness. J Addict Dis 19:61–69, 2000

McDougle CJ, Epperson CN, Pelton GH, et al: A double-blind, placebo-controlled study of risperidone addition in serotonin reuptake inhibitor-refractory obsessive-compulsive disorder. Arch Gen Psychiatry 57:794–801, 2000

McGlashan TH, Carpenter WT: Postpsychotic depression in schizophrenia. Arch Gen Psychiatry 33:231–239, 1976

Meltzer HY: Suicidality in schizophrenia: a review of the evidence for risk factors and treatment options. Curr Psychiatry Rep 4:279–283, 2002

Meltzer HY, Okayli G: Reduction of suicidality during clozapine treatment of neuroleptic-resistant schizophrenia: impact of risk-benefit assessment. Am J Psychiatry 152:183–190, 1995

Meltzer HY, Alphs L, Green AI, et al: Clozapine treatment for suicidality in schizophrenia: International Suicide Prevention Trial (InterSePT). Arch Gen Psychiatry 60:82–91, 2003

Messias E, Kirkpatrick B, Ram R, et al: Suspiciousness as a specific risk factor for major depressive episodes in schizophrenia. Schizophr Res 47:159–165, 2001

Miller WR, Rollnick S: Motivational Interviewing. New York, Guilford, 2002

Moller HJ, Muller H, Borison R, et al: A path analytic approach to differentiate between direct and indirect drug effects on negative symptoms in schizophrenia patients: a re-evaluation of the North American risperidone study. Eur Arch Psychiatry Clin Neurosci 245:45–49, 1995

Moorey H, Soni SD: Anxiety symptoms in stable chronic schizophrenia. J Ment Health Adm 3:257–262, 1994

Morrison D, Clark D, Goldfarb E, et al: Worsening of obsessive-compulsive symptoms following treatment with olanzapine. Am J Psychiatry 155:855, 1998

Morrison RL, Bellack AS: Social functioning of schizophrenic patients: clinical and research issues. Schizophr Bull 13:715–725, 1987

Mueser KT, Yarnold PR, Levinson DF, et al: Prevalence of substance abuse in schizophrenia: demographic and clinical correlates. Schizophr Bull 16:31–56, 1990

Mueser KT, Drake RE, Clark RE, et al: Toolkit for Evaluating Substance Abuse in Persons With Severe Mental Illness. Cambridge, MA, Evaluation Center at Human Service Research Institute, 1995

Mueser KT, Goodman LA, Trumbetta SL, et al: Trauma and posttraumatic stress disorder in severe mental illness. J Consult Clin Psychol 66:493–499, 1998

Mueser KT, Noordsy DL, Drake RE, et al: Integrated Treatment for Dual Disorders: A Guide to Effective Practice. New York, Guilford, 2003a

Mueser KT, Noordsy DL, Fox M, et al: Disulfiram treatment for alcoholism in severe mental illness. Am J Addict 12:242–252, 2003b

Mueser KT, Salyers MP, Rosenberg SD, et al: Interpersonal trauma and posttraumatic stress disorder in patients with severe mental illness. Schizophr Bull 30:45–57, 2004

Mueser KT, Rosenberg SD, Xie H, et al: A randomized controlled trial of cognitive-behavioral treatment for posttraumatic stress disorder in severe mental illness. J Consult Clin Psychol 76:259–271, 2008

Muller-Siecheneder F, Muller MJ, Hillert A: Risperidone versus haloperidol and amitriptyline in the treatment of patients with a combined psychotic and depressive syndrome. J Clin Psychopharmacol 18:111–120, 1998

Mulholland C, Lynch G, King DJ, et al: A double-blind, placebo-controlled trial of sertraline for depressive symptoms in patients with stable, chronic schizophrenia. J Psychopharmacol 17(1):107–112, 2003

Nechmad A, Ratzoni G, Poyurovsky M, et al: Obsessive-compulsive disorder in adolescent schizophrenia patients. Am J Psychiatry 160:1002–1004, 2003

Neria Y, Bromet EJ, Sievers S, et al: Trauma exposure and posttraumatic stress disorder in psychosis: findings from a first-admission cohort. J Consult Clin Psychol 70:246–251, 2002

Nino-Gomez J, Carlini S, Nemani K, et al: Safety and efficacy of varenicline in schizophrenia: preliminary data from 12-week trial. 16th Annual Meeting of the Society for Research on Nicotine and Tobacco, Baltimore, MD, 2010, p 163

Noordsy DL, Green AI: Pharmacotherapy for schizophrenia and co-occurring substance use disorders. Curr Psychiatry Rep 5:340–346, 2003

Noordsy DL, Torrey WC, Mead S, et al: Recovery-oriented pharmacology: redefining the goals of antipsychotic treatment. J Clin Psychiatry 61 (suppl 3):22–29, 2000

Noordsy DL, O'Keefe CD, Mueser KT, et al: Six-month outcomes for patients who switched to olanzapine treatment. Psychiatr Serv 52:501–507, 2001

Nordentoft M, Jeppesen P, Abel M, et al: OPUS Study: suicidal behavior, suicidal ideation and hopelessness among patients with first-episode psychosis. Br J Psychiatry 181 (suppl 43):S98–S106, 2002

Norman RMG, Malla AK, Cortese L, et al: Aspects of dysphoria and symptoms of schizophrenia. Psychol Med 28:1433–1441, 1998

Ohta M, Kokai M, Morita Y: Features of obsessive-compulsive disorder in patients primarily diagnosed with schizophrenia. Psychiatry Clin Neurosci 57:67–74, 2003

Oosthuizen P, Emsley RA, Roberts M, et al: Depressive symptoms at baseline predict fewer negative symptoms at follow-up in patients with first-episode schizophrenia. Schizophr Res 58:247–252, 2002

Osby U, Correia N, Brandt L, et al: Mortality and causes of death in schizophrenia in Stockholm County, Sweden. Schizophr Res 45:21–28, 2000

Owen RR, Fischer EP, Booth BM, et al: Medication noncompliance and substance abuse among patients with schizophrenia. Psychiatr Serv 47:853–858, 1996

Pallanti S, Quercioli L, Rossi A, et al: The emergence of social phobia during clozapine treatment and its response to fluoxetine augmentation. J Clin Psychiatry 60:819–823, 1999

Pallanti S, Quercioli L, Hollander E: Social anxiety in outpatients with schizophrenia: a relevant cause of disability. Am J Psychiatry 161:53–58, 2004

Palmer BA, Pankratz S, Bostwick JM: The lifetime risk of suicide in schizophrenia: a reexamination. Arch Gen Psychiatry 62:247–253, 2005

Patel JK, Salzman C, Green AI, et al: Chronic schizophrenia: response to clozapine, risperidone and paroxetine. Am J Psychiatry 154:543–546, 1997

Penn DL, Hope DA, Spaulding W, et al: Social anxiety in schizophrenia. Schizophr Res 11:277–284, 1994

Petrakis IL, O'Malley SS, Rounsaville B, et al: Naltrexone augmentation of neuroleptic treatment in alcohol abusing patients with schizophrenia. Psychopharmacology (Berl) 172:291–297, 2004

Petrakis IL, Poling J, Levinson C, et al: Naltrexone and disulfiram in patients with alcohol dependence and comorbid psychiatric disorders. Biol Psychiatry 57:1128–1137, 2005

Peuskens J: Risperidone in the treatment of patients with chronic schizophrenia: a multinational, multi-center, double-blind, parallel group study versus haloperidol. Br J Psychiatry 166:712–726, 1995

Potvin S, Stip E, Lipp O, et al: Quetiapine in patients with comorbid schizophrenia-spectrum and substance use disorders: an open-label trial. Curr Med Res Opin 22:1277–1285, 2006

Poyurovsky M, Hermesh H, Weizman A: Fluvoxamine treatment in clozapine-induced obsessive-compulsive symptoms in schizophrenic patients. Clin Neuropharmacol 19:305–313, 1996

Poyurovsky M, Bergman Y, Shoshani D, et al: Emergence of obsessive-compulsive symptoms and tics during clozapine withdrawal. Clin Neuropharmacol 21:97–100, 1998

Poyurovsky M, Fuchs C, Weizman A: Obsessive-compulsive disorder in patients with first-episode schizophrenia. Am J Psychiatry 156:1998–2000, 1999a

Poyurovsky M, Isakov V, Hromnikov S, et al: Fluvoxamine treatment of obsessive-compulsive symptoms in schizophrenic patients: an add-on open study. Int Clin Psychopharmacol 14:95–100, 1999b

Poyurovsky M, Dorfman-Etrog P, Hermesh H, et al: Beneficial effects of olanzapine in schizophrenia patients with obsessive-compulsive symptoms. Int Clin Psychopharmacol 15:169–173, 2000

Poyurovsky M, Hramenkov S, Isakov V, et al: Obsessive-compulsive disorder in hospitalized patients with chronic schizophrenia. Psychiatry Res 102:49–57, 2001

Poyurovsky M, Kurs R, Weizman A: Olanzapine-sertraline combination in schizophrenia with obsessive-compulsive disorder. J Clin Psychiatry 64:611, 2003

Priebe S, Broker M, Gunkel S: Involuntary admission and posttraumatic stress disorder symptoms in schizophrenia patients. Compr Psychiatry 39:220–224, 1998

Provencher HL, Gregg R, Mead S, et al: The role of work in the recovery of persons with psychiatric disabilities. Psychiatr Rehabil J 26:132–144, 2002

Prusoff BA, Williams DH, Weissman MM, et al: Treatment of secondary depression in schizophrenia. Arch Gen Psychiatry 36:569–575, 1979

Read J, Argyle N: Hallucinations, delusions, and thought disorder among adult psychiatric inpatients with a history of child abuse. Psychiatr Serv 50:1467–1472, 1999

Regier DA, Farmer ME, Rae DS, et al: Comorbidity of mental disorders with alcohol and other drug abuse. JAMA 264:2511–2518, 1990

Reid WH, Mason M, Hogan T: Suicide prevention effects associated with clozapine therapy in schizophrenia and schizoaffective disorder. Psychiatr Serv 49:1029–1033, 1998

Ridgely MS, Goldman HH, Willenbring M: Barriers to care of persons with dual diagnoses: organizational and financing issues. Schizophr Bull 16:123–132, 1990

Rosenberg SD, Drake RE, Wolford GL, et al: Dartmouth Assessment of Lifestyle Instrument (DALI): a substance use disorder screen for people with severe mental illness. Am J Psychiatry 155:232–238, 1998

Rosenberg SD, Goodman LA, Osher FC, et al: Prevalence of HIV, hepatitis B, and hepatitis C in people with severe mental illness. Am J Public Health 91:31–37, 2001a

Rosenberg SD, Mueser KT, Friedman MJ, et al: Developing effective treatments for posttraumatic stress disorders among people with severe mental illness. Psychiatr Serv 52:1453–1461, 2001b

Ross CA, Anderson G, Clark P: Childhood abuse and the positive symptoms of schizophrenia. Hosp Community Psychiatry 45:489–491, 1994

Rossau CD, Mortensen PB: Risk factors for suicide in patients with schizophrenia: nested case-control study. Br J Psychiatry 171:355–359, 1997

Roy A: Risk factors for suicide in psychiatric patients. Arch Gen Psychiatry 39:1089–1095, 1982

Saarinen PI, Lehtonen J, Lonnqvist J: Suicide risk in schizophrenia: an analysis of 17 consecutive suicides. Schizophr Bull 25:533–542, 1999

Salyers MP, Mueser KT: Social functioning, psychopathology, and medication side effects in relation to substance use and abuse in schizophrenia. Schizophr Res 48:109–123, 2001

Sax KW, Strakowski SM, Keck PE, et al: Relationship among negative, positive, and depressive symptoms in schizophrenia and psychotic depression. Br J Psychiatry 168:68–71, 1996

Schmidtke L, Schorb A, Winkelmann G, et al: Cognitive frontal lobe dysfunction in obsessive-compulsive disorder. Biol Psychiatry 43:666–673, 1998

Schwartz RC, Cohen BN: Psychosocial correlates of suicidal intent among patients with schizophrenia. Compr Psychiatry 42:118–123, 2001

Selzer JA, Lieberman JA: Schizophrenia and substance abuse. Psychiatr Clin North Am 16:401–412, 1993

Shepherd M, Watt D, Falloon IR, et al: The natural history of schizophrenia: a five-year follow-up study of outcome and prediction in a representative sample of schizophrenics. Psychol Med 15:1–46, 1989

Singh AN, Saxena B, Nelson HL: A controlled clinical study of trazodone in chronic schizophrenic patients with pronounced depressive symptomatology. Curr Ther Res Clin Exp 23:485–501, 1978

Siris SG: Akinesia and postpsychotic depression: a difficult differential diagnosis. J Clin Psychiatry 38:240–243, 1987

Siris S: Pharmacological treatment of substance-abusing schizophrenic patients. Schizophr Bull 16:111–122, 1990

Siris SG: Depression in schizophrenia: perspective in the era of "atypical" antipsychotics. Am J Psychiatry 157:1379–1389, 2000a

Siris SG: Management of depression in schizophrenia. Psychiatr Ann 30:13–19, 2000b

Siris S, Morgan V, Fagerstrom R, et al: Adjunctive imipramine in the treatment of post-psychotic depression: a controlled trial. Arch Gen Psychiatry 44:533–539, 1987

Siris S, Cutler J, Owen K: Adjunctive imipramine maintenance in schizophrenic patients with remitted post-psychotic depressions. Am J Psychiatry 146:1495–1497, 1989a

Siris SG, Aronson A, Sellew AP: Imipramine-responsive panic-like symptomatology in schizophrenia/schizoaffective disorder. Biol Psychiatry 25:485–488, 1989b

Siris SG, Bermanzohn PC, Mason SE, et al: Adjunctive imipramine for dysphoric schizophrenic patients with past histories of cannabis abuse. Prog Neuropsychopharmacol Biol Psychiatry 16:539–547, 1992

Siris SG, Mason SE, Bermanzohn PC, et al: Adjunctive imipramine in substance-abusing dysphoric schizophrenic patients. Psychopharmacol Bull 29:127–133, 1993

Smelson D, Losonczy M, Davis CW, et al: Risperidone decreases craving and relapses in individuals with schizophrenia and cocaine dependence. Can J Psychiatry 47:671–675, 2002

Stratkowsky SM, Tohen M, Stoll AL, et al: Comorbidity in psychosis at first hospitalization. Am J Psychiatry 150:752–757, 1993

Strous RD, Patel JK, Zimmet SV, et al: Clozapine and paroxetine in the treatment of schizophrenia with obsessive-compulsive features. Am J Psychiatry 156:973–974, 1999

Tamminga CA, Buchanan RW, Gold J: The role of negative symptoms and cognitive dysfunction in schizophrenia outcome. Int Clin Psychopharmacol 13:S21–S26, 1998

Tibbo P, Swainson J, Chue P, et al: Prevalence and relationship to delusions and hallucinations of anxiety disorders in schizophrenia. Depress Anxiety 17:65–72, 2003

Tollefson GD, Sanger TM, Lu Y, et al: Depressive signs and symptoms in schizophrenia: a prospective blinded trial of olanzapine and haloperidol. Arch Gen Psychiatry 55:250–258, 1998

Tollefson GD, Andersen SW, Tran PV: The course of depressive symptoms in predicting relapse in schizophrenia: a double-blind, randomized comparison of olanzapine and risperidone. Biol Psychiatry 46:365–373, 1999

Tsuang MT, Fleming JA, Simpson JC: Suicide and schizophrenia, in The Harvard Medical School Guide to Suicide Assessment and Intervention. Edited by Jacobs DG. San Francisco, CA, Jossey-Bass, 1999, pp 287–299

Tsuang MT, Marder SR, Han A, et al: Olanzapine treatment for patients with schizophrenia and cocaine abuse. J Clin Psychiatry 63(12):1180–1181, 2002

Vlokh I, Mikhnyak S, Kachura O: Zoloft in management of depression in schizophrenia (abstract). Schizophr Res 41:209, 2000

Waehrens J, Gerlach J: Antidepressant drugs in anergic schizophrenia: a double-blind cross-over study with maprotiline and placebo. Acta Psychiatr Scand 61:438–444, 1980

Walker A, Lanaza L, Arellano F, et al: Mortality in current and former users of clozapine. Epidemiology 8:671–677, 1997

Warsi M, Sattar SP, Bhatia SC, et al: Aripiprazole reduces alcohol use. Can J Psychiatry 50:244, 2005

Weiner E, Ball MP, Summerfelt A, et al: Effects of sustained-release bupropion and supportive group therapy on cigarette consumption in patients with schizophrenia. Am J Psychiatry 158:635–637, 2001

Weiss R, Hufford M: Substance abuse and suicide, in The Harvard Medical School Guide to Suicide Assessment and Intervention. Edited by Jacobs DG. San Francisco, CA, Jossey-Bass, 1999, pp 300–310

Westermeyer JF, Harrow M, Marengo JT: Risk for suicide in schizophrenia and other psychotic and nonpsychotic disorders. J Nerv Ment Dis 179:259–266, 1991

Wilkins JN: Pharmacotherapy of schizophrenia patients with comorbid substance abuse. Schizophr Bull 23:215–228, 1997

Ziedonis D, Richardson T, Lee E, et al: Adjunctive desipramine in the treatment of cocaine abusing schizophrenics. Psychopharmacol Bull 28:309–314, 1992

Zimmet SV, Strous RD, Burgess ES, et al: Effects of clozapine on substance use in patients with schizophrenia and schizoaffective disorder: a retrospective survey. J Clin Psychopharmacol 20:94–98, 2000

Zisook S, McAdams LA, Kuck J, et al: Depressive symptoms in schizophrenia. Am J Psychiatry 156:1736–1743, 1999

MEDICAL COMORBIDITIES

ERICK MESSIAS, M.D., M.P.H., PH.D.

LISA DIXON, M.D., M.P.H.

Several studies have documented markedly increased mortality rates among persons with schizophrenia. The life expectancy of persons with schizophrenia is, on average, reduced by 9–10 years (Tsuang et al. 1980). Although suicide is responsible for a significant share of this increased mortality, most of the extra mortality is from natural causes (Brown et al. 2010). Such comorbidities influence the care of patients with schizophrenia by complicating treatment and affecting prognosis. In improving the health status and quality of life of persons with schizophrenia, it is imperative to enhance our understanding and management of comorbidity. In this chapter, we review the findings regarding the presence of medical conditions among patients with schizophrenia and discuss how these issues affect the treatment of schizophrenia.

MEDICAL ILLNESSES IN SCHIZOPHRENIA

Persons with schizophrenia are at higher risk for many medical illnesses, particularly diabetes, cardiovascular disease, infectious diseases (especially sexually transmitted diseases), liver disease, and respiratory conditions such as emphysema, chronic obstructive pulmonary disease, asthma, and chronic bronchitis (Carney et al. 2006; Dixon et al. 1999; Sokal et al. 2004). Contributors to this increased risk include higher rates of obesity (Allison et al. 1999), cigarette smoking (Dalack et al. 1998), and medication side effects (Jeste et al. 1996). Even in patients who do not yet have cardiovascular disease or diabetes, a high proportion will have abnormal lipid profiles (triglycerides and cholesterol), elevated fasting glucose levels, and truncal obesity consistent with a "metabolic syndrome" and indicating an elevated risk for cardiovascular disease and diabetes (Ryan and Thakore 2002).

Research indicates that patients with schizophrenia are less likely to receive preventive medical care and make fewer visits for chronic medical conditions (Folsom et al. 2002). One possible reason is that the social withdrawal associated with schizophrenia prevents self-care and treatment-seeking behavior for physical complaints (Goldman 1999). Also, patients with schizophrenia perceive more barriers to treatment of medical conditions (Dickerson et al. 2003), which may lead to lack of preventive services that could have affected the prevalence of certain conditions.

DIABETES MELLITUS AND CARDIOVASCULAR DISEASE

While type 2 diabetes is a highly prevalent chronic medical condition diagnosed in approximately 4.5% of the U.S. population (Centers for Disease Control and Prevention 2005), those with schizophrenia are more often affected, with an estimated prevalence of 16%–25% (Dixon et al. 2000; Mukherjee et al. 1996; Newcomer et al. 2002; Subramaniam et al. 2003). Factors that contribute to diabetes risk include use of antipsychotic medications that cause metabolic abnormalities associated with diabetes risk (e.g., elevated lipids, glucose, and truncal obesity) (Koro et al. 2002; Sernyak et al. 2002). Other risk factors for diabetes in persons with schizophrenia include sedentary lifestyle, obesity, poor diet, and high smoking rates. Furthermore, drug-naive patients have been shown to have more highly impaired fasting glucose tolerance, to be more insulin resistant, and to have higher levels of plasma glucose, insulin, and cortisol than do healthy comparison subjects (Fernandez-Egea et al. 2009; Ryan et al. 2003), suggesting that schizophrenia itself may be associated with a biological vulnerability to diabetes through some as yet unknown mechanism. Diabetes also may have additional consequences for persons with schizophrenia, as shown in its role as a risk factor for tardive dyskinesia (Mukherjee et al. 1989; Woerner et al. 1993).

Acute Complications

Severe hyperglycemia is associated with symptoms such as polyuria, poly-dipsia, weight loss, and blurred vision. The most important acute compli-cation of diabetes mellitus is diabetic ketoacidosis, defined as low serum pH (≤7.35), low serum bicarbonate (≤15), and an anion gap, concomitant with ketonemia (Henderson and Ettinger 2003). Diabetic ketoacidosis is a life-threatening situation and requires immediate action on the part of the clinician.

Chronic Complications

Long-term complications of diabetes include retinopathy (with potential loss of vision), nephropathy (leading to renal failure), peripheral neuropathy (increased risk of foot ulcers, amputation, and Charcot's joints), autonomic neuropathy (cardiovascular, gastrointestinal, and genitourinary dysfunc-tion), and greatly increased risk of atheroma affecting large vessels (increased risk of macrovascular complications of stroke, myocardial infarction, or periph-eral vascular disease).

Metabolic Syndrome

Problems with glucose metabolism are one component of the metabolic syn-drome, which encompasses three or more of the following (National Insti-tutes of Health 2001):

1. Abdominal obesity: waist circumference >102 cm in men and >88 cm in women
2. Elevated serum triglycerides: ≥150 mg/dL
3. Low high-density lipoprotein cholesterol: <40 mg/dL in men and <50 mg/dL in women
4. High blood pressure: ≥130/85 mm Hg
5. Impaired fasting glucose: ≥110 mg/dL

Clinicians treating schizophrenia should be aware of and screen for the metabolic syndrome because it appears to be more prevalent in persons with schizophrenia and has been associated with increased all-cause mortality rate, and coronary heart disease, in middle-aged men (Lakka et al. 2002).

Treatment Implications: Importance of Intensive Glucose Control

Intensive glucose control has been shown to reduce the rate of complications from diabetes (UK Prospective Diabetes Study Group 1998). A 10-year follow-up has shown that intensive glucose control in diabetes reduces risk for myocardial infarction and death from any cause (Holman et al. 2008). Much like schizophrenia treatment, diabetes care should be thought of in an integrative and multicomponent fashion. Diabetes treatment should have a multidimensional approach that may include education, counseling, monitoring, self-management, and pharmacological treatment with insulin or oral antidiabetic agents.

HIV AND AIDS

Concern has been growing about the rates at which HIV and other sexually transmitted diseases have spread among those with chronic and severe mental illness (McKinnon et al. 1997). Individuals with schizophrenia are at an increased risk for HIV infection compared with the general population. The current best estimates of HIV prevalence among individuals with a severe mental illness vary according to location, being highest in large urban centers (5%) versus nonmetropolitan areas (2%) (Rosenberg et al. 2001). A national sample of veterans found an HIV prevalence of 1% among veterans with serious mental illness as compared with 0.5% among those without. An interaction between schizophrenia diagnosis and substance abuse was also found, whereby those with schizophrenia and substance abuse had a higher HIV risk while those with schizophrenia without substance abuse had a decreased risk, when compared with those without serious mental illness or substance abuse (Himelhoch et al. 2007). This prevalence estimate is about eight times the overall estimated prevalence in the U.S. general population (Rosenberg et al. 2001). Women with schizophrenia are at particularly high risk for HIV infection—the male-to-female ratio is 4:3, in contrast with the 5:1 ratio reported in the general population (Rosenberg et al. 2001).

Contributing factors to this increased prevalence include injection drug use and unsafe sexual practices (Rosenberg et al. 2001). Data suggest that persons with severe mental illness are more likely to engage in high-risk sexual behavior and less likely to change their health behaviors (Davidson et al. 2001; McDermott et al. 1994). Persons with severe mental illness are able to participate in HIV treatment and, when receiving HAART therapy, are less likely to discontinue treatment (Himelhoch et al. 2009a).

VIRAL HEPATITIS

The seroprevalence of hepatitis B virus (HBV) and hepatitis C virus (HCV) among those with severe mental illness is much higher than in the general population. Current estimates are 23.4% for HBV and 19.6% for HCV; these rates are 5 and 11 times the prevalence rates in the general population for these infections, respectively (Rosenberg et al. 2001). A national sample of veterans found a 7.1% recorded prevalence of hepatitis C in veterans with schizophrenia, as compared with 2.5% among those without serious mental illness, with an increased risk in those with comorbid substance abuse (Himelhoch et al. 2009b). Contributing factors to the increased prevalence of these infections include unsafe sexual practices and comorbid substance abuse (Davidson et al. 2001).

Chronic Complications

Hepatocellular carcinoma is a long-term complication of hepatitis B and C (Kaplan and Reddy 2003). Hepatitis C infection also increases the risk of cirrhosis (Yoho et al. 2003). The simultaneous infection with hepatitis B and C, for which injection drug users are at increased risk, is associated with further increases in cirrhosis risk. Other complications of viral hepatitis include fulminant hepatitis (massive hepatic necrosis), spontaneous reactivations, and chronic hepatitis.

Clinicians must think of long-term monitoring of hepatitis viruses in persons with schizophrenia, particularly because this population is exposed to other hepatotoxic agents, such as alcohol and some antipsychotic medications. As an example, 1% of the patients taking chlorpromazine will develop intrahepatic cholestasis with jaundice 1–4 weeks into the treatment (Dienstag and Isselbacher 2005).

OTHER CONDITIONS ASSOCIATED WITH SCHIZOPHRENIA

Osteoporosis

Patients with schizophrenia are more likely to have osteoporosis than the general population (Halbreich and Palter 1996). Reasons for this decrease in bone mineral densities include increased level of smoking, antipsychotic-induced hyperprolactinemia that in turn may cause decreases in estrogen and testosterone, and hypercortisolemia (Halbreich and Palter 1996). Up to three-quarters of adults in the general population may be vitamin D deficient, with lack of sun exposure and smoking contributing risk factors (Audran and Briot 2010). In addition persons with schizophrenia may be more likely to have a sedentary lifestyle and so not engage in weight-bearing activity.

Respiratory Diseases

Persons with schizophrenia have a higher prevalence of respiratory diseases, such as asthma, emphysema, and chronic bronchitis, when compared with the general population (Sokal et al. 2004). Some studies have reported that individuals with schizophrenia have higher mortality rates from all respiratory diseases compared with the general population (Buda et al. 1988; Joukamaa et al. 2001). Part of this association is likely to come from the higher rates of cigarette smoking, which points to opportunities of preventive strategies in this population.

Polydipsia and Hyponatremia

Polydipsia is the intake of more than 3 L/day of fluid, and it may be primary or secondary to medical conditions or medication side effects (Brookes and Ahmed 2002). The estimated prevalence for psychiatric populations is between 5% and 20% (Brookes and Ahmed 2002; de Leon et al. 1994). Polydipsia may lead to serious metabolic imbalances, such as water intoxication (i.e., severe *hyponatremia*—serum sodium < 120 mmol/L), which is potentially fatal because the cerebral edema can result in delirium, seizures, coma, and death. Characteristics associated with the risk of polydipsia among psychiatric populations include chronicity, schizophrenia diagnosis, smoking, some medications, male gender, and white race (de Leon et al. 1994).

Before a diagnosis of psychosis-induced polydipsia is reached, other causes, such as diabetes mellitus, diabetes insipidus, chronic renal failure, malignancy, pulmonary disease, hypocalcemia, and hypokalemia, should be excluded.

Pharmacological interventions to treat polydipsia are few and of questionable efficacy (Brookes and Ahmed 2002), although there is some indication that clozapine may help (Verghese et al. 1996). Fluid restriction, along with sodium replacement, is the most recommended treatment (Verghese et al. 1996).

CONDITIONS NEGATIVELY ASSOCIATED WITH SCHIZOPHRENIA

Rheumatoid Arthritis

There have been several reports of a lower than expected prevalence rate of rheumatoid arthritis in patients with schizophrenia. A review of the epidemiological evidence supported this finding (Eaton et al. 1992). This association points to the hypothesis of there being an autoimmune component to schizophrenia. The proper identification of rheumatoid arthritis, a condition linked with autoimmune pneumonia, as opposed to the much more prevalent arthritic syndrome, more associated with degenerative joint disease, is one of the main limitations to studies on this relation. A recent community-based study failed to show an association between arthritis and schizophrenia (Sokal et al. 2004).

Cancer

There had been some initial indication that patients with schizophrenia might have a lower than expected cancer incidence (Allebeck 1989; Mortensen 1994), but larger epidemiological studies have failed to reach a definite conclusion regarding cancer risk in schizophrenia (Bushe et al. 2009; Dalton et al. 2005; Goldacre et al. 2005; Tran et al. 2009).

TREATMENT CONSIDERATIONS

MEDICAL COMORBIDITIES: REDUCING BARRIERS TO HEALTH CARE

As reviewed in this chapter, persons with schizophrenia are at higher risk for specific somatic diseases compared with the general population. Among these diseases are diabetes, cardiovascular disease, chronic respiratory disorders, and sexually transmitted diseases. These conditions share two features: they are potentially preventable, and they demand lifelong monitoring and treatment after they develop. Reducing barriers to health care to persons with schizophrenia is necessary to address both of these features. In this context, psychiatrists and the mental health team should strive to work in conjunction and coordination with their counterparts in medical care.

Besides reducing barriers to primary care, clinicians treating schizophrenia should remain alert because of the high presence of multiple risk factors in this population. For example, clinicians should consider regular (e.g., semiannual) monitoring of fasting glucose or hemoglobin A_{1C}, as well as triglycerides and HDL cholesterol, to detect emerging diabetes, especially in patients with obesity. Prevention of weight gain should be a high priority, because losing weight is difficult for many patients. Interventions that reduce or eliminate tobacco consumption are key to reducing risk of respiratory disorders. A summary of recommended monitoring and psychoeducational measures is presented in Table 7–1. Medical management can be integrated with community mental health, leading to improved quality and better primary care outcomes (Druss et al. 2010).

TABLE 7–1. Summary of recommended monitoring and psychoeducational measures for patients with schizophrenia

Issue	Recommendation
Weight gain	• Regular monitoring of weight and body mass index (BMI). • The relative risk of weight gain for the different antipsychotic medications should be a consideration in drug selection for patients who have a BMI>25. • Unless a patient is underweight (BMI<18.5), a weight gain of 1 BMI unit (about 5 lbs.) indicates a need for an intervention (e.g., diet and exercise counseling). • Consider providing or referring patients with BMI>27 for diet and activity level modification counseling. • Recent clinical trial data suggest that pharmacological interventions, such as metformin, may stabilize weight and prevent further weight gain in patients with antipsychotic-associated weight gain (Maayan et al. 2010).
Diabetes	• A baseline measure of glucose and/or hemoglobin A_{1C} should be obtained for all patients before starting a new antipsychotic. • Patients who have significant risk factors for diabetes should have fasting glucose or hemoglobin A_{1C} monitored 4 months after starting an antipsychotic and then yearly. • Be aware of the symptoms of new-onset diabetes (including weight change, polyuria, polydipsia), inform patients about the warning signs of diabetes, and monitor their presence at regular intervals.
HIV and viral hepatitis	• Ask about sexual practices and injection drug use. • Educate patients about safe sexual practices and needle use. • Inquire about and address drug use.
Hyperlipidemia	• Monitor, or collaborate with a primary healthcare provider who monitors, lipid profiles, especially triglycerides and HDL cholesterol. • As a group, individuals with schizophrenia should be considered to be at high risk for coronary heart disease. • Follow National Cholesterol Education Program guidelines (http://www.nhlbi.nih.gov/about/ncep/) or U.S. Preventive Services Task Force guidelines (http://www.ahcpr.gov/clinic/ajpmsuppl/lipidrr.htm) for screening and treating patients who are at high risk for cardiovascular disease.

TABLE 7–1. Summary of recommended monitoring and psychoeducational measures for patients with schizophrenia *(continued)*

Issue	Recommendation
Chronic lung disease	• Assess level of cigarette smoking, and ask patients who smoke if they are interested in smoking cessation interventions. • Inquire about respiratory symptoms.
Osteoporosis	• When prescribing antipsychotics that elevate prolactin (especially risperidone), inquire about menstrual cycle irregularities (that may occur if elevated prolactin levels have lowered estrogen levels). • Consider obtaining vitamin D [25(OH)D] level. (For patients with vitamin D deficiency, replacement with a prescription for 50,000 IU per week for 6 weeks is safe and usually effective. 50,000 IU once or twice a month usually will typically maintain adequate vitamin D levels.)
QT prolongation	• Clinicians should *not* prescribe thioridazine, mesoridazine, or pimozide for patients with known heart disease, a personal history of syncope, a family history of sudden death at an early age (younger than 40, especially if both parents had sudden death), or prolonged QTc syndrome. • If ziprasidone is prescribed for patients with the risk factors described in the previous recommendation, an electrocardiogram should be evaluated at baseline, and a subsequent electrocardiogram is indicated if a patient presents with symptoms (e.g., syncope).

Source. Adapted from Marder et al. 2004.

HIV AND HEPATITIS: RISK REDUCTION STRATEGIES

Elements shown to be effective in risk reduction programs for HIV and hepatitis include the following (Wainberg et al. 2003):

• Information and skills training in sexual assertiveness, negotiation, problem solving, use of condoms, and risk self-management
• Intensive sessions (6–15 hours) to achieve reduction in risk behavior
• Training of participants to become AIDS educators or advocates

- Booster or maintenance sessions
- Gender sensitivity training
- Inclusion of sexually abstinent patients in training programs as a way to validate this choice for other patients choosing to remain abstinent

CONCLUSION

Medical comorbidities play a substantial role in the lives of persons with schizophrenia, and a comprehensive approach to the care of persons with schizophrenia is needed. These comorbidities pose substantial challenges for the treatment system in the care of persons with a core disease that is itself socially and cognitively disabling. The care system and physicians must be mindful of the higher rate of medical problems among persons with schizophrenia. Although more research is necessary, such attention is likely to positively influence long-term outcomes for the schizophrenia population.

REFERENCES

Allebeck P: Schizophrenia: a life-shortening disease. Schizophr Bull 15:81–89, 1989

Allison DB, Fontaine KR, Heo M, et al: The distribution of body mass index among individuals with and without schizophrenia. J Clin Psychiatry 60:215–220, 1999

Audran M, Briot K: Critical reappraisal of vitamin D deficiency. Joint Bone Spine 77:115–119, 2010

Brookes G, Ahmed AG: Pharmacological treatments for psychosis-related polydipsia. Cochrane Database Syst Rev (3): CD003544, 2002

Brown S, Kim M, Mitchell C, et al: Twenty-five year mortality of a community cohort with schizophrenia. Br J Psychiatry 196:116–121, 2010

Buda M, Tsuang MT, Fleming JA: Causes of death in DSM-III schizophrenics and other psychotics (atypical group): a comparison with the general population. Arch Gen Psychiatry 45:283–285, 1988

Bushe CJ, Bradley AJ, Wildgust HJ, et al: Schizophrenia and breast cancer incidence: a systematic review of clinical studies. Schizophr Res 114:6–16, 2009

Carney CP, Jones L, Woolson RF: Medical comorbidity in women and men with schizophrenia: a population-based controlled study. J Gen Intern Med 21:1133–1137, 2006

Centers for Disease Control and Prevention: National Diabetes Fact Sheet. Atlanta, GA, National Center for Chronic Disease Prevention and Health Promotion, 2005. Available at: http://www.cdc.gov/diabetes/pubs/estimates.htm Accessed September 21, 2005.

Dalack GW, Healy DJ, Meador-Woodruff JH: Nicotine dependence in schizophrenia: clinical phenomena and laboratory findings. Am J Psychiatry 155:1490–1501, 1998

Dalton SO, Mellemkjaer L, Thomassen L, et al: Risk for cancer in a cohort of patients hospitalized for schizophrenia in Denmark, 1969–1993. Schizophr Res 75:315–324, 2005

Davidson S, Judd F, Jolley D, et al: Risk factors for HIV/AIDS and hepatitis C among the chronic mentally ill. Aust N Z J Psychiatry 35:203–209, 2001

de Leon J, Verghese C, Tracy JI, et al: Polydipsia and water intoxication in psychiatric patients: a review of the epidemiological literature. Biol Psychiatry 35:408–419, 1994

Dickerson FB, McNary SW, Brown CH, et al: Somatic healthcare utilization among adults with serious mental illness who are receiving community psychiatric services. Med Care 41:560–570, 2003

Dienstag J, Isselbacher K: Toxic and drug-induced hepatitis, in Harrison's Principles of Internal Medicine, 16th Edition. Edited by Kasper DL, Fauci AS, Longo DL, et al. New York, McGraw-Hill, 2005, pp 1838–1844

Dixon L, Postrado L, Delahanty J, et al: The association of medical comorbidity in schizophrenia with poor physical and mental health. J Nerv Ment Dis 187:496–502, 1999

Dixon L, Weiden P, Delahanty J, et al: Prevalence and correlates of diabetes in national schizophrenia samples. Schizophr Bull 26:903–912, 2000

Druss BG, von Esenwein SA, Compton MT, et al: A randomized trial of medical care management for community mental health settings: the Primary Care Access, Referral, and Evaluation (PCARE) study. Am J Psychiatry 167:151–159, 2010

Eaton WW, Hayward C, Ram R: Schizophrenia and rheumatoid arthritis: a review. Schizophr Res 6:181–192, 1992

Fernandez-Egea E, Bernardo M, Donner T, et al: Metabolic profile of antipsychotic-naive individuals with non-affective psychosis. Br J Psychiatry 194:434–438, 2009

Folsom DP, McCahill M, Bartels SJ, et al: Medical comorbidity and receipt of medical care by older homeless people with schizophrenia or depression. Psychiatr Serv 53:1456–1460, 2002

Goldacre MJ, Kurina LM, Wotton CJ, et al: Schizophrenia and cancer: an epidemiological study. Br J Psychiatry 187:334–338, 2005

Goldman LS: Medical illness in patients with schizophrenia. J Clin Psychiatry 60 (suppl 21):10–15, 1999

Halbreich U, Palter S: Accelerated osteoporosis in psychiatric patients: possible pathophysiological processes. Schizophr Bull 22:447–454, 1996

Henderson D, Ettinger E: Glucose intolerance and diabetes in schizophrenia, in Medical Illness and Schizophrenia. Edited by Meyer J, Nasrallah H. Washington, DC, American Psychiatric Publishing, 2003, pp 99–114

Himelhoch S, McCarthy JF, Ganoczy D, et al: Understanding associations between serious mental illness and HIV among patients in the VA Health System. Psychiatr Serv 58:1165–1172, 2007

Himelhoch S, Brown CH, Walkup J, et al: HIV patients with psychiatric disorders are less likely to discontinue HAART. AIDS 23:1735–1742, 2009a

Himelhoch S, McCarthy JF, Ganoczy D, et al: Understanding associations between serious mental illness and hepatitis C virus among veterans: a national multivariate analysis. Psychosomatics 50:30–37, 2009b

Holman RR, Paul SK, Bethel MA, et al: 10-year follow-up of intensive glucose control in type 2 diabetes. N Engl J Med 359:1577–1589, 2008

Jeste DV, Gladsjo JA, Lindamer LA, et al: Medical comorbidity in schizophrenia. Schizophr Bull 22:413–430, 1996

Joukamaa M, Heliovaara M, Knekt P, et al: Mental disorders and cause-specific mortality. Br J Psychiatry 179:498–502, 2001

Kaplan DE, Reddy KR: Rising incidence of hepatocellular carcinoma: the role of hepatitis B and C: the impact on transplantation and outcomes. Clin Liver Dis 7:683–714, 2003

Koro CE, Fedder DO, L'Italien GJ, et al: Assessment of independent effect of olanzapine and risperidone on risk of diabetes among patients with schizophrenia: population based nested case-control study. BMJ 325(7358):243, 2002

Lakka H, Laaksonen D, Lakka T, et al: The metabolic syndrome and total and cardiovascular disease mortality in middle-aged men. JAMA 288:2709–2716, 2002

Maayan L, Vakhrusheva J, Correll CU: Effectiveness of medications used to attenuate antipsychotic-relted weight gain and metabolic abnormalities: a system review and meta-analysis. Neuropsychopharmacology 35:1520–1530, 2010

Marder SR, Essock SM, Miller AL, et al: Physical health monitoring of patients with schizophrenia. Am J Psychiatry 161:1334–1349, 2004

McDermott BE, Sautter FJ Jr, Winstead DK, et al: Diagnosis, health beliefs, and risk of HIV infection in psychiatric patients. Hosp Community Psychiatry 45:580–585, 1994

McKinnon K, Carey MP, Cournos F: Research on HIV, AIDS, and severe mental illness: recommendations from the NIMH National Conference. Clin Psychol Rev 17:327–331, 1997

Mortensen PB: The occurrence of cancer in first admitted schizophrenic patients. Schizophr Res 12:185–194, 1994

Mukherjee S, Roth SD, Sandyk R, et al: Persistent tardive dyskinesia and neuroleptic effects on glucose tolerance. Psychiatry Res 29:17–27, 1989

Mukherjee S, Decina P, Bocola V, et al: Diabetes mellitus in schizophrenic patients. Compr Psychiatry 37:68–73, 1996

National Institutes of Health: Third Report of the National Cholesterol Education Program Expert Panel on Detection, Evaluation and Treatment of High Blood Cholesterol in Adults (Adult Treatment Panel III). Bethesda, MD, National Institutes of Health, 2001

Newcomer JW, Haupt DW, Fucetola R, et al: Abnormalities in glucose regulation during antipsychotic treatment of schizophrenia. Arch Gen Psychiatry 59:337–345, 2002

Rosenberg SD, Goodman LA, Osher FC, et al: Prevalence of HIV, hepatitis B, and hepatitis C in people with severe mental illness. Am J Public Health 91:31–37, 2001

Ryan MC, Thakore JH: Physical consequences of schizophrenia and its treatment: the metabolic syndrome. Life Sci 71:239–257, 2002

Ryan MC, Collins P, Thakore JH: Impaired fasting glucose tolerance in first-episode, drug-naive patients with schizophrenia. Am J Psychiatry 160:284–289, 2003

Sernyak MJ, Leslie DL, Alarcon RD, et al: Association of diabetes mellitus with use of atypical neuroleptics in the treatment of schizophrenia. Am J Psychiatry 159:561–566, 2002

Sokal J, Messias E, Dickerson FB, et al: Comorbidity of medical illnesses among adults with serious mental illness who are receiving community psychiatric services. J Nerv Ment Dis 192:421–427, 2004

Subramaniam M, Chong SA, Pek E: Diabetes mellitus and impaired glucose tolerance in patients with schizophrenia. Can J Psychiatry 48:345–347, 2003

Tran E, Rouillon F, Loze JY, et al: Cancer mortality in patients with schizophrenia: an 11-year prospective cohort study. Cancer 115:3555–3562, 2009

Tsuang MT, Woolson RF, Fleming JA: Premature deaths in schizophrenia and affective disorders: an analysis of survival curves and variables affecting the shortened survival. Arch Gen Psychiatry 37:979–983, 1980

UK Prospective Diabetes Study Group: Intensive blood-glucose control with sulphonylureas or insulin compared with conventional treatment and risk of complications in patients with type 2 diabetes. Lancet 352:837–853, 1998

Verghese C, de Leon J, Josiassen RC: Problems and progress in the diagnosis and treatment of polydipsia and hyponatremia. Schizophr Bull 22:455–464, 1996

Wainberg M, Cournos F, McKinnon K, et al: HIV and hepatitis C in patients with schizophrenia, in Medical Illness and Schizophrenia. Edited by Meyer J, Nasrallah H. Washington, DC, American Psychiatric Publishing, 2003, pp 115–140

Woerner MG, Saltz BL, Kane JM, et al: Diabetes and development of tardive dyskinesia. Am J Psychiatry 150:966–968, 1993

Yoho RA, Cruz LL, Mazaheri R, et al: Hepatitis C: a review. Plast Reconstr Surg 112:597–605, 2003

PHARMACOTHERAPIES

T. SCOTT STROUP, M.D., M.P.H.

STEPHEN R. MARDER, M.D.

JEFFREY A. LIEBERMAN, M.D.

Pharmacological treatments are an essential component of a comprehensive approach to the treatment of schizophrenia. Rational pharmacotherapies can contribute greatly to symptom relief and to a broader psychosocial recovery for affected individuals. However, antipsychotic drugs do not cure schizophrenia. Moreover, if not used judiciously, drug therapies can create significant financial, side-effect, and medical morbidity burdens that may hinder progress toward personal and treatment goals. Importantly, evidence-based plans of care should be individualized and should integrate both appropriate pharmacotherapies and psychosocial interventions (Buchanan et al. 2010b; Dixon et al. 2010).

In this chapter, we discuss drugs commonly used in the treatment of schizophrenia. The goal of pharmacological treatment of schizophrenia is to minimize symptoms and functional impairments to allow individuals to pursue personal goals as best as possible. Antipsychotic drugs are commonly and effectively used to treat positive symptoms, such as hallucinations, delusions, and disorganized speech and behavior. Antipsychotics are only partially effective for treating negative symptoms, including anhedonia, avolition, alogia, affective flattening, and social withdrawal. Antipsychotic drugs are also used to treat behavioral disturbances such as aggression and hostility and to reduce anxiety and suicidal behaviors. Anxiolytics, antidepressants, and mood-stabilizing drugs are often used as adjunctive treatments for mood symptoms. Because cognitive impairments are common in schizophrenia and are related to functional outcomes, cognitive functioning is now an important focus of research and a possible target of pharmacotherapies; however, there are neither U.S. Food and Drug Administration (FDA)–approved nor commonly used drugs available for this purpose in schizophrenia.

ANTIPSYCHOTIC DRUGS

Modern drug treatment for schizophrenia dates to the early 1950s, when Deniker and Delay reported the antipsychotic effects of chlorpromazine (Healy 2002). Chlorpromazine was introduced in the United States in 1954, followed over the next three decades by several drugs, including fluphenazine, haloperidol, perphenazine, and thioridazine, with similar therapeutic effects. These and all subsequently developed antipsychotics block postsynaptic dopamine receptors in the brain, with the dopamine blockade in frontal cortical and limbic regions thought to account for the antipsychotic effect. Antipsychotics also interact with other neurotransmitter systems that cause side effects and may affect their therapeutic effects.

Antipsychotic medicines ameliorate psychotic symptoms such as hallucinations, delusions, and disorganized speech or behavior. The drugs reduce the intensity of the symptoms, shorten exacerbations of illness, and reduce the risk of relapse. An early landmark study led by the U.S. National Institute of Mental Health (NIMH) found that approximately 60% of the subjects who received antipsychotic drugs, as compared with 20% of placebo-treated subjects, had a nearly complete resolution of acute positive symptoms during a 6-week trial (Guttmacher 1964). Only 8% of the medication-treated subjects showed no improvement or worsening, whereas almost half of the placebo-treated subjects did not improve or their symptoms worsened. Positive and negative symptoms improved with antipsychotic treatment, but positive symptoms responded to a greater degree and more consistently than did negative symptoms. The antipsychotics studied (fluphenazine, perphenazine, and thioridazine) did not appear to differ in efficacy. Subsequent research showed that patients with schizophrenia who achieve remission and then consistently take antipsychotic drugs are about three times less likely to relapse than patients who do not take the medicines consistently (Hogarty et al. 1976).

From early in the history of modern antipsychotic use, adverse effects were important considerations. Rigidity, bradykinesia, and tremor resembling Parkinson's disease were particularly prominent, along with a sometimes severe restlessness known as akathisia, and persistent, involuntary choreoathetoid movements called *tardive dyskinesia* (TD). These adverse effects, together known as *extrapyramidal side effects* (EPS), were an extremely significant problem in the early decades of antipsychotic use, and tardive dyskinesia was the source of several prominent lawsuits (Healy 2002).

In the late 1980s clozapine, a drug first tested in the late 1950s, was shown to have greater efficacy than chlorpromazine in patients with refractory symptoms. In the critical study of clozapine in patients with treatment-resistant symptoms, 30% of clozapine-treated patients met response criteria compared with only 4% of chlorpromazine-treated patients (Kane et al. 1988). Clozapine was remarkable not only for its superior efficacy for patients with refractory symptoms, but also for its very low risk of EPS and TD. However, clozapine had a significant risk of agranulocytosis and other life-threatening side effects that greatly limited its use.

Clozapine's unique clinical benefits and pharmacological profile led to the development of many drugs with pharmacological similarities. In particular, clozapine has prominent effects on neurotransmitter receptors other than dopamine and a different side-effect profile from that of the chlorpromazine-like drugs. The goal of drug developers was to achieve clozapine's efficacy advantages and very low risk of EPS and TD without the risk of agranulocytosis. The very low risks of EPS and of TD were key to its influence on antipsychotic development in the wake of lawsuits over liability for TD (Healy 2002).

The older (first-generation) antipsychotic drugs introduced before clozapine all block dopamine receptors and have side effects that tend to vary according to drug potency. High-potency drugs have a stronger affinity for dopamine receptors than low-potency drugs; lower dosages of the high-potency drugs achieve the same antipsychotic effect as higher dosages of low-potency drugs. The (second-generation) antipsychotics also block postsynaptic dopamine receptors. Antagonism of central serotonin receptors and perhaps relatively loose binding to dopamine$_2$ (D$_2$) receptors are common features in their actions. The different effects of antipsychotics on dopamine receptors and on other neurotransmitter systems determine their pharmacological actions and side effects.

Although the drugs introduced after clozapine, including risperidone, olanzapine, quetiapine, ziprasidone, aripiprazole, paliperidone, asenapine, and iloperidone, are often known as atypical or second-generation antipsychotics, they are heterogeneous in many ways (Leucht et al. 2009a, 2009b). In general, these drugs cause fewer extrapyramidal side effects than the drugs that came before clozapine, but there is considerable variation of this risk within both groups. Similarly, there is variation within the older and newer groups, and overlap between them in the propensity to cause sedation, anticholinergic effects, weight gain, and dyslipidemias. Therefore, when possible, we avoid the terms *first-* and *second-generation*, and *typical* and *atypical*, and *conventional* and *novel* when referring to antipsychotic medications. This decision is based on recent research that has brought into question the validity and helpfulness of the distinction, as well as considerable evidence of heterogeneity within both of the groupings (Leucht et al. 2009a).

Below we describe the key clinical features of several antipsychotics that are of interest because they are in common use, represent a group of antipsychotics, or have been recently introduced.

LOW-POTENCY ANTIPSYCHOTICS

Low-potency drugs (e.g., chlorpromazine and thioridazine) have a relatively low risk of EPS, high risk of sedation, and high risk of anticholinergic (e.g., dry mouth, constipation, blurred vision) and antiadrenergic (e.g., orthostatic hypotension) side effects. Chlorpromazine, the first antipsychotic approved for use, has been available since 1954. It is effective in treating schizophrenic psychopathology but is associated with substantial weight gain, sedation, orthostatic hypotension, anticholinergic side effects, and modest EPS when used at currently recommended doses. Because of its effect in prolonging cardiac repolarization (i.e., the QT interval of the electrocardiogram), thioridazine should be reserved for patients who cannot be treated with other antipsychotics. The use of doses above those recommended in Table 8–1 is not associated with better outcomes but has an increased risk of adverse effects, including TD.

MEDIUM-POTENCY ANTIPSYCHOTICS

Medium-potency drugs (e.g., loxapine, molindone, perphenazine, thiothixene) tend to have a moderate risk of common side effects. For example, perphenazine, which has been available since 1958, is effective in treating schizophrenic psychopathology but is associated with moderate hypotension and EPS when used at currently recommended doses. A large clinical trial initiated by the National Institute of Mental Health, known as the Clinical Antipsychotic Trials of Intervention Effectiveness (CATIE) study, brought increased attention to perphenazine because it worked well and caused only moderate EPS and little or no weight gain (Lieberman et al. 2005). The use of doses above those recommended in Table 8–1 are not associated with better outcomes but have an increased risk of adverse effects, including TD.

TABLE 8–1. Selected information on commonly used oral antipsychotic medications

Antipsychotic	Recommended dosage range (mg/day)	Half-life (hours)	Weight/Metabolic side effects	EPS/TD	Prolactin elevation	Sedation	Anticholinergic side effects	Hypotension
Aripiprazole	10–30	75	−	+	−	+	−	−
Asenapine	10–20	24	+	+	++	++	−	+
Chlorpromazine	300–1,000	6	+++	+	++	+++	+++	+++
Clozapine	150–600	12	+++	−	−	+++	+++	+++
Fluphenazine	5–20	33	+	+++	+++	+	−	−
Haloperidol	5–20	21	+	+++	+++	++	−	−
Iloperidone	12–24	14	++	+	+	+	+	+++
Loxapine	30–100	4	++	++	++	++	+	+
Molindone	30–100	24	−	++	++	++	+	−
Olanzapine	10–30	33	+++	+	+	++	++	−
Paliperidone	6–12	23	++	++	+++	+	−	+
Perphenazine	12–48	10	++	++	++	++	−	−
Quetiapine	300–750	6	++	−	−	++	+	++
Risperidone	2–8	20	++	++	+++	+	−	++
Thioridazine	300–800	24	+++	+	++	+++	+++	+++
Thiothixene	15–50	34	++	+++	++	+	−	−
Trifluoperazine	15–50	24	++	+++	++	+	−	+
Ziprasidone	120–160	7	−	+	+	+	−	+

Note. −=minimal risk; +=low risk; ++=moderate risk; +++=high risk. EPS/TD=extrapyramidal side effects and tardive dyskinesia.

HIGH-POTENCY ANTIPSYCHOTICS

High-potency drugs (e.g., haloperidol and fluphenazine) have a high risk of EPS, moderate risk of sedation, and low risk of anticholinergic and antiadrenergic effects. Haloperidol, available since 1967 and widely used, is effective in reducing schizophrenic psychopathology and in reducing acutely agitated behaviors. It is associated with a high risk of EPS but with little risk of sedation, orthostatic hypotension, weight gain, or anticholinergic side effects. Haloperidol's short-acting injections are commonly used in emergency situations when rapid effects are needed, whereas a long-acting haloperidol formulation that allows monthly injections is used when patients have trouble regularly taking oral antipsychotic medications. High-potency antipsychotics pose an especially high risk of TD that is dose related; therefore it is important to limit the dosage of these medications to the lowest dose that is effective in controlling symptoms well (Buchanan et al. 2010b)

CLOZAPINE

Clozapine was approved for use in the United States in 1990, despite a significant risk of the potentially lethal side effect agranulocytosis, because of its unique efficacy in patients with symptoms that were resistant to treatment. The key study in its approval by the FDA found that among patients with rigorously defined treatment resistance, 30% of the clozapine-treated group but only 4% of the chlorpromazine-treated group met a priori response criteria after 6 weeks of double-blind treatment. (Treatment resistance was defined as failure to respond to at least three prior antipsychotics, with no period of good functioning in the past 5 years, then having no response to haloperidol in a 6-week lead-in trial.)

A meta-analysis of randomized, double-blind trials comparing clozapine with an antipsychotic drug (usually haloperidol or chlorpromazine) in patients with treatment-refractory schizophrenia showed an advantage for clozapine with regard to total psychopathology, categorical response to treatment, extrapyramidal symptoms, TD, and study completion rates (Chakos et al. 2001). The CATIE study provided additional evidence to support use of clozapine in patients with persistent symptoms (McEvoy et al. 2006). Furthermore, clozapine has been found to be effective in reducing suicidal behaviors in patients with schizophrenia or schizoaffective disorder at high risk for suicide (Meltzer et al. 2003) and in reducing hostility and aggression among patients with treatment-resistant symptoms (Chengappa et al. 2002; Citrome et al. 2001). Additional meta-analyses of the effectiveness of antipsychotics have found that clozapine has the largest effect in reducing symptoms of schizophrenia (Leucht 2009a, 2009c).

Unfortunately, 0.5%–1% of patients develop clozapine-induced agranulo-cytosis (Alvir et al. 1993), and this risk has limited clozapine's use. In addition to agranulocytosis, seizures occur in up to 2% of patients, and a small but increased risk of myocarditis, cardiomyopathy, and pancreatitis is seen. Common side effects of clozapine include sedation, hypotension, hypersalivation, and tachycardia. Furthermore, clozapine is associated with substantial weight gain and a higher risk of glucose and lipid abnormalities compared with most other antipsychotic drugs (American Diabetes Association et al. 2004). Nevertheless, because of its efficacy in reducing refractory positive symptoms, with virtually no acute EPS or TD, clozapine represents a unique and important treatment option for severely ill patients for whom adequate medical supervision is available. Furthermore, the success of clozapine provided the impetus for the development of other antipsychotic drugs and hope for better outcomes.

RISPERIDONE

Risperidone was approved for use in the United States in 1994. Meta-analyses have shown risperidone to be slightly more efficacious than some (e.g., halo-peridol, quetiapine, ziprasidone) but not all (e.g., clozapine, olanzapine) antipsychotics (Leucht 2009a, 2009c). At typical dosages (2–6 mg/day), risperi-done has a low risk of EPS, but this risk increases at higher doses. Risperidone frequently causes high elevations in serum prolactin, especially in women and children, and sometimes causes weight gain, glucose abnormalities, and lipid abnormalities. Risperidone occasionally causes orthostatic hypotension. A long-acting, injectable microsphere formulation of risperidone is available to help enhance treatment adherence.

OLANZAPINE

The FDA approved olanzapine in 1996 for the treatment of schizophrenia. In acute treatment studies, olanzapine was effective in reducing positive and negative symptoms. Meta-analyses have shown olanzapine to be slightly to modestly more efficacious than other antipsychotics with the exception of ris-peridone and clozapine (Leucht 2009a, 2009c).

Olanzapine frequently causes sedation and weight gain at therapeutic doses and is thought to cause more glucose and lipid abnormalities than do first-generation antipsychotics and other second-generation antipsychotics except clozapine (American Diabetes Association et al. 2004). Olanzapine does not increase prolactin levels. Olanzapine has a low risk of causing EPS. The association of olanzapine with weight gain and adverse metabolic effects is so significant that the evidence-based Schizophrenia Patient Outcomes Research Team (PORT) treatment recommendations excluded olanzapine as a first-line choice for individuals experiencing a first episode of psychosis (Buchanan et al. 2010b).

Olanzapine is also available as an extended-release intramuscular suspension (olanzapine pamoate) that can be administered every 2 or 4 weeks. Patients receiving this formulation are at risk for a post-injection delirium/sedation syndrome. As a result, olanzapine pamoate is only available through a restricted distribution program, and patients must be observed in a registered healthcare facility for at least 3 hours after each injection.

QUETIAPINE

Quetiapine was approved for the treatment of schizophrenia in the United States in 1998. Two meta-analyses showed quetiapine to have efficacy similar to that of haloperidol in treating symptoms of schizophrenia (Davis et al. 2003; Leucht et al. 1999), but its efficacy is slightly less than that of olanzapine and risperidone (Leucht 2009a). Because of a half-life of only 6 hours, doses of quetiapine should be given two or three times daily, although a small study suggested that once-daily dosing may be feasible (Chengappa et al. 2003). A once-daily, sustained-release oral preparation was introduced in 2007. At recommended dosages, quetiapine causes no elevation in prolactin levels and little or no EPS. It often causes sedation and sometimes causes hypotension, weight gain, and lipid and glucose abnormalities. Because of its sedative properties, quetiapine is sometimes selected for patients with prominent insomnia.

ZIPRASIDONE

The FDA approved ziprasidone in 2001 for the treatment of schizophrenia. With a half-life of 7 hours, it is recommended as a twice-daily drug. Ziprasidone causes little or no weight gain, a feature that distinguishes it from most other antipsychotics. It very rarely causes sedation. Ziprasidone rarely causes EPS (except possibly akathisia). It is rarely associated with glucose or lipid abnormalities but sometimes causes prolactin elevations. Because of substantial food effects on drug absorption, ziprasidone should be taken with meals.

Approval of ziprasidone was delayed by the FDA in 1998 because of clinical trial data that showed that it delayed cardiac repolarization, as measured by the QT interval on electrocardiograms (ECGs). Because QT prolongation is associated with torsades de pointes, a potentially fatal ventricular arrhythmia, additional safety data were required. Ziprasidone was approved when it was shown that 4,000 patients had been treated in clinical trials with ziprasidone without evidence of torsades de pointes or sudden death. The FDA issued a warning about QT prolongation and instructed prescribers to avoid coadministration with other QT-prolonging drugs and to avoid prescribing ziprasidone to other patients with histories of or at significant risk for cardiac arrhythmias. The FDA did not, however, require pretreatment ECGs. A large simple trial designed to evaluate the impact of ziprasidone's QT-prolonging effect on cardiovascular events found no differences among patients treated with ziprasidone and those treated with olanzapine in nonsuicide mortality over one year (Strom et al. 2008). Clinical use over several years now indicates that ziprasidone can be safely used with current labeling related to QT prolongation.

ARIPIPRAZOLE

Aripiprazole was approved by the FDA for treatment of schizophrenia in 2002. Unlike other approved antipsychotics, aripiprazole has partial agonist activity at dopamine D_2 receptors. This has the theoretical advantage of agonist activity when dopamine levels are relatively low and antagonist activity when dopamine levels are high (Lieberman 2004). Meta-analyses have found aripiprazole to have efficacy similar to that of most antipsychotics but slightly lower than that of olanzapine (Leucht et al. 2009a, 2009c).

Of the common antipsychotic side effects, aripiprazole is associated with only occasional or mild sedation. It is very rarely associated with weight gain, glucose or lipid abnormalities, or hypotension. Aripiprazole sometimes causes an akathisia-like syndrome, but it rarely causes other forms of EPS. Headache, insomnia, and nausea early in treatment are relatively more common for aripiprazole than for other antipsychotics.

PALIPERIDONE

Paliperidone (9-hydroxy-risperidone) is an active metabolite of risperidone that is available in a once-daily oral preparation and a monthly injectable preparation. The oral version was approved by the FDA in 2007, and the long-acting injectable formulation was approved in 2009. Its pharmacologic profile is similar to that of risperidone, but paliperidone appears to cause somewhat more prolactin elevation at typical doses. It is not extensively metabolized in the liver and thus may be suitable for individuals with hepatic impairment. The long-acting injectable formulation is given every 4 weeks following two initial injections 1 week apart, without a need for supplementation by an oral antipsychotic medication.

ILOPERIDONE

Iloperidone was approved by the FDA for the treatment of schizophrenia in 2009 after an extended drug development process. The results of clinical trials conducted to achieve approval suggest that iloperidone has low risk of EPS and prolactin elevation but significant risk of orthostatic hypotension. Because of the risk of orthostatic hypotension during the initial treatment period, a slow titration schedule is recommended that achieves the recommended target dose after 1 week. Iloperidone is associated with QT prolongation similar in magnitude to that of ziprasidone and should not be prescribed to patients also taking other QT-prolonging drugs and/or those at significant risk for cardiac arrhythmias or with electrolyte disturbances.

ASENAPINE

Asenapine was approved by the FDA for the treatment of schizophrenia in 2009. Because bioavailability is extremely low if asenapine is swallowed, asenapine is provided as sublingual dissolvable tablets. The recommended starting dose (5 mg twice daily) is the same as the target dose for treating schizophrenia. In clinical trials, asenapine was associated with weight gain, EPS (particularly akathisia), oral hypoesthesia, and dizziness (presumed to be orthostatic hypotension).

TABLE 8–2.   Selected medications for treating extrapyramidal side effects (EPS)

Generic name	Dosage (mg/day)	Elimination half-life (hours)	Targeted EPS
Benztropine mesylate[a]	0.5–6.0	24	Akathisia, dystonia, parkinsonism
Trihexyphenidyl hydrochloride	1–15	4	Akathisia, dystonia, parkinsonism
Amantadine	100–300	10–14	Akathisia, parkinsonism
Propranolol	30–90	3–4	Akathisia
Lorazepam[a]	1–6	12	Akathisia
Clonazepam	1–3	20–50	Akathisia
Diphenhydramine[a]	25–50	4–8	Akathisia, dystonia, parkinsonism

[a]Available in oral and parenteral forms.
Source.   Adapted from Lehman et al. 2004b.

COMMON SIDE EFFECTS: MONITORING AND MANAGEMENT RECOMMENDATIONS

Extrapyramidal Side Effects

Antipsychotic-induced EPS may occur acutely or after long-term treatment. High-potency antipsychotics (e.g., haloperidol, fluphenazine) are more likely than other antipsychotics to cause EPS when the drugs are used at usual therapeutic doses. However, as noted in Table 8–1, considerable variation in the incidence of EPS is seen. Common acute EPS include akathisia, parkinsonism, and dystonia. Importantly, each of these side effects often responds to medication treatment (Table 8–2). Each type of acute EPS has a characteristic time of onset. Akathisia typically occurs a few hours to days after medication administration, dystonia within the first few days, and parkinsonism within a few days to weeks after starting a new drug or after a dosage increase (Casey 1993).

Akathisia. Akathisia, a subjective feeling of restlessness accompanied by restless movements, usually in the legs or feet, is the most common form of EPS. Severe akathisia can be diagnosed when frequent pacing, restless foot movements, or an inability of patients to sit still is present. This condition must be differentiated from *psychotic agitation*, which is often a response to disturbing hallucinations or delusions, but also may represent hostility related to acute psychosis or increased motor activity associated with excited catatonia. Patients who experience milder akathisia may not have any evidence of increased motor activity but may experience an unpleasant sensation of restlessness subjectively similar to anxiety.

Patients should be closely monitored for akathisia when starting a new antipsychotic drug or when the dosage is increased. Severe, unrelenting akathisia has been associated with an increased risk of suicidal behaviors. If symptoms of schizophrenia are adequately treated, lowering the antipsychotic dose is a feasible first approach to reduce akathisia. Another common approach is to change to an antipsychotic less likely to cause akathisia. Drug treatments for akathisia include β-blockers, anticholinergic agents, or benzodiazepines (Table 8–2). Evidence from controlled trials is inadequate to compare the efficacy of the various treatments for akathisia.

Drug-induced parkinsonism (pseudoparkinsonism). Drug-induced parkinsonism (pseudoparkinsonism) may include the classic Parkinson's disease symptoms of tremor, muscular rigidity, and a decrease in spontaneous movements (bradykinesia), as well as cognitive slowing and apathy. Milder forms of parkinsonism may include decreased expressive gestures, decreased facial expressiveness, or diminished arm swing. Recognition and management of parkinsonism is important because parkinsonism is frequently associated with poor adherence to antipsychotic medication regimens (Perkins 2002; Robinson et al. 2002). The initial approach to parkinsonian side effects is to lower the dose of antipsychotic if feasible. Common drug treatments for parkinsonism include anticholinergic medications, such as benztropine or trihexyphenidyl (Table 8–2). Another common approach is to change to an antipsychotic less likely to cause parkinsonism.

Dystonias. Dystonias are intermittent or sustained muscular spasms and abnormal postures affecting mainly the musculature of the head and neck but sometimes the trunk and lower extremities. Common forms of dystonia include abnormal positioning of the neck (torticollis), impaired swallowing (dysphagia), hypertonic or enlarged tongue, and deviations of the eyes (oculogyric crisis). These reactions usually appear within the first few days of treatment with antipsychotic drugs and sometimes occur within minutes to hours. These reactions can be painful and dramatic. They occur most commonly with high-potency antipsychotics, particularly when these medications are given in substantial doses (e.g., haloperidol 5–10 mg) to drug-naïve patients. For this reason, prophylactic treatment with benztropine 1–2 mg is recommended if starting high-potency antipsychotics at these substantial doses, which may be required in emergency situations. The antihistamine antiemetic promethazine provided at a dose of 50 mg intramuscularly has also been shown to prevent acute dystonic reactions when given with intramuscular haloperidol, although use of promethazine in this way is not common practice in the United States (Huf et al. 2007; Raveendran et al. 2007). Acute dystonic reactions are treated with diphenhydramine 25–50 mg or benztropine 1–2 mg. Usually these treatments are given intramuscularly to provide rapid relief for the considerable discomfort of dystonias.

Neuroleptic malignant syndrome. Neuroleptic malignant syndrome (NMS), another neurological side effect, is characterized by rigidity, hyperthermia, mental status changes, and autonomic instability. NMS has a lifetime incidence of approximately 0.2% among antipsychotic users (Caroff 2003). Hyperthermia and severe muscle rigidity may lead to rhabdomyolysis and renal failure. Serum levels of creatine kinase may rise dramatically. Risk factors for NMS include rapid dose escalation of high-potency antipsychotics, parenteral administration, and underlying neurological impairment. NMS is thought to be less common with drugs that have decreased risk of EPS, but the incidence with older-generation antipsychotics may be decreasing because lower doses than in the past are now commonly used.

NMS may be fatal if untreated. Treatment includes discontinuation of the antipsychotic and supportive care. Temperature reduction by cooling blankets if necessary and correction of fluid imbalances are crucial. The dopamine agonist bromocriptine (2.5 mg every 8 hours) has been shown to reduce NMS duration and mortality. The muscle relaxant dantrolene (1–2.5 mg/kg intravenously every 6 hours) is also commonly used, although there is no strong evidence of its effectiveness. Electroconvulsive therapy is indicated if catatonia related to NMS persists or response is otherwise inadequate with drugs and supportive care. If NMS occurs, need for an antipsychotic medication should be carefully assessed before antipsychotic treatment is resumed. When another trial of an antipsychotic drug is attempted, drugs with low risk of EPS (in particular, clozapine) are preferred. A rechallenge should begin with low doses and slow titration.

Tardive dyskinesia and other tardive syndromes.   Tardive dyskinesia and other tardive (late-onset) syndromes are involuntary, repetitive, purposeless, hyperkinetic, abnormal movements of the mouth, face and tongue, trunk, and extremities that occur during or following the cessation of long-term antipsychotic drug therapy. According to DSM-IV-TR (American Psychiatric Association 2000) diagnostic criteria, the abnormal movements should be present for at least 4 weeks, and patients should have been exposed to an antipsychotic for at least 3 months. The onset of the abnormal movements should occur either while the patient is receiving an antipsychotic or within 4 weeks of discontinuing an oral or 8 weeks after the withdrawal of a long-acting injectable antipsychotic. Oral-facial movements occur in about three-fourths of TD patients and can include lip smacking, sucking, puckering, and grimacing. Other movements include irregular movements of the limbs, particularly choreoathetoid-like movements of the fingers and toes and slow, writhing movements of the trunk. When severe, TD is disfiguring. In addition to TD, tardive dystonias and tardive akathisia have been described.

The incidence of tardive dyskinesia was estimated to be 4%–5% per year in non-elderly adults with older antipsychotics, with these estimates based on data collected when these medications were used at relatively high doses and before drugs were developed with lower risk of EPS (Glazer et al. 1993; Kane et al. 1985; Morgenstern and Glazer 1993). The risk of TD may be five to six times higher in the elderly (Jeste et al. 1999). A systematic review of 1-year studies that grouped amisulpride, olanzapine, quetiapine, risperidone, and ziprasidone as second-generation antipsychotics, found a lower risk of TD in patients taking these antipsychotics (annual risk=2.1%) than in patients taking the high-potency antipsychotic haloperidol at relatively high doses (annual risk=5.2%) (Correll et al. 2004). This review did not include clozapine, but clozapine-induced TD is thought to be extremely rare. Nor did the review include low- or medium-potency antipsychotics, which cause fewer acute EPS than haloperidol and may thus have a lower risk of TD. Risk factors for TD include increased age, female gender, higher dosages of antipsychotics, presence of parkinsonism, and longer periods of treatment.

Treatment of TD has largely been unsuccessful, although symptoms may diminish over time. The antioxidant vitamin E may be useful in less chronic cases, but any benefit seems to be restricted to reducing worsening of dyskinesia (Soares-Weiser et al. 2011). Clozapine has been used to treat TD, but there have been no methodologically rigorous trials to support this practice. The recommended clinical approach is to use the lowest possible dose of antipsychotic that is effective and to consider changing to a medication with lower risk of TD (i.e., an antipsychotic with low risk of EPS) if TD is present or is an important concern.

Monitoring for EPS.   Guidelines from the Mount Sinai Conference on physical health monitoring of patients with schizophrenia, which were derived by consensus from a group of mental health clinicians and researchers and medical experts who reviewed data on the side effects of antipsychotics, recommend an assessment of EPS prior to starting an antipsychotic and at weekly intervals until the dose has been stabilized for at least 2 weeks (Marder et al. 2004). Although the risk of EPS varies, it is not uncommon for patients receiving any antipsychotic—with the possible exception of clozapine—to experience mild akathisia or rigidity.

The examination for EPS includes observing patients for restlessness movements and inquiring if patients feel restless. Asking patients if they are having difficulty sitting still can be helpful. Parkinsonism is evaluated by observing patients' gait and examining for rigidity in the elbow and wrist. Dystonias usually present as urgent events reported by patients.

Regular monitoring for TD should be a component of management strategies with antipsychotics. We recommend examining patients for TD before starting an antipsychotic and at 6-month intervals. Patients who are at high risk, including the elderly and those who are sensitive to EPS, should be examined more frequently. The Abnormal Involuntary Movement Scale (AIMS; 1988) provides instructions for examining patients as well as means for recording the results of the examination.

Metabolic Effects

Physicians prescribing antipsychotics should screen carefully and monitor patients who take antipsychotic drugs for signs of rapid weight gain or other problems that could lead to diabetes, obesity, and heart disease. Although Table 8–1 indicates that risk of weight gain and metabolic problems varies among medications, the importance of this problem is such that all patients taking antipsychotics should be monitored carefully. Table 8–3 is adapted from the recommendations of a joint panel of the American Diabetes Association, American Psychiatric Association, American Association of Clinical Endocrinologists, and the North American Association for the Study of Obesity (2004), and those of the Mount Sinai Conference on physical health monitoring (Marder et al. 2004).

Weight gain.   Individuals with schizophrenia are more likely than the population at large to be overweight or obese (Allison et al. 1999a). Antipsychotics vary in their association with weight gain. A meta-analysis by Allison et al. (1999b) estimated the amount of weight gain associated with moderate doses of several antipsychotics over 10 weeks. When the meta-analysis was expanded by Newcomer (2005) to cover additional drugs, the mean increases were less than 1 kilogram with aripiprazole, ziprasidone, molindone, and fluphenazine, 1–2 kilograms with haloperidol, 2–3 kilograms with risperidone and chlorpromazine, and more than 4 kilograms with olanzapine and clozapine. These differences in weight gain liabilities are consistent with findings from other studies (Correll et al. 2009; Lieberman et al. 2005; Wirshing et al. 1999).

The Mount Sinai consensus recommendation is that mental health providers should monitor and chart the body mass index (BMI: weight in kg/height in m^2) of every patient with schizophrenia, regardless of the antipsychotic medication prescribed (Marder et al. 2004). Patients should be weighed at every visit for the first 6 months following a medication change. BMI monitoring should be supplemented by measurement and recording of the patient's waist circumference. A waist circumference greater than 40 inches for men or greater than 35 inches for women is a criterion of the metabolic syndrome and places a person at elevated risk for diabetes. The relative risk of weight gain for the different antipsychotic medications should be a consideration in drug selection for patients who have a BMI greater than 25. Interventions for patients who gain weight may include closer monitoring of weight, engagement in a weight management program, or a change in antipsychotic medication. If a patient is taking a medication that is associated with a high risk for weight gain, the clinician should consider switching to medication with less weight gain liability, although it is also important to consider the impact of such a change on the patient's overall clinical status. Another approach with growing evidence of effectiveness is the use of adjunctive metformin to reduce weight (Maayan et al. 2010).

Diabetes.   Diabetes is more prevalent in individuals with schizophrenia than in the general population (Dixon et al. 2000). This may be related to the high rates of obesity associated with schizophrenia or to a possible association of

TABLE 8–3. Suggested protocol for monitoring metabolic effects of antipsychotics

	Baseline	4 weeks	8 weeks	12 weeks	Quarterly	Annually	At least every 5 years
Personal or family history	X					X	
Weight (body mass index)	X	X	X	X	X		
Waist circumference	X			X		X	
Blood pressure	X			X		X	
Fasting plasma glucose	X			X		X	
Fasting lipid profile	X			X			X

Note. More frequent assessments may be warranted based on clinical status.
Source. American Diabetes Association, American Psychiatric Association, American Association of Clinical Endocrinologists, et al. 2004; Marder et al. 2004.

schizophrenia with insulin resistance (American Diabetes Association et al. 2004). Other evidence suggests that antipsychotics have the potential for increasing the risk of diabetes. This could be either a result of antipsychotic-associated weight gain or a direct effect of antipsychotic drugs on insulin resistance. In 2004 the FDA issued a warning that all second-generation antipsychotics increase the risk of hyperglycemia and diabetes (U.S. Food and Drug Administration 2004). However, it is likely that all drugs that are associated with weight gain are also associated to some extent with an increased risk of diabetes.

Mental health practitioners should be aware of risk factors for diabetes and the symptoms of new-onset diabetes (including weight change, polyuria, and polydipsia) and should inform patients about these symptoms and monitor for their presence at regular intervals. Furthermore, a baseline measure of glucose should be collected for all patients before starting a new antipsychotic. A fasting glucose level is preferred, but a hemoglobin A_{1C} level is sufficient if fasting glucose is not feasible. The Mount Sinai guidelines (Marder et al. 2004) and the American Diabetes Association, American Psychiatric Association, American Association of Clinical Endocrinologists, et al. (2004) recommend measuring fasting blood glucose level before starting an antipsychotic, 3 or 4 months later, and then annually. Patients who are gaining weight should have fasting glucose or hemoglobin A_{1C} levels monitored every 4 months.

Mental health providers should ensure that patients who are diagnosed with diabetes receive follow-up with an appropriate medical provider. The patient's psychiatrist and medical care provider should communicate when medication changes are instituted that may affect the control of the patient's diabetes. If symptoms of diabetes are reported, a random blood glucose level should be collected, and if the level is elevated ($\geq$126 if fasting or $\geq$200 if nonfasting), then the patient should be referred to a medical care provider who manages diabetes.

Dyslipidemia. Elevated levels of total cholesterol, low-density lipoprotein (LDL) cholesterol, and triglycerides may, in part, account for the high risk of coronary heart disease in schizophrenia. Studies of second-generation antipsychotics indicate that the tendency of these agents to cause weight gain is also associated with their risk for worsening serum lipid levels. Table 8–1 summarizes the associations between antipsychotics and dyslipidemias.

Mental health providers should be aware of the lipid profiles for all patients with schizophrenia. The National Cholesterol Education Program (Grundy et al. 2004) and the U.S. Preventive Services Task Force (2001) guidelines provide direction for screening and treating patients who are at high risk for cardiovascular disease. If a lipid panel is not available, one should be obtained and reviewed. As noted in Table 8–3, lipid levels should be checked before medication changes, after 12 weeks, and then at least every 5 years. Patients who fulfill criteria for the metabolic syndrome should be carefully monitored by a medical care provider.

Prolactin. Many antipsychotics, in particular high-potency antipsychotics. risperidone, paliperidone, sulpiride, and amisulpride, elevate serum prolactin levels through blockade of dopamine receptors in the anterior pituitary. Consequences may include decreased libido, anorgasmia, amenorrhea, galactorrhea, and gynecomastia. Dopamine receptor antagonists, such as first-generation antipsychotics, have been associated with an increased risk of breast cancer, possibly related to elevated prolactin levels (Wang et al. 2002). Growing evidence suggests that high levels of prolactin increase the risk of osteoporosis by reducing estrogen levels (Abraham et al. 2003; Becker et al. 2003; Meaney et al. 2004). Aripiprazole, which has agonist effects on pituitary dopamine receptors, can be associated with decreases in serum prolactin levels that are not thought to have clinical significance.

The Mount Sinai guidelines recommend yearly monitoring of patients taking antipsychotics for symptoms of prolactin elevation, including galactorrhea, decreased libido, or menstrual disturbances in women and decreased libido or erectile or ejaculatory disturbances in men (Marder et al. 2004). Patients who are receiving an agent that is associated with prolactin elevation should be asked about symptoms of prolactin elevation at each visit after starting the agent until they are receiving a stable dose. If any symptoms of prolactin elevation are present, prolactin should be measured and, if possible, other medical causes ruled out. Consideration also should be given to a medication change to a prolactin-sparing antipsychotic. If, after a change in antipsychotic, the signs and symptoms disappear and the prolactin level declines to normal, an endocrine workup is not needed. For patients with symptomatic antipsychotic-induced hyperprolactinemia, hormone replacement therapy (estrogen/progestogen for women and testosterone in men) is considered the first choice for medication treatment (Miller 2004). As a last resort, treatment with a dopamine agonist (e.g., cabergoline or bromocriptine) may effectively lower prolactin levels, but psychotic exacerbation is a risk warranting careful monitoring.

Other Side Effects

Antipsychotics can also cause varying amounts of sedation and postural hypotension, as noted in Table 8–1. Patients should be asked about these side effects at each visit after starting an antipsychotic until tolerance develops. If the side effects do not resolve, a change to an antipsychotic with a lower risk of sedation or hypotension is indicated.

Tachycardia may be a side effect of certain agents, particularly clozapine. In addition, mental health providers are often in the best position to diagnose hypertension. Guidelines recommend measuring blood pressure and pulse at baseline, 12 weeks, and annually (Table 8–3). In addition, we recommend monitoring blood pressure and pulse at each visit after starting an antipsychotic until the dosage is stable.

Neuroleptic dysphoria, an unpleasant subjective response to antipsychotic medicines, is associated with poor adherence to antipsychotic medication regimens (Perkins 2002; Van Putten et al. 1984; Weiden et al. 1989). Neuroleptic dysphoria has been associated with akathisia and parkinsonism and thus may be more common among drugs most associated with these side effects (Perkins 2002).

Maintenance Treatment Effects and Relapse Prevention

Many studies have reported that maintenance antipsychotic treatment for schizophrenia that has responded to antipsychotic medication reduces symptom relapse and rehospitalization (Davis 1975; Kane and Lieberman 1987). A reasonable estimate, based on controlled clinical trials of drug discontinuation, is that stopping antipsychotics after 1 year of maintenance treatment will result in relapse in about two-thirds of patients, whereas only one-third of the patients who continue to take antipsychotic medicines will relapse. Hogarty and colleagues (1976) found a relapse rate of 66% within 1 year of treatment discontinuation even among patients who had been successfully maintained in the community for 2–3 years with antipsychotic drugs. First-episode patients who meet symptom response criteria may have lower relapse rates. During the year following initial recovery, a relapse rate of 40% has been reported for patients taking placebo as compared with 0% for patients taking medication (Kane et al. 1982). Furthermore, Robinson and colleagues (1999a) showed that discontinuing drug therapy increased the risk of relapse almost five times in a sample of patients with first-episode schizophrenia or schizoaffective disorder over several years of follow-up.

The benefits of maintenance antipsychotic drug treatment are tempered by the risk of long-term side effects, such as the development of TD as well as obesity, diabetes, hyperlipidemias, and other factors associated with heart disease. Targeted, intermittent antipsychotic medication strategies that involve slowly titrating stabilized patients off medication and reintroducing medication when signs or symptoms of imminent relapse occur have not been found to reduce the risk of TD and are associated with risks of symptom exacerbation and relapse (Carpenter et al. 1990; Gaebel et al. 1993; Herz et al. 1991; Jolley et al. 1990; Schooler 1993). The Schizophrenia PORT (Buchanan et al. 2010b) and the American Psychiatric Association "Practice Guideline for the Treatment of Patients With Schizophrenia" (Lehman et al. 2004b) recommend continuous maintenance treatment for all patients with chronic schizophrenia. Targeted, intermittent therapy is acceptable only for those patients who cannot tolerate or will not accept continuous antipsychotic treatment.

CHOICE OF ANTIPSYCHOTICS

The antipsychotics introduced after clozapine were developed with the hope that they would lead to improved outcomes for individuals with schizophrenia, in part by reducing negative symptoms and the burden of extrapyramidal side effects. Although advantages for clozapine have been shown in many studies, only some of the drugs that have followed have advantages in efficacy over the older antipsychotics when they are prescribed at appropriate doses. Meta-analyses of randomized controlled trials consistently show modest advantages for clozapine and small advantages for amisulpride, olanzapine, and risperidone over other antipsychotics in reducing psychotic symptoms (Leucht et al. 2003, 2009c). Side effects vary considerably among the medications and have an impact on overall effectiveness by affecting patients' willingness to continue taking them. The most recent Schizophrenia PORT recommendations, based on exhaustive reviews of the literature, suggest that any antipsychotic other than clozapine is an appropriate treatment for people with multi-episode schizophrenia (Buchanan et al. 2010b). For patients experiencing a first episode of psychosis, the PORT recommendation is for any antipsychotic other than clozapine or olanzapine. Clozapine is excluded in both instances because of its risk of agranulocytosis; olanzapine is not recommended in first-episode psychosis because of its association with weight gain and other metabolic risk factors for cardiovascular disease (Buchanan et al. 2010b).

LONG-ACTING INJECTABLE (DEPOT) ANTIPSYCHOTIC MEDICATIONS

Long-acting injectable antipsychotics, also known as *depot antipsychotics,* are commonly thought to have important advantages over oral medications in some situations, although the evidence to support this is weak (Buchanan et al. 2010b). The primary reason long-acting formulations are used is to improve adherence with treatment regimens; thus, they are recommended for individuals who do not regularly take medications or who are expected not to do so. Another purported advantage is less fluctuation in drug levels than with oral medications, which is thought to lower the incidence of side effects (Ereshefsky et al. 1990). Other advantages are a clear knowledge of an individual's treatment adherence because of the need for injections and improved surveillance for missed medicine doses. Another possible advantage is increased contact with caregivers, because injections are needed every 2–4 weeks instead of on the typical monthly or less frequent appointment schedules. Disadvantages are that some patients do not like regular injections, the injections can be painful, and the requirement for regular injections can be inconvenient for clinicians as well as patients. Table 8–4 contains summary information on the long-acting injectable antipsychotics available in the United States.

IMPLEMENTING AND MONITORING ANTIPSYCHOTIC DRUG TREATMENT

DOSING

Recommended dose ranges for commonly used oral antipsychotics appear in Table 8–1. Few data support the usefulness of doses beyond these recommendations, but a greater incidence of side effects is likely. Some reports of positive results with high doses of olanzapine have not been confirmed in rigorous studies (Conley et al. 2003; Sheitman et al. 1997). The administration of large parenteral doses of antipsychotics within a 24-hour period ("rapid neuroleptization") has not shown any gains in efficacy over standard treatment and is not a recommended strategy (Lehman et al. 2004a).

During the treatment of an acute episode of schizophrenia, antipsychotic drugs usually have a therapeutic effect within 1–3 weeks, with most gains in the first 6–8 weeks (Davis et al. 1989). Some evidence suggests that antipsychotic effects begin within the first week of treatment (Agid et al. 2003). Some patients, however, may require several months to achieve a full clinical response and symptom remission. This also applies to first-episode patients, whose symptoms typically respond relatively rapidly to modest doses of antipsychotic medications (Lieberman 1993). When patients' symptoms do not respond to a standard course of treatment, clinicians generally increase the dose, switch to another antipsychotic drug, or maintain the initial treatment for an extended period. Little evidence from controlled clinical trials supports the efficacy of any of these strategies (Kinon et al. 1993; Levinson et al. 1990; Rifkin et al. 1991; Van Putten et al. 1990; Volavka et al. 1992), although an individual patient may show a better response to one particular drug than to another (Gardos 1974). Another common approach, also without strong evidence for effectiveness, is simultaneous use of more than one

TABLE 8–4. Long-acting antipsychotic drugs (all given intramuscularly)

	How supplied	Half-life (days)	Starting dose (mg)	Second dose (mg)	Maintenance dose (mg)
Fluphenazine decanoate	25 mg/mL	6–10	12.5	12.5–25 (6–14 days later)	12.5–50 every 2–3 weeks
Haloperidol decanoate	50 mg/mL or 100 mg/mL	21	50	50–100 (3–28 days later)	50–200 every 3–4 weeks
Risperidone microspheres	Prepared packages of 25, 37.5, and 50 mg	3–6	25	25–50 (2 weeks later)	25–50 every 2 weeks
Paliperidone palmitate	Prefilled syringes containing 39, 78, 117, 156, or 234 mg	25–49	234	156 (7 days later)	39–234 every 4 weeks
Olanzapine pamoate	Prepared packages of 210, 300, or 405 mg	30	210–300	210–300 (2 weeks later)	150–300 every 2 weeks or 300–405 every 4 weeks

antipsychotic. This strategy, known as *antipsychotic polypharmacy* or *combination antipsychotic treatment*, is discussed later in this chapter (see subsection "Antipsychotic Polypharmacy").

ROUTE OF ADMINISTRATION

Oral pills are the most commonly used form of antipsychotic medication and are suitable for most patients in most situations. Liquids and dissolvable tablets are useful for patients who cannot or will not swallow pills or who prefer this form. Short-acting injections that are rapidly active are available for emergency treatment of agitated, psychotic patients or others in need of rapid decreases in symptoms or dangerous behavior.

Long-acting injections are recommended for patients with frequent relapses on oral medications, poor adherence to oral medication regimens, or a preference for injections (Buchanan et al. 2010b). Despite limited evidence from well-conducted clinical trials, this recommendation is supported by the experience of clinicians who believe that long-acting injections work well for patients who cannot or will not consistently take oral medications and that adherence with injectable regimens is easier to monitor than with oral regimens.

IMPLEMENTING CLOZAPINE TREATMENT

A complete blood count with differential should be obtained before starting clozapine to make sure the patient is not granulocytopenic (white blood cell count $<3,000/mm^3$). General and cardiovascular health should be assessed because of the side effects of orthostatic hypotension and tachycardia and the rare occurrence of life-threatening cardiovascular side effects. The initial dosage should be 12.5–25 mg once or twice daily. Increases should be made gradually (increase by 25–50 mg/day) because risks of sedation, hypotension, and seizures are higher with rapid dose escalation. The target dosage is 300–800 mg/day. The minimum effective dose should be used. If response is inadequate once 600 mg/day is reached, a blood level should be obtained, because there appears to be a therapeutic threshold of about 350 ng/mL. If this level has not been obtained, slow upward titration of the clozapine dosage to 800 mg/day is recommended. One important drug interaction is with selective serotonin reuptake inhibitors and other drugs that are metabolized by the cytochrome P450 2D6 isozyme (e.g., fluoxetine, fluvoxamine), which can lead to significant increases in clozapine plasma levels.

To limit the risk of agranulocytosis, a complete blood count must be repeated weekly for the first 6 months and biweekly after that. Clozapine should not be given if the white blood cell count declines below $2,000/mm^3$

or the absolute neutrophil count declines below $1,000/mm^3$. Drugs known to suppress bone marrow function (e.g., carbamazepine) should not be used with clozapine.

There is no clear consensus on how to monitor for myocarditis. One recommended approach is to monitor carefully for chest discomfort, shortness of breath, flu-like symptoms, peripheral edema, or unusual fatigue during the first 2 months of treatment, when the risk is greatest. If any of these signs or symptoms are present, then an electrocardiogram and laboratory tests (including creatinine kinase, CK-MB, complete blood count with differential, and troponin) are examined (Annamraju et al. 2007). Clozapine should be stopped if substantial evidence of a new cardiac problem is found early in treatment, but if signs and symptoms are nonspecific, then a cardiology consultation may be helpful in determining the diagnosis and may prevent unnecessary discontinuation of this very useful medication.

Because clozapine is the best available drug treatment for refractory symptoms, a trial should last 8–12 weeks at an effective dosage. Clinical benefits may continue to accrue for up to 12 months. If effective, clozapine should be continued as a maintenance treatment. However, because of its side effects and the need for continued white blood cell monitoring, if clozapine does not offer advantages over previous treatments, then it should be slowly discontinued after 6 months of treatment and replaced with a new or previously helpful treatment.

TREATMENT TARGETS: RESPONSE CRITERIA

Although drugs classified as antipsychotics may have a wide range of therapeutic effects, the primary standard of efficacy has been the reduction of positive psychotic symptoms such as delusions, hallucinations, and disorganization. Antipsychotic drugs that have been approved by regulatory agencies are all superior to placebo in reducing positive psychotic symptoms. Antipsychotic drugs also reduce negative symptoms (i.e., affective flattening, alogia, and avolition), but the magnitude of the effect is smaller than the effect on positive symptoms (Leucht et al. 1999), and any effect on residual negative symptoms or the deficit syndrome is small (Carpenter 1996; Kirkpatrick et al. 2000). The clearest types of negative symptoms that can be reduced with antipsychotic medicines are those secondary to positive symptoms, such as social withdrawal and avoidance due to delusions or paranoia (Carpenter et al. 1988). As positive symptoms decrease in response to antipsychotic drugs, the secondary negative symptoms also diminish.

Because cognitive impairments are common in schizophrenia and have been shown to relate more strongly to functional outcomes than to positive symptom severity, cognitive functioning is now an important focus of research and a target for drug development (Buchanan et al. 2010a; Green et al. 2004; see also Chapter 4, "Neurocognitive Impairments" in this book). The cognitive domains under study include learning and secondary memory, motor function, verbal fluency, attention, and executive functioning. Studies of antipsychotic drugs have failed to demonstrate significant cognitive function–enhancing effects of these medications, nor is there evidence to support the use of any adjunctive treatment for this purpose (Buchanan et al 2010a; Keefe et al. 2006).

Factors Influencing Antipsychotic Response

Significant efforts are under way to identify factors that may be associated with antipsychotic treatment refractoriness because preventive measures may offer more hope than new drugs. For example, a delay in treatment of the first episode of schizophrenia (Addington et al. 2004; Loebel et al. 1992) and in the treatment of acute exacerbations (May et al. 1976; Wyatt 1995) is associated with poorer clinical outcomes. Robinson and colleagues (1999b) reported that 87% of their sample of first-episode patients with schizophrenia or schizoaffective disorder responded to treatment within 1 year. Male gender, a history of obstetric complications, poorer attention at baseline, more severe hallucinations and delusions, and the development of EPS during antipsychotic treatment were associated with a significantly lower likelihood of response.

OTHER PHARMACOLOGICAL TREATMENTS

Because antipsychotic medications often fail to resolve the full range of schizophrenic psychopathology and other common symptoms (e.g., anxiety, depression, mood instability), adjunctive treatments are commonly tried. Adjunctive pharmacological treatments in patients with schizophrenia have been the subject of numerous reviews (Christison et al. 1991; Donaldson et al. 1983; Farmer and Blewett 1993; Johns and Thompson 1995; Lehman et al. 2004b; Leucht et al. 2007a, 2007b; Lindenmayer 1995; Meltzer 1992; Rifkin 1993; Siris 1993; Whitehead et al. 2003). In addition, some psychotropic medications other than antipsychotics have been used alone to treat schizophrenia. Below we summarize information on the use of anxiolytics/hypnotics, antidepressants, and mood stabilizers to treat either symptoms of schizophrenia or common comorbid conditions.

ANTIANXIETY OR HYPNOTIC DRUGS

Although benzodiazepines have long been prescribed for patients with schizophrenia to treat anxiety, depression, or hostility, little evidence from research supports their use for this purpose. The systematic review conducted by the Schizophrenia PORT and a meta-analysis conducted for the Cochrane Collaboration each concluded that there is insufficient evidence to reach a conclusion about the usefulness of benzodiazepines for schizophrenia (Buchanan et al. 2010b; Volz et al. 2007). The lack of systematic research on benzodiazepines may be due to the potential for dependency and reluctance to prescribe these drugs to patients with comorbid substance use disorders. Given the lack of evidence supporting their use, benzodiazepines are probably best used for short-term treatment of specific symptoms such as insomnia or anxiety.

ANTIDEPRESSANTS

Because depression among patients with schizophrenia is common, antidepressants are widely used to treat depression among persons with schizophrenia, although the evidence for the effectiveness of this strategy is modest. A meta-analysis that included 11 randomized controlled trials comparing adjunctive antidepressants to placebo in persons with schizophrenia and depression found small advantages in symptom improvement and response rates for adjunctive antidepressants (Whitehead et al. 2003). Although a previous report suggested that antidepressants may worsen psychotic symptoms in people suffering an acute episode (Plasky 1991), this was not confirmed in the review by Whitehead and colleagues (2003). These authors concluded that the use of adjunctive antidepressants for depression in patients with schizophrenia is unproven. A reasonable recommendation is to use antidepressants when depressive symptoms persist in spite of adequate treatment with an antipsychotic or when patients develop postpsychotic depression.

Adjunctive antidepressants have also been tried as treatment for negative symptoms, which respond only somewhat to antipsychotic medications. A meta-analysis for the Cochrane Collaboration found higher rates of clinically significant improvement in negative symptoms among patients treated with antipsychotics and antidepressants than among those treated with antipsychotics and placebo (Rummel-Kluge et al. 2006). However, the Schizophrenia PORT concluded that there are no treatments for negative symptoms that warrant a recommendation (Buchanan et al. 2010b).

Important practical issues must be considered when antidepressants are used in combination with clozapine. Selective serotonin reuptake inhibitors—in particular, fluvoxamine, fluoxetine, and sertraline—inhibit the metabolism of clozapine and can cause large increases in clozapine levels that are potentially toxic. Serum clozapine levels and side effects, particularly anticholinergic side effects, should be monitored when using the combination of selective serotonin reuptake inhibitors and clozapine. Because bupropion and clozapine both increase the risk of seizures, this combination is not recommended.

LITHIUM AND ANTICONVULSANTS

Lithium

Lithium is not an effective monotherapy for people with schizophrenia (Leucht et al. 2007b). As an adjunct to antipsychotic treatment, there is inadequate evidence to support its use for people with residual positive symptoms (Buchanan et al. 2010b). In a Cochrane Collaboration meta-analysis, lithium augmentation was associated with a higher response rate than augmentation with placebo, but there was a suggestion that the benefit of lithium was mainly seen in patients with schizoaffective disorder (Leucht et al. 2007b). Thus, it remains unclear if lithium has benefits for the core symptoms of schizophrenia or if the benefit is restricted to those with affective symptoms. Furthermore, it appears that lithium plus an antipsychotic is less well tolerated than an antipsychotic alone (Leucht et al. 2007b).

Carbamazepine

Carbamazepine is not effective as a sole treatment for schizophrenia and is not recommended for routine use to augment antipsychotics (Leucht et al. 2007a). A trial of carbamazepine may be warranted for those with a history of response to carbamazepine or for patients with associated electroencephalogram abnormalities (Leucht et al. 2007a). In clinical practice carbamazepine is sometimes used as an adjunct to antipsychotics to treat aggressive, agitated patients, although strong evidence supporting this use is lacking.

Because of carbamazepine's ability to upregulate hepatic enzymes, plasma antipsychotic levels may be lowered when carbamazepine is used. If antipsychotic efficacy is lost, antipsychotic levels can be checked or the dosage can be increased (Christison et al. 1991). Because of carbamazepine's risk of bone marrow toxicity, including agranulocytosis, it should not be used in combination with clozapine.

Valproate

Valproate, the active component of valproic acid and divalproex, is widely used as an adjunctive treatment for schizophrenia, but both the Schizophrenia PORT and the Cochrane Collaboration reviewers concluded that there is inadequate evidence to support its routine use (Buchanan et al. 2010b; Schwarz et al. 2008). In addition, there is no strong evidence that valproate is effective when used as an adjunctive treatment for patients with treatment-refractory schizophrenia (Conley et al. 2003).

ANTIPSYCHOTIC POLYPHARMACY

Although the use of antipsychotic polypharmacy is a common practice, there is little evidence that suggests greater effectiveness as compared with antipsychotic monotherapy. A recent meta-analysis of randomized trials comparing combination antipsychotic therapy with monotherapy concluded that there is insufficient evidence from the available research findings to derive "conclusive clinical recommendations" (Correll et al. 2008). However, this review found that certain study characteristics seemed to predict favorable outcomes for polypharmacy: specifically, studies using combinations that included clozapine, those that began with two medications rather than adding a second after a period of non-response on a single drug, and those that lasted at least 10 weeks were most likely to demonstrate benefits.

We recommend clozapine monotherapy prior to antipsychotic polypharmacy for the treatment of schizophrenia. Unfortunately, in the event of clozapine refusal or intolerance, few data are available to guide the use of specific antipsychotic combinations.

REFERENCES

Abnormal Involuntary Movement Scale (AIMS). Psychopharmacol Bull 24:781–783, 1988

Abraham G, Paing WW, Kaminski J, et al: Effects of elevated serum prolactin on bone mineral density and bone metabolism in female patients with schizophrenia: a prospective study. Am J Psychiatry 160:1618–1620, 2003

Addington J, Van Mastrigt S, Addington D: Duration of untreated psychosis: impact on 2-year outcome. Psychol Med 34:277–284, 2004

Agid O, Kapur S, Arenovich T, et al: Delayed-onset hypothesis of antipsychotic action: a hypothesis tested and rejected. Arch Gen Psychiatry 60:1228–1235, 2003

Allison DB, Fontaine KR, Heo M, et al: The distribution of body mass index among individuals with and without schizophrenia. J Clin Psychiatry 60:215–220, 1999a

Allison DB, Mentore JL, Heo M, et al: Antipsychotic-induced weight gain: a comprehensive research synthesis. Am J Psychiatry 156:1686–1696, 1999b

Alvir JM, Lieberman JA, Safferman AZ, et al: Clozapine-induced agranulocytosis: incidence and risk factors in the United States. N Engl J Med 329:162–167, 1993

American Diabetes Association, American Psychiatric Association, American Association of Clinical Endocrinologists, et al: Consensus development conference on antipsychotic drugs and obesity and diabetes. J Clin Psychiatry 65:267–272, 2004

American Psychiatric Association: Diagnostic and Statistical Manual of Mental Disorders, 4th Edition, Text Revision. Washington, DC, American Psychiatric Association, 2000

Annamraju S, Sheitman B, Saik S, et al: Early recognition of clozapine-induced myocarditis. J Clin Psychopharmacol 27:479–483, 2007

Becker D, Liver O, Mester R, et al: Risperidone, but not olanzapine, decreases bone mineral density in female premenopausal schizophrenia patients. J Clin Psychiatry 64:761–766, 2003

Buchanan RW, Keefe RS, Umbricht D, et al: The FDA-NIMH-MATRICS Guidelines for Clinical Trial Design of Cognitive-Enhancing Drugs: what do we know 5 years later? Schizophr Bull July 13, 2010a [Epub ahead of print]

Buchanan RW, Kreyenbuhl J, Kelly DL, et al: Schizophrenia Patient Outcomes Research Team (PORT): the 2009 Schizophrenia PORT psychopharmacological treatment recommendations and summary statements. Schizophr Bull 36:71–93, 2010b

Caroff S: Neuroleptic malignant syndrome: still a risk, but which patients may be in danger? Current Psychiatry 2:36–42, 2003

Carpenter WT Jr: The treatment of negative symptoms: pharmacological and methodological issues. Br J Psychiatry Suppl (29):17–22, 1996

Carpenter WT Jr, Heinrichs DW, Wagman AM: Deficit and nondeficit forms of schizophrenia: the concept. Am J Psychiatry 145:578–583, 1988

Carpenter WT Jr, Hanlon TE, Heinrichs DW, et al: Continuous versus targeted medication in schizophrenic outpatients: outcome results. Am J Psychiatry 147:1138–1148, 1990

Casey DE: Neuroleptic-induced acute extrapyramidal syndromes and tardive dyskinesia. Psychiatr Clin North Am 16:589–610, 1993

Chakos M, Lieberman J, Hoffman E, et al: Effectiveness of second-generation antipsychotics in patients with treatment-resistant schizophrenia: a review and meta-analysis of randomized trials. Am J Psychiatry 158:518–526, 2001

Chengappa KN, Vasile J, Levine J, et al: Clozapine: its impact on aggressive behavior among patients in a state psychiatric hospital. Schizophr Res 53:1–6, 2002

Chengappa KN, Parepally H, Brar JS, et al: A random-assignment, double-blind, clinical trial of once- vs twice-daily administration of quetiapine fumarate in patients with schizophrenia or schizoaffective disorder: a pilot study. Can J Psychiatry 48:187–194, 2003

Christison GW, Kirch DG, Wyatt RJ: When symptoms persist: choosing among alternative somatic treatments for schizophrenia. Schizophr Bull 17:217–245, 1991

Citrome L, Volavka J, Czobor P, et al: Effects of clozapine, olanzapine, risperidone, and haloperidol on hostility among patients with schizophrenia. Psychiatr Serv 52:1510–1514, 2001

Conley RR, Kelly DL, Richardson CM, et al: The efficacy of high-dose olanzapine versus clozapine in treatment-resistant schizophrenia: a double-blind crossover study. J Clin Psychopharmacol 23:668–671, 2003

Correll CU, Leucht S, Kane JM: Lower risk for tardive dyskinesia associated with second-generation antipsychotics: a systematic review of 1-year studies. Am J Psychiatry 161:414–425, 2004

Correll CU, Rummel-Kluge C, Corves C, et al: Antipsychotic combinations vs monotherapy in schizophrenia: a meta-analysis of randomized controlled trials. Schizophr Bull 35:443–457, 2009

Correll CU, Manu P, Olshanskiy V, et al: Cardiometabolic risk of second-generation antipsychotic medications during first-time use in children and adolescents. JAMA 302:1765–1773, 2009

Davis JM: Overview: maintenance therapy in psychiatry, I: schizophrenia. Am J Psychiatry 132:1237–1245, 1975

Davis JM, Barter JT, Kane JM (eds): Antipsychotic Drugs. Baltimore, MD, Williams & Wilkins, 1989

Davis JM, Chen N, Glick ID: A meta-analysis of the efficacy of second-generation antipsychotics. Arch Gen Psychiatry 60:553–564, 2003

Dixon L, Weiden PJ, Delahanty J, et al: Prevalence and correlates of diabetes in national schizophrenia samples. Schizophr Bull 26:903–912, 2000

Dixon LB, Dickerson F, Bellack AS, et al: Schizophrenia Patient Outcomes Research Team (PORT): the 2009 Schizophrenia PORT psychosocial treatment recommendations and summary statements. Schizophr Bull 36:48–70, 2010

Donaldson SR, Gelenberg AJ, Baldessarini RJ: The pharmacologic treatment of schizophrenia: a progress report. Schizophr Bull 9:504–527, 1983

Ereshefsky L, Saklad SR, Tran-Johnson T, et al: Kinetics and clinical evaluation of haloperidol decanoate loading dose regimen. Psychopharmacol Bull 26:108–114, 1990

Farmer AE, Blewett A: Drug treatment of resistant schizophrenia: limitations and recommendations. Drugs 45:374–383, 1993

Gaebel W, Frick U, Kopcke W, et al: Early neuroleptic intervention in schizophrenia: are prodromal symptoms valid predictors of relapse? Br J Psychiatry Suppl September(21):8–12, 1993

Gardos G: Are antipsychotic drugs interchangeable? J Nerv Ment Dis 159:343–348, 1974

Glazer WM, Morgenstern H, Doucette JT: Predicting the long-term risk of tardive dyskinesia in outpatients maintained on neuroleptic medications. J Clin Psychiatry 54:133–139, 1993

Green MF, Nuechterlein KH, Gold JM, et al: Approaching a consensus cognitive battery for clinical trials in schizophrenia: the NIMH-MATRICS Conference to Select Cognitive Domains and Test Criteria. Biol Psychiatry 56:301–307, 2004

Grundy SM, Cleeman JI, Merz CN, et al: Implications of recent clinical trials for the National Cholesterol Education Program Adult Treatment Panel III guidelines. Circulation 110(2):227–239, 2004

Guttmacher MS: Phenothiazine treatment in acute schizophrenia; effectiveness: the National Institute of Mental Health Psychopharmacology Service Center Collaborative Study Group. Arch Gen Psychiatry 10:246–261, 1964

Healy D: The Creation of Psychopharmacology. Cambridge, MA, Harvard University Press, 2002

Herz MI, Glazer WM, Mostert MA, et al: Intermittent vs maintenance medication in schizophrenia: two-year results. Arch Gen Psychiatry 48:333–339, 1991

Hogarty GE, Ulrich RF, Mussare F, et al: Drug discontinuation among long term, successfully maintained schizophrenic outpatients. Dis Nerv Syst 37:494–500, 1976

Huf G, Coutinho ESF, Adams CE; TREC Collaborative Group: Rapid tranquillisation of violent or agitated people in psychiatric emergency settings: pragmatic randomised controlled trial of intramuscular haloperidol versus intramuscular haloperidol plus promethazine. BMJ 335(7625):86, 2007

Jeste DV, Rockwell E, Harris MJ, et al: Conventional vs. newer antipsychotics in elderly patients. Am J Geriatr Psychiatry 7:70–76, 1999

Johns CA, Thompson JW: Adjunctive treatments in schizophrenia: pharmacotherapies and electroconvulsive therapy. Schizophr Bull 21:607–619, 1995

Jolley AG, Hirsch SR, Morrison E, et al: Trial of brief intermittent neuroleptic prophylaxis for selected schizophrenic outpatients: clinical and social outcome at two years. BMJ 301:837–842, 1990

Kane J, Lieberman J (eds): Maintenance Pharmacotherapy in Schizophrenia. New York, Raven, 1987

Kane JM, Rifkin A, Quitkin F, et al: Fluphenazine vs placebo in patients with remitted, acute first-episode schizophrenia. Arch Gen Psychiatry 39:70–73, 1982

Kane JM, Woerner M, Lieberman J: Tardive dyskinesia: prevalence, incidence, and risk factors. Psychopharmacology Suppl 2:72–78, 1985

Kane J, Honigfeld G, Singer J, et al: Clozapine for the treatment-resistant schizophrenic: a double-blind comparison with chlorpromazine. Arch Gen Psychiatry 45:789–796, 1988

Keefe RS, Bilder RM, Harvey PD, et al: Baseline neurocognitive deficits in the CATIE schizophrenia trial. Neuropsychopharmacology 31:2003–2046, 2006

Kinon BJ, Kane JM, Johns C, et al: Treatment of neuroleptic-resistant schizophrenic relapse. Psychopharmacol Bull 29:309–314, 1993

Kirkpatrick B, Kopelowicz A, Buchanan RW, et al: Assessing the efficacy of treatments for the deficit syndrome of schizophrenia. Neuropsychopharmacology 22:303–310, 2000

Lehman AF, Kreynbuhl J, Buchanan RW, et al: The Schizophrenia Patient Outcomes Research Team (PORT): updated treatment recommendations 2003. Schizophr Bull 30:193–217, 2004a

Lehman AF, Lieberman JA, Dixon LB, et al: Practice guideline for the treatment of patients with schizophrenia (second edition). Am J Psychiatry 161:1–56, 2004b

Leucht S, Pitschel-Walz G, Abraham D, et al: Efficacy and extrapyramidal side-effects of the new antipsychotics olanzapine, quetiapine, risperidone, and sertindole compared to conventional antipsychotics and placebo: a meta-analysis of randomized controlled trials. Schizophr Res 35:51–68, 1999

Leucht S, Wahlbeck K, Hamann J, et al: New generation antipsychotics versus low-potency conventional antipsychotics: a systematic review and meta-analysis. Lancet 361:1581–1589, 2003

Leucht S, Kissling W, McGrath J, et al: Carbamazepine for schizophrenia. Cochrane Database of Systematic Reviews Issue 3. Art No: CD001258. DOI: 10.1002/14651858.CD001258.pub2, 2007a

Leucht S, Kissling W, McGrath J: Lithium for schizophrenia. Cochrane Database of Systematic Reviews Issue 3. Art No: CD003834. DOI: 10.1002/14651858. CD003834.pub2, 2007b

Leucht S, Corves C, Arbter C, et al: Second-generation versus first-generation antipsychotic drugs for schizophrenia: a meta-analysis. The Lancet 373(9657):31–41, 2009a

Leucht S, Kissling W, Davis JM: Second-generation antipsychotics for schizophrenia: can we resolve the conflict? Psychol Med 39:1591–1602, 2009b

Leucht S, Komossa K, Rummel-Kluge C, et al: A meta-analysis of head-to-head comparisons of second-generation antipsychotics in the treatment of schizophrenia. Am J Psychiatry 166:152–163, 2009c

Levinson DF, Simpson GM, Singh H, et al: Fluphenazine dose, clinical response, and extrapyramidal symptoms during acute treatment. Arch Gen Psychiatry 47:761–768, 1990

Lieberman JA: Prediction of outcome in first-episode schizophrenia. J Clin Psychiatry 54 (suppl):13–17, 1993

Lieberman JA: Dopamine partial agonists: a new class of antipsychotic. CNS Drugs 18:251–267, 2004

Lieberman JA, Stroup TS, McEvoy JP, et al: Effectiveness of antipsychotic drugs in patients with chronic schizophrenia. N Engl J Med 353:1209–1223, 2005

Lindenmayer JP: New pharmacotherapeutic modalities for negative symptoms in psychosis. Acta Psychiatr Scand Suppl 388:15–19, 1995

Loebel AD, Lieberman JA, Alvir JM, et al: Duration of psychosis and outcome in first-episode schizophrenia. Am J Psychiatry 149:1183–1188, 1992

Maayan L, Vakhrusheva J, Correll CU: Effectiveness of medications to attenuate antipsychotic-related weight gain and metabolic abnormalities: a systematic review and meta-analysis. Neuropsychopharmacology 35:1520–1530, 2010 2010

Marder SR, Essock SM, Miller AL, et al: Physical health monitoring of patients with schizophrenia. Am J Psychiatry 161:1334–1349, 2004

May PR, Tuma AH, Yale C, et al: Schizophrenia—a follow-up study of results of treatment. Arch Gen Psychiatry 33:481–486, 1976

McEvoy JP, Lieberman JA, Stroup TS, et al: Effectiveness of clozapine versus olanzapine, quetiapine, and risperidone in patients with chronic schizophrenia who did not respond to prior atypical antipsychotic treatment. Am J Psychiatry 163:600–610, 2006

Meaney AM, Smith S, Howes OD, et al: Effects of long-term prolactin-raising antipsychotic medication on bone mineral density in patients with schizophrenia. Br J Psychiatry 184:503–508, 2004

Meltzer HY: Treatment of the neuroleptic-nonresponsive schizophrenic patient. Schizophr Bull 18:515–542, 1992

Meltzer HY, Alphs L, Green AI, et al: Clozapine treatment for suicidality in schizophrenia: International Suicide Prevention Trial (InterSePT). Arch Gen Psychiatry 60:82–91, 2003

Miller KK: Management of hyperprolactinemia in patients receiving antipsychotics. CNS Spectr 9 (8 suppl 7):28–32, 2004

Morgenstern H, Glazer WM: Identifying risk factors for tardive dyskinesia among long-term outpatients maintained with neuroleptic medications: results of the Yale Tardive Dyskinesia Study. Arch Gen Psychiatry 50:723–733, 1993

Newcomer JW: Second-generation (atypical) antipsychotics and metabolic effects : a comprehensive literature review. CNS Drugs 19 (suppl 1):1–93, 2005

Perkins DO: Predictors of noncompliance in patients with schizophrenia. J Clin Psychiatry 63:1121–1128, 2002

Plasky P: Antidepressant usage in schizophrenia. Schizophr Bull 17:649–657, 1991

Raveendran NS, Tharyan P, Alexander J, et al: Rapid tranquillisation in psychiatric emergency settings in India: pragmatic randomised controlled trial of intramuscular olanzapine versus intramuscular haloperidol plus promethazine. BMJ 335(7625):865, 2007

Rifkin A: Pharmacologic strategies in the treatment of schizophrenia. Psychiatr Clin North Am 16:351–363, 1993

Rifkin A, Doddi S, Karajgi B, et al: Dosage of haloperidol for schizophrenia. Arch Gen Psychiatry 48:166–170, 1991

Robinson D, Woerner MG, Alvir JM, et al: Predictors of relapse following response from a first episode of schizophrenia or schizoaffective disorder. Arch Gen Psychiatry 56:241–247, 1999a

Robinson DG, Woerner MG, Alvir JM, et al: Predictors of treatment response from a first episode of schizophrenia or schizoaffective disorder. Am J Psychiatry 156:544–549, 1999b

Robinson DG, Woerner MG, Alvir JM, et al: Predictors of medication discontinuation by patients with first-episode schizophrenia and schizoaffective disorder. Schizophr Res 57:209–219, 2002

Rummel-Kluge C, Kissling W, Leucht S: Antidepressants for the negative symptoms of schizophrenia. Cochrane Database of Systematic Reviews, Issue 3. Art No: CD005581. DOI: 10.1002/14651858.CD005581.pub2, 2006

Schooler NR: Reducing dosage in maintenance treatment of schizophrenia: review and prognosis. Br J Psychiatry Suppl December (22):58–65, 1993

Schwarz C, Volz A, Li C, Leucht S: Valproate for schizophrenia. Cochrane Database of Systematic Reviews, Issue 3. Art No: CD004028. DOI: 10.1002/14651858. CD004028.pub3, 2008

Sheitman BB, Lindgren JC, Early J, et al: High-dose olanzapine for treatment-refractory schizophrenia. Am J Psychiatry 154:1626, 1997

Siris SG: Adjunctive medication in the maintenance treatment of schizophrenia and its conceptual implications. Br J Psychiatry Suppl (22):66–78, 1993

Soares-Weiser K, Maayan N, McGrath J: Vitamin E for neuroleptic-induced tardive dyskinesia. Cochrane Database of Systematic Reviews, Issue 2. Art No: CD000209. DOI: 10.1002/14651858.CD000209.pub2, 2011

Strom BL, Faich G, Eng SM, et al: Comparative mortality associated with ziprasidone vs. olanzapine in real-world use: the Ziprasidone Observational Study of Cardiac Outcomes (ZODIAC). Eur Psychiatry 23(2):S158, 2008

U.S. Food and Drug Administration: Warning about hyperglycemia and atypical antipsychotic drugs. FDA Patient Safety News, Show #28, June 2004. Available at: http://www.accessdata.fda.gov/scripts/cdrh/cfdocs/psn/printer.cfm?id=229. Accessed December 6, 2005.

U.S. Preventive Services Task Force: Screening adults for lipid disorders: recommendations and rationale. Am J Prev Med 20:73–76, 2001

Van Putten T, May PR, Marder SR: Response to antipsychotic medication: the doctor's and the consumer's view. Am J Psychiatry 141:16–19, 1984

Van Putten T, Marder SR, Mintz J: A controlled dose comparison of haloperidol in newly admitted schizophrenic patients. Arch Gen Psychiatry 47:754–758, 1990

Volavka J, Cooper T, Czobor P, et al: Haloperidol blood levels and clinical effects. Arch Gen Psychiatry 49:354–361, 1992

Volz A, Khorsand V, Gillies D, et al: Benzodiazepines for schizophrenia. Cochrane Database of Systematic Reviews, Issue 1, Art No: CD006391. DOI: 10.1002/14651858.CD006391, 2007

Wang PS, Walker AM, Tsuang MT, et al: Dopamine antagonists and the development of breast cancer. Arch Gen Psychiatry 59:1147–1154, 2002

Weiden PJ, Mann JJ, Dixon L, et al: Is neuroleptic dysphoria a healthy response? Compr Psychiatry 30:546–552, 1989

Whitehead C, Moss S, Cardno A, et al: Antidepressants for the treatment of depression in people with schizophrenia: a systematic review. Psychol Med 33:589–599, 2003

Wirshing DA, Wirshing WC, Kysar L, et al: Novel antipsychotics: comparison of weight gain liabilities. J Clin Psychiatry 60:358–363, 1999

Wyatt RJ: Early intervention for schizophrenia: can the course of the illness be altered? Biol Psychiatry 38:1–3, 1995

PSYCHOSOCIAL THERAPIES

MARVIN S. SWARTZ, M.D.

NORA R. FROHBERG, M.D.

ROBERT E. DRAKE, M.D., PH.D.

JOHN LAURIELLO, M.D.

Major advances in the treatment of schizophrenia were heralded by the development of antipsychotic drugs in the 1950s and 1960s, which are clearly effective for the treatment of acute symptomatology and the prevention of relapse (Lauriello et al. 2003). However, long-term follow-up studies have consistently shown that the great majority of persons with schizophrenia continue to be plagued by residual psychotic symptoms, cognitive deficits, and other psychosocial problems.

Antipsychotic medications, including the new generation of antipsychotics, reduce positive symptoms and, to some extent, negative symptoms, but medications to date have had a limited effect on cognitive impairment and social and vocational functioning. Moreover, 20% or more of patients with schizophrenia have psychotic symptoms that do not respond to antipsychotic medications, and many other patients have residual symptoms. As a result of the limited effectiveness of antipsychotics, it is clear that most patients will need psychosocial therapies to address disabling residual symptoms, impaired social and vocational functioning, or risk of future relapse (Lauriello et al. 2003).

In this chapter, we review the current state of key psychosocial interventions designed to augment and complement treatment with medications. Effective psychosocial treatments should not merely reduce overt psychotic symptoms or rates of hospitalization but also lead to gains in cognitive abilities and social skills, quality of life, and sustained competitive employment; reduction of comorbid substance abuse; and improvements in other domains. We also highlight psychosocial treatment recommendations and summary statements by the 2009 Schizophrenia Patient Outcomes Research Team (PORT). This evidence-based review process supports the following eight treatment interventions: Assertive Community Treatment, supported employment, cognitive-behavioral therapy, family-based services, token economy, skills training, psychosocial interventions for alcohol/substance use disorders, and weight management (Dixon et al. 2010).

INDIVIDUAL PSYCHOTHERAPIES FOR SCHIZOPHRENIA

Although individual psychodynamic psychotherapy for schizophrenia has largely been abandoned, a summary of its role will provide a historical context for the discussion of other psychosocial treatments.

The effectiveness of individual psychodynamic psychotherapy for schizophrenia was tested in two landmark studies. May (1968) and colleagues sought to show the effectiveness of psychotherapy alone or in combination with medications. Unexpectedly, the combination of antipsychotic medication and individual therapy conferred no advantage over antipsychotic medication alone. This study, however, was criticized for using relatively inexperienced therapists and a possibly inadequate dose of weekly psychotherapy.

Stanton and colleagues (1984) sought to address the criticisms of the May study by deploying experienced psychotherapists in more intensive treatment. The intensive psychotherapy conditions showed no superiority compared with supportive psychotherapy and were associated with greater attrition, particularly with more severely symptomatic patients. Even among less symptomatic patients, the outcome favored the nonpsychodynamic treatment. The results of these studies and the growing influence of alternative models of psychotherapy have diminished the interest in the psychodynamic treatment of schizophrenia.

More recent approaches to individual therapy, informed by the "stress-vulnerability" hypothesis of schizophrenia, have received study and include individual personal therapy and cognitive-behavioral therapy (CBT). These psychotherapies attempt to ameliorate residual psychotic symptoms and prevent relapse by modifying individual patterns of stress and response to the illness.

PERSONAL THERAPY

Hogarty and colleagues (1995), at the University of Pittsburgh, developed *personal therapy*. They believed that patients with psychotic disorders could benefit by learning to anticipate and manage their episode-related affective arousal and sources of stress. The individualized therapeutic approach used in personal therapy includes stress reduction and cognitive reframing techniques as well as vocational rehabilitation principles.

A 3-year trial of personal therapy (Hogarty et al. 1997a, 1997b) contrasted four treatment conditions: personal therapy, family therapy, supportive therapy, and family therapy combined with personal therapy. The trial found that personal therapy was no more effective than the other therapies in the primary outcome of relapse prevention. However, personal therapy was superior in social adjustment outcomes, with the greatest benefit occurring during the last 2 years of treatment. The study reported that only 60% of the patients in the personal therapy condition were able to progress to the third phase of therapy, in which skills were tested in real-world settings.

COGNITIVE-BEHAVIORAL THERAPY

CBT approaches to schizophrenia draw on previous work in depression and anxiety disorders. Largely led by investigators in the United Kingdom, studies have focused on the use of CBT to address residual psychotic symptoms, whereas more recent studies have sought to apply CBT to acute episodes. One approach, *coping strategy enhancement*, is used to decrease distress by teaching coping mechanisms by which the patient can distract himself or herself and ignore the content of some residual psychotic symptoms. The 2009 PORT psychosocial treatment review recommends offering CBT to persons with schizophrenia who have persistent psychotic symptoms despite adequate pharmacotherapy. Characteristics of successful CBT include 4–9 months of individual or group therapy focusing on both identification and strategies to cope with target symptoms or problems. Controlled trials of CBT treatment support decreasing the severity of delusions, hallucinations, positive symptoms, negative symptoms, and overall symptoms and improving social function (Dixon et al. 2010).

A study by Kuipers and colleagues (1998) randomly assigned 60 individuals with schizophrenia to receive either a 9-month course of CBT plus usual care or usual care alone. Patients receiving CBT had a significant reduction in overall symptom scores (29% for CBT group vs. 2% for control group), delusional distress, and frequency of hallucinations at the end of treatment; these differences continued to be significant 9 months after treatment ended.

Another study by Tarrier and colleagues (1998) compared CBT with supportive counseling and routine care alone and found significant reductions in delusions and hallucinations in the CBT group and at 12-month follow-up (Tarrier et al. 1999). However, at 24 months, the CBT group had lost its advantage over the supportive therapy condition (Tarrier et al. 2000). Sensky and colleagues (2000) compared patients who received routine care in addition to CBT with a befriending intervention of equal intensity. In this study, both groups showed reduced psychotic symptoms after 9 months of treatment. However, at 9-month follow-up, symptom reduction was sustained in the CBT group but not in the comparison condition.

Psychoeducational medication management training, cognitive psychotherapy, cognitive therapy addressed to family members, and standard care were contrasted in various combinations in a study by Buchkremer and colleagues (1997). The intervention lasted 8 months, with follow-up assessments at 1 and 2 years. The treatment group combinations did not show a significant difference in psychopathological symptoms, compliance, or rehospitalization rates compared with the control group. However, the group that received all three interventions showed a trend toward fewer hospitalizations.

Drury and colleagues (1996) attempted to test the efficacy of CBT in acute episodes and found that acutely psychotic inpatients receiving CBT in addition to antipsychotic medication experienced a significantly faster and more complete remission compared with a control group that spent equal hours with a therapist doing structured or supportive activities. At 9-month follow-up, the CBT group continued to report significantly fewer symptoms. One limitation of this study was that psychopathology measures were rated by unblinded treatment staff.

A brief CBT-based intervention known as compliance therapy, targeted at improved adherence to antipsychotic medication regimens in acutely psychotic inpatients, resulted in significant improvements in compliance, attitudes toward drug treatment, and insight into illness compared with control subjects receiving standard treatment (Kemp et al. 1996), although a recent review called for further study to validate its effectiveness (McIntosh et al. 2006).

To date, CBT has not been shown to improve vocational functioning (Kuipers et al. 1997, 1998) or relapse rates (Tarrier et al. 1998). Other areas where CBT effectiveness is not clearly established with limited studies include depression, suicidality, hopelessness, illness insight, relapse, and rehospitalization. Patients with recent-onset schizophrenia or patients who are experiencing an acute exacerbation of psychotic symptoms are not as well studied for adjunctive CBT, and the results seen with these two patient groups are inconsistent (Dixon et al. 2010).

ILLNESS MANAGEMENT AND RECOVERY RESOURCE TOOL KIT

Psychoeducational programs provide individually based information about mental illness, symptoms, the roles of stress and vulnerability, and approaches to treatment. Mueser and colleagues (2002) reviewed the controlled trials of psychoeducational models and found that three out of four controlled studies improved knowledge about mental illness, but only one of these had an appreciable effect on treatment adherence. The authors concluded that psychoeducation should play a role in other interventions but should not be expected to improve treatment outcomes without additional interventions.

Mueser and colleagues (2002) also reviewed other promising approaches to individual treatment and noted that four complementary approaches have a strong evidence base: 1) psychoeducational progams increase knowledge and awareness of illness, 2) behavioral tailoring approaches reduce behavioral barriers to adherence behaviors, 3) warning sign recognition treatment helps avert relapse, and 4) CBT reduces residual psychotic symptomatology. Mueser and colleagues combined these four approaches in a manualized combined intervention termed *Illness Management and Recovery*. The approach also has been developed into an evidence-based resource tool kit and is being disseminated as part of the national Implementing Evidence-Based Practices Project (see http://www.mentalhealthpractices.org).

FAMILY TREATMENT

It is now widely accepted that familial dysfunction is largely secondary to the stress of living with a seriously ill relative. Nevertheless, family stress and distressed interactions do appear to have a significant effect on the course of illness. These distressed family interactions have been defined and referred to as *expressed emotion*. Brown and Rutter (1966) developed the concept of expressed emotion to explain why some hospitalized patients with schizophrenia who had had a good response to pharmacological treatment relapsed soon after returning home. The construct of expressed emotion was empirically derived and refers to three related family behaviors: high frequency of critical comments, hostility, and emotional overinvolvement. Patients with extensive contact with families with high expressed emotion have been found to have significantly higher rates of relapse despite adequate medication compliance (Kavanagh 1992; Leff et al. 1982).

The 2009 PORT study recommends that persons with schizophrenia who interact with family or significant others be ideally offered a family intervention of at least 6–9 months. Most studies of adjunctive family therapy focus on patients with recent illness exacerbation with a goal to reduce rates of relapse and rehospitalization. Important facets of effective family interventions include illness education, crisis intervention, emotional support, and training for addressing illness symptoms and related problems. Patients may experience reduced psychiatric symptoms, improved treatment adherence as well as functional and vocational status. Families may benefit from reduced family burden and improved satisfaction with family relationships (Dixon et al. 2010). Most controlled clinical interventions have documented the effectiveness of various family interventions for reducing relapse in the index patient (Leff 1996). Relapse rates for patients with schizophrenia whose families undergo psychoeducational and stress-modifying family treatment are approximately 24% compared with 64% for routine treatment (Mueser and Glynn 1998), similar to the magnitude of treatment effect seen with maintenance antipsychotic medication. Interventions that are longer in duration (typically longer than 9 months) appear to provide long-term relapse prevention and have been found to persist for 2 years (Mueser and Glynn 1998) or longer (Tarrier et al. 1994).

Reduction of high expressed emotion has been hypothesized to be the key ingredient in the efficacy of family interventions. In interventions with families with high expressed emotion, nonrelapsing patients were more likely to reside in families that had changed from high to low expressed emotion during treatment (Falloon et al. 1982; Hogarty et al. 1986; Leff et al. 1982; Tarrier et al. 1988).

The Treatment Strategies for Schizophrenia Study (Schooler et al. 1997) was one of the few large-scale studies investigating the efficacy of maintenance medication treatment combined with family intervention. The study showed that relatively nonintensive multifamily psychoeducational monthly groups provided equal long-term relapse prevention compared with more intensive family treatment.

McFarlane and colleagues (1996) studied schizophrenia patients at high risk for relapse because of histories of poor compliance, violence, and homelessness. Half of the patients and families received biweekly multifamily group treatment, and half received family intervention only during crises. No differences in relapse were seen for the two treatment groups (27% at

2 years), again suggesting that more intensive family treatment is not necessarily better.

Family intervention studies also have yielded negative findings. In a study of adolescent patients early in the illness, Linszen and colleagues (Linszen et al. 1996; Nugter et al. 1997) found that both the group receiving family treatment and the control group had equally low (16%–20%) overall relapse rates at 1 year, although the active comparison intervention involved a fairly intensive individual treatment approach. Similarly, in Hogarty and colleagues' (1997b) study of personal therapy, their family therapy arm offered no advantage over supportive therapy in preventing relapse, which was relatively low at 29% over 3 years. In studies with newer antipsychotic regimens with potentially lower relapse rates (Csernansky et al. 2002), the effects of family intervention may be more difficult to detect.

Family intervention studies also have improved outcomes in family stress, coping, and knowledge of schizophrenia (Barrowclough and Tarrier 1990; Dixon et al. 2001; Falloon et al. 1987; McFarlane et al. 1996; Zhang and Yan 1993). However, these improved outcomes may be highly correlated with reduced relapse, suggesting no independent effect of family intervention on these outcomes. Interest in family treatment approaches should be stimulated by dissemination of a "Family Psychoeducation" resource tool kit through the national Implementing Evidence-Based Practices Project (Dixon et al. 2001).

SOCIAL SKILLS TRAINING

Even with the anticipated development of more efficacious medication regimens, most patients with schizophrenia will likely continue to have residual symptoms, cognitive impairments, and impaired social skills. Systematic research over the past several decades has sought to use psychosocial interventions to reduce functional impairments in schizophrenia. Social skills training (SST) is a carefully defined set of interventions specifically targeted toward acquisition of social functioning skills. There are currently three models of SST:

1. *Basic*—entails identifying and "overlearning" components of social interactions through repetition.
2. *Social problem solving*—attempts to correct deficits in receptive learning, processing, and sending skills.
3. *Cognitive remediation*—targets more fundamental cognitive impairments, including attention and planning.

BASIC MODEL

The basic SST model entails breaking down complex social repertoires into their basic elements, such as eye contact, speech volume, length of response, questioning, and other behaviors. Through repetitive practice and modeling by the therapist, new skills are acquired and then developed into a functional repertoire. The patient uses role-playing to practice integrating the social repertoires with the therapist and peers and is directed to practice in a real-world setting.

This model can be successfully implemented, with acquisition of social skills that persist anywhere between 6 and 12 months (Bellack and Mueser 1993). It is unclear whether the improvement in these social skills generalizes to improved symptomatology and reduced relapse rates. Investigators in Pittsburgh, Pennsylvania (Hogarty et al. 1986, 1991), found that patients receiving an intensive trial of SST combined with antipsychotic medications had a significantly lower relapse rate than did a group receiving only medications (30% vs. 46%). These gains persisted at 21 months but not at 24 months. This finding suggests that SST and other psychosocial interventions may require booster sessions or ongoing treatment in order to maintain a favorable effect.

SOCIAL PROBLEM-SOLVING MODEL

The social problem-solving model assumes that impairments in information processing underlie the limited social competence present in many patients with schizophrenia. Specific domains of skill acquisition are broken down into modules on medication management, symptom management, recreation, basic conversation, and self-care. Patients can be assigned the modules that are the most salient. It is hoped that greater durability and generalization of social skills will be acquired through emphasis on learning, receiving, processing, and retaining skills. Marder and colleagues (1996) found a small but statistically significant advantage for the problem-solving intervention over supportive therapy in two of six measures of social adjustment after 2 years. Liberman and colleagues (1998) found that a problem-solving group had superior outcomes over occupational therapy in 3 of 10 independent living skills that were maintained up to 18 months after completion of the intervention.

COGNITIVE REMEDIATION

Although patients with schizophrenia clearly have a wide range of cognitive impairments (Braff 1993), some deficits have been attributed to psychotic symptoms or medication side effects. Cognitive impairments associated with schizophrenia have not been definitively characterized, but some particular functions such as attention, memory, and planning appear to be more affected than others. Psychopharmacological interventions to ameliorate or prevent cognitive deficits are active areas of investigation. In addition, the practice of cognitive remediation of schizophrenia is an area of intensive investigation.

Given the limitations on the durability and generalizability of SST, researchers have sought to improve the impairments in elementary cognitive functions before teaching social skills as a way to "boost" the effectiveness of SST. Cognitive remediation shows some promise in improving performance and measures of vigilance and planning. However, insufficient evidence shows that these improvements generalize to other cognitive tests or particular social skills.

Integrated psychological treatment (Brenner et al. 1992), developed by researchers in Switzerland, is based on the theory that dysfunctions in lower and higher levels of cognitive deficits interact to diminish social competence, leading to increased stress resulting from difficult social interactions and to further impairment in cognitive functioning. Integrated psychological treatment includes sequential subprograms targeted to cognitive social functioning: the cognitive differentiation subprogram emphasizes treatment of basic cognitive skills through computer-based training in card sorting and concept formation; social perception and verbal communication subprograms refine these skills into verbal and social responses through social problem-solving exercises; and social skills and interpersonal problem-solving subprograms address more complex interpersonal problems through similar techniques to the motor skills models.

Outcome studies of cognitive remediation have been mixed. A study by Wykes and colleagues (1999) comparing intensive cognitive remediation and comparably intensive occupational therapy targeting deficits in executive functioning showed improvements in 3 of 12 cognitive measures but no direct improvements in social or vocational functioning or symptomatology. In a study of cognitive remediation before skills training, compared with a mirror image regimen, Hodel and Brenner (1994) found no advantage to initial treatment with cognitive remediation. In contrast, a recent meta-analysis by McGurk and colleagues (2007) reported improved outcomes across the domains of cognitive performance, symptoms, and psychosocial functioning.

Ninety severely impaired long-term hospital patients were offered equally intensive 6-month duration cognitive remediation plus social problem-solving modules compared with supportive therapy also paired with social problem-solving modules (Spaulding et al. 1999). The cognitive remediation group had better outcomes in two of four measures of social competence and showed better acquisition of skills in two of four of the social problem-solving modules, suggesting that the cognitive remediation approach can enhance response to more standard skills training in very ill institutionalized patients.

An additional approach to SST is embodied by the clubhouse model of psychosocial rehabilitation. Originated in 1948 at Fountain House in New York City, the clubhouse model was developed as a collaborative community of professional staff and persons with mental illness (Anderson 1998; Macias et al. 2001). Community activities within the clubhouse focus on the work-ordered day, in which staff and patients work together to maintain clubhouse functions, with the expectation that patients will gain social and vocational skills and ultimately transition to competitive employment with the support of clubhouse-related transitional vocational programs. The clubhouse model has been widely disseminated, and efforts since the late 1970s have focused on enhancing program fidelity. Clubhouses are highly regarded among patients but have been subject to little empirical study. Nonetheless, they represent an important and likely predominant method of social skills enhancement in the United States.

Newly developing programs run by consumers based on self-help principles are also spreading rapidly in many states (Yanos et al. 2001). Many patients with serious mental illness have highlighted the importance of their participation in peer-run or self-help programs. Patients point to the role of self-help and peer-led services in promoting psychological well-being, empowerment, and sense of self-efficacy. There has been little empirical research on the effectiveness of self-help organizations and related interventions. Emerging empirical work on consumer-run and self-help services will elucidate the role of these services in community programs.

SUPPORTED EMPLOYMENT

The proportion of persons with chronic schizophrenia with competitive employment is 20% or lower (Bond et al. 2001a). Lack of sustainable living wages increases dependence on families and public assistance, contributes to low self-esteem and stigma, and often leads to a lack of daily structure and sense of purpose. With ever-shortening hospital stays, hospital-based vocational rehabilitation programs are no longer feasible, and vocational rehabilitation is largely community-based. Unfortunately, many approaches to vocational rehabilitation are not well suited to address the long-term impairment often associated with schizophrenia. In contrast to vocational rehabilitation programs in which patients are trained and then placed in the job, newer vocational models reverse that process.

A standardized approach to supported employment has been termed *individual placement and support*. The principles of individual placement and support have evolved as research shows how to improve employment outcomes (Becker and Drake 2003; Bond et al. 2001a, 2001b; Dixon et al. 2010; Drake et al. 1999; Lehman et al. 2002).

Key principles of the individual placement and support model include

1. *Competitive employment*—The goal of supported employment is competitive employment in work settings integrated into the community.
2. *Rapid job search*—Searching for jobs occurs early in the process of supported employment rather than following lengthy pre-employment assessment, training, or work trials.
3. *Integration of rehabilitation and mental health*—Vocational rehabilitation is considered an integral component of mental health treatment rather than a separate service. Optimally, employment specialists are integrated into multidisciplinary teams.
4. *Patient preferences*—Services are based on patients' preferences and choices rather than on providers' judgments.
5. *Continuous and comprehensive assessment*—Assessment occurs primarily in the course of community work experiences.
6. *Ongoing support*—Follow-along supports are tailored to the individual patient's needs and continued indefinitely.

Traditional vocational rehabilitation programs had limited success because workshop-based or sheltered employment skills were not generalizable to competitive employment settings (Bond et al. 2001a). In contrast, findings from studies of the supported employment model have been consistently positive. RCTs consistently demonstrate supported employment as effective in helping persons with schizophrenia achieve competitive employment, work more hours, and earn more than individuals without this intervention. The PORT 2009 treatment recommendations include offering supported employment to any person with schizophrenia who expresses this goal (Dixon et al. 2010). Individual placement and support has shown effectiveness in diverse patient samples in New Hampshire and Washington, D.C. (Drake et al. 1999). An additional study compared individual placement and support with a standard psychosocial rehabilitation program in a population with severe mental illness and high rates of substance abuse and reported that the individual placement and support group was significantly more likely to obtain employment—42% vs. 1%—although job retention was low, leveling off at 15%–20% (Lehman et al. 2002). The availability of a treatment manual for individual placement and support (Becker and Drake 1993) and a supported employment resource tool kit (Bond et al. 2001a) should stimulate further research into this treatment modality.

ASSERTIVE COMMUNITY TREATMENT

As a response to service fragmentation, the Assertive Community Treatment (ACT) program was originally developed by researchers in Madison, Wisconsin (Stein and Test 1980). ACT is currently the most carefully studied, defined, documented, and successful program being used in the delivery of services for persons with severe mental illness. In most ACT programs, patients are served by a multidisciplinary team that has a fixed caseload of patients and a high staff-to-patient ratio (1:10–12). ACT programs provide treatment, rehabilitation, and supports in the community 24 hours a day, 7 days a week. Services often provided include home delivery of medications, monitoring of physical and mental health, SST in the patient's natural environment, and support for family reintegration.

The landmark ACT study in Wisconsin (Stein and Test 1980) examined outcomes in a group of severely mentally ill patients assigned to ACT compared with a group discharged from the hospital to standard community care. The ACT group showed significant advantages in rates of hospitalization, employment, independent living, and family burden, with essentially no difference in costs; however, the advantages conferred by ACT did not persist after the patients were discharged from the experimental program. More than 25 control trials have shown the effectiveness of ACT in reducing hospitalization and other adverse outcomes and increasing patients' and their families' satisfaction (Burns and Santos 1995). A meta-analysis (Coldwell and Bender 2007) including six RCTs revealed that ACT also decreased homelessness 37% more than standard care.

Bond and co-workers (2001b) reviewed the evidence on outcomes for ACT services. Twenty-three controlled studies examined hospital outcomes for ACT patients and for those served by comparison programs. Seventeen trials found ACT to be superior in reducing hospital use. Similarly, of 12 studies examining residential stability, 8 studies found superior housing stability in the ACT condition, although one study found poorer outcomes for ACT patients. Of 16 studies that examined symptomatic outcomes in ACT programs, 7 trials found ACT to be superior. Quality of life was demonstrably superior in 7 of 12 control trials, and social adjustment improved in 3 of 13 trials. Jail or arrests were reduced in only 2 of 10 trials, and in one trial, poorer outcomes were found in the ACT condition. Substance abuse was improved in 2 of 6 trials. Medication adherence was improved in 2 of 4 studies. Vocational outcomes were improved in 3 of 8 studies. Consumer satisfaction was improved in 7 of 8 studies. Despite these impressive outcomes, these studies show that several outcome domains remain in which the performance of ACT could be improved, specifically in the areas of substance abuse, medication adherence, and vocational outcomes. New models of ACT, which integrate substance abuse treatment and supported employment, hold promise for improving these outcomes.

Because of the complexity of the services provided by ACT, it is difficult to answer several questions about its effectiveness, including

- What are the key ingredients that prevent relapse and hospitalization?
- Is ACT more cost-effective than other high-intensity services or modified ACT models?
- What minimum program intensity is needed to maintain gains?
- Which special populations of patients may require indefinite treatment?

It is clear, however, that programs that maintain good fidelity to the original ACT model have better outcomes (Scott and Dixon 1995). Dissemination of an ACT resource tool kit (Phillips et al. 2001) should strengthen interest in the fidelity of ACT in community programs.

PSYCHOSOCIAL APPROACHES FOR SUBSTANCE ABUSE

The 2009 PORT study (Dixon et al. 2010) recommends that persons with schizophrenia and a comorbid alcohol or drug use disorder should be offered treatments for their substance use disorders. Effective interventions generally include motivational therapies, coping skills and relapse prevention training, and integration with mental health care. The most consistently effective interventions are professional-led dual diagnosis groups and residential treatments, suggesting that peer supports are critical (Drake et al. 2008). Most studies include clients with serious mental illnesses, not just those with schizophrenia. RCTs of persons receiving integrated interventions for co-occurring substance use disorders support improved treatment attendance, decreased substance use/relapse, decreased symptoms, and increased functioning. One critical finding is that clients with co-occurring disorders benefit from supported employment and typically begin working several months before they attain full remissions of their substance use disorders (Xie et al. 2010).

CONCLUSION

Although antipsychotic medications were major advancements in schizophrenia therapeutics and helped make possible the era of deinstitutionalization, merely preventing rehospitalization can no longer be viewed as the final goal of treatment. Many patients can be maintained as outpatients despite persistent psychotic symptoms, pervasive negative symptoms, and poor social competence, but these residual impairments can no longer be regarded as acceptable outcomes. Newer antipsychotic drugs may significantly improve compliance, treatment of symptoms, and possibly relapse rates and overall outcome compared with the first generation of antipsychotics. Pharmacological interventions aimed at deficit symptoms may become available in the future as well.

Psychosocial interventions clearly will retain a pivotal place in the modern therapeutic armamentarium. Relatively simple interventions such as sustained family interventions and more comprehensive ACT programs are demonstrably effective in preventing relapse and hospital recidivism, and patients with treatment-resistant psychotic symptoms may benefit from new modalities of CBT. For patients with persistent negative symptoms and impaired social competence, SST shows great promise and should be more broadly available to such patients. As empirically validated therapies continue to emerge, implementation of these new treatment strategies in usual care settings will require careful attention.

It is also important to acknowledge emerging trends in psychosocial services and research—even though many newer approaches have not been definitively studied. Newer interventions are based on commonsense approaches to helping patients adapt and adjust to serious psychiatric disorders. These approaches generally involve use of education, skills training, and natural supports to help people learn to manage their own illnesses, to improve their functioning in normal adult roles, to reintegrate into their communities, and to pursue improved quality of life. These model approaches also place a primary focus on developing trusting, collaborative relationships between practitioners and patients to help patients pursue their own goals. Even though these approaches are termed *recovery-oriented* treatments, they share a hopeful outlook regarding long-term outcomes, a focus on patient preferences for outcomes and choice of interventions, and a focus on helping people to achieve community integration and to function in the real-life settings of their choice.

REFERENCES

Anderson SB: We Are Not Alone: Fountain House and the Development of Clubhouse Culture. New York, Fountain House, 1998

Barrowclough C, Tarrier N: Social functioning in schizophrenic patients, I: the effects of expressed emotion and family intervention. Soc Psychiatry Psychiatr Epidemiol 25:125–129, 1990

Becker DR, Drake RE: A Working Life: The Individual Placement and Support (IPS) Program. Concord, New Hampshire–Dartmouth Psychiatric Research Center, 1993

Becker DR, Drake RE: A Working Life for People With Severe Mental Illness. New York, Oxford University Press, 2003

Bellack AS, Mueser KT: Psychosocial treatment for schizophrenia. Schizophr Bull 19:317–336, 1993

Bond GR, Becker DR, Drake RE, et al: Implementing supported employment as an evidence-based practice. Psychiatr Serv 52:313–322, 2001a

Bond GR, Drake RE, Mueser KT, et al: Assertive community treatment for people with severe mental illness. Disease Management and Health Outcomes 9:141–159, 2001b

Braff DL: Information processing and attention dysfunctions in schizophrenia. Schizophr Bull 19:233–259, 1993

Brenner HD, Hodel B, Roder V, et al: Treatment of cognitive dysfunctions and behavioral deficits in schizophrenia. Schizophr Bull 18:21–26, 1992

Brown GW, Rutter M: The measurement of family activities and relationships: a methodological study. Hum Relat 2 (suppl):10–15, 1966

Buchkremer G, Klingberg S, Holle R, et al: Psychoeducational psychotherapy for schizophrenic patients and their key relatives or care-givers: results of a 2-year follow-up. Acta Psychiatr Scand 96:483–491, 1997

Burns BJ, Santos AB: Assertive community treatment: an update of randomized trials. Psychiatr Serv 46:669–675, 1995

Coldwell CM, Bender WS: The effectiveness of assertive community treatment for homeless populations with severe mental illness: a meta-analysis. Am J Psychiatry 164:393–399, 2007

Csernansky JG, Mahmoud R, Brenner R: A comparison of risperidone and haloperidol for the prevention of relapse in patients with schizophrenia. N Engl J Med 346:16–22, 2002

Dixon L, McFarlane WR, Lefley H, et al: Evidence-based practices for services to families of people with psychiatric disabilities. Psychiatr Serv 52:903–910, 2001

Dixon L, Dickerson F, Bellack AS, et al: The 2009 schizophrenia PORT psychosocial treatment recommendations and summary statements. Schizophr Bull 36:48–70, 2010

Drake RE, McHugo GJ, Bebout RR, et al: A randomized clinical trial of supported employment for inner-city patients with severe mental disorders. Arch Gen Psychiatry 56:627–633, 1999

Drake RE, O'Neal EL, Wallach MA: A systematic review of psychosocial interventions for people with co-occurring substance use and severe mental disorders. J Subst Abuse Treat 34:123–138, 2008

Drury V, Birchwood M, Cochrane R, et al: Cognitive therapy and recovery from acute psychosis: a controlled trial, I: impact on psychotic symptoms. Br J Psychiatry 169:593–601, 1996

Falloon IR, Boyd JL, McGill CW, et al: Family management in the prevention of exacerbations of schizophrenia: a controlled study. N Engl J Med 306:1437–1440, 1982

Falloon IR, McGill CW, Boyd JL, et al: Family management in the prevention of morbidity of schizophrenia: social outcome of a two-year longitudinal study. Psychol Med 17:59–66, 1987

Hodel B, Brenner HD: Cognitive therapy with schizophrenic patients: conceptual basis, present state, future directions. Acta Psychiatr Scand Suppl 384:108–115, 1994

Hogarty GE, Anderson CM, Reiss DJ, et al: Family psychoeducation, social skills training, and maintenance chemotherapy in the aftercare treatment of schizophrenia, I: one-year effects of a controlled study on relapse and expressed emotion. Arch Gen Psychiatry 43:633–642, 1986

Hogarty GE, Anderson CM, Reiss DJ, et al: Family psychoeducation, social skills training, and maintenance chemotherapy in the aftercare treatment of schizophrenia, II: two-year effects of a controlled study on relapse and adjustment. Environmental-Personal Indicators in the Course of Schizophrenia (EPICS) Research Group. Arch Gen Psychiatry 48:340–347, 1991

Hogarty GE, Kornblith SJ, Greenwald D, et al: Personal therapy: a disorder-relevant psychotherapy for schizophrenia. Schizophr Bull 21:379–393, 1995

Hogarty GE, Greenwald D, Ulrich RF, et al: Three-year trials of personal therapy among schizophrenic patients living with or independent of family, II: effects on adjustment of patients. Am J Psychiatry 154:1514–1524, 1997a

Hogarty GE, Kornblith SJ, Greenwald D, et al: Three-year trials of personal therapy among schizophrenic patients living with or independent of family, I: description of study and effects on relapse rates. Am J Psychiatry 154:1504–1513, 1997b

Kavanagh DJ: Recent developments in expressed emotion and schizophrenia. Br J Psychiatry 160:601–620, 1992

Kemp R, Hayward P, Applewhaite G, et al: Compliance therapy in psychotic patients: randomized controlled trial. BMJ 312:345–349, 1996

Kuipers E, Garety P, Fowler D, et al: London-East Anglia randomized controlled trial of cognitive-behavioural therapy for psychosis, I: effects of the treatment phase. Br J Psychiatry 171:319–327, 1997

Kuipers E, Fowler D, Garety P, et al: London-East Anglia randomized controlled trial of cognitive-behavioural therapy for psychosis, III: follow-up and economic evaluation at 18 months. Br J Psychiatry 173:61–68, 1998

Lauriello J, Lenroot R, Bustillo JR: Maximizing the synergy between pharmacotherapy and psychosocial therapies for schizophrenia. Psychiatr Clin North Am 26:191–211, 2003

Leff J: First perceptions of treatment: the physician-family patient network. Journal of Practical Psychiatry and Behavioral Health 2:10–15, 1996

Leff J, Kuipers L, Berkowitz R, et al: A controlled trial of social intervention in the families of schizophrenia patients. Br J Psychiatry 141:121–134, 1982

Lehman AF, Goldberg R, Dixon LB, et al: Improving employment outcomes for persons with severe mental illnesses. Arch Gen Psychiatry 59:165–172, 2002

Liberman RP, Wallace CJ, Blackwell G, et al: Skills training versus psychosocial occupational therapy for persons with persistent schizophrenia. Am J Psychiatry 155:1087–1091, 1998

Linszen D, Dingemans P, Van der Does JW, et al: Treatment, expressed emotion and relapse in recent onset schizophrenic disorders. Psychol Med 26:333–342, 1996

Macias C, Barreira P, Alden M, et al: The ICCD benchmarks for clubhouses: a practical approach to quality improvement in psychiatric rehabilitation. Psychiatr Serv 52:207–213, 2001

Marder SR, Wirshing WC, Mintz J, et al: Two-year outcome of social skills training and group psychotherapy for outpatients with schizophrenia. Am J Psychiatry 153:1585–1592, 1996

May PRA: Treatment of Schizophrenia: A Comparative Study of Five Treatment Models. New York, Science House, 1968

McFarlane WR, Dushay RA, Stastny P, et al: A comparison of two levels of family aided assertive community treatment. Psychiatr Serv 47:744–750, 1996

McGurk SR, Twamley EW, Sitzer DI, et al: A meta-analysis of cognitive remediation in schizophrenia. Am J Psychiatry 164:1791–1802, 2007

McIntosh A, Conlon L, Lawrie S, et al: Compliance therapy for schizophrenia. Cochrane Database Syst Rev 2006;3:CD003442

Mueser KT, Glynn SM: Family intervention for schizophrenia, in Best Practice: Developing and Promoting Empirically Supported Interventions. Edited by Dobson KS, Craig KE. Newbury Park, CA, Sage, 1998, pp 157–186

Mueser KT, Corrigan PW, Hilton DW, et al: Illness management and recovery: a review of the research. Psychiatr Serv 53:1272–1284, 2002

Nugter A, Dingemans P, Van der Does JW, et al: Family treatment, expressed emotion and relapse in recent onset schizophrenia. Psychiatry Res 72:23–31, 1997

Phillips SD, Burns BJ, Edgar ER, et al: Moving assertive community treatment into standard practice. Psychiatr Serv 52:771–779, 2001

Schooler NR, Keith SJ, Severe JB, et al: Relapse and rehospitalization during maintenance treatment of schizophrenia: the effects of dose reduction and family treatment. Arch Gen Psychiatry 54:453–463, 1997

Scott JE, Dixon LB: Assertive community treatment and case management for schizophrenia. Schizophr Bull 21:657–668, 1995

Sensky T, Turkington D, Kingdon D, et al: A randomized controlled trial of cognitive-behavioral therapy for persistent symptoms in schizophrenia resistant to medication. Arch Gen Psychiatry 57:165–172, 2000

Spaulding WD, Reed D, Sullivan M, et al: Effects of cognitive treatment in psychiatric rehabilitation. Schizophr Bull 25:657–676, 1999

Stanton AH, Gunderson JG, Knapp PH, et al: Effects of psychotherapy in schizophrenia, I: designed implementation of a controlled study. Schizophr Bull 10:520–563, 1984

Stein LI, Test MA: Alternative to mental hospital treatment, I: conceptual model, treatment program, and clinical evaluation. Arch Gen Psychiatry 37:392–397, 1980

Tarrier N, Barrowclough C, Vaughn C, et al: The community management of schizophrenia: a controlled trial of a behavioural intervention with families to reduce relapse. Br J Psychiatry 153:532–542, 1988

Tarrier N, Barrowclough C, Porceddu K, et al: The Salford Family Intervention Project: relapse rates of schizophrenia at five and eight years. Br J Psychiatry 165:829–832, 1994

Tarrier N, Yusupoff L, Kinney C, et al: Randomised controlled trial of intensive cognitive behaviour therapy for patients with chronic schizophrenia. BMJ 317:303–307, 1998

Tarrier N, Wittkowski A, Kinney C, et al: Durability of the effects of cognitive-behavioural therapy in the treatment of chronic schizophrenia: 12-month follow-up. Br J Psychiatry 174:500–504, 1999

Tarrier N, Kinney C, McCarthy E, et al: Two-year follow-up of cognitive-behavioral therapy and supportive counseling in the treatment of persistent symptoms in chronic schizophrenia. J Consult Clin Psychol 68:917–922, 2000

Wykes T, Reeder C, Corner J, et al: The effects of neurocognitive remediation on executive processing in patients with schizophrenia. Schizophr Bull 25:291–307, 1999

Xie H, Drake RE, McHugo GJ, et al: The 10-year course of remission, abstinence, and recovery in dual diagnosis. J Subst Abuse Treat 39:132–140, 2010

Yanos PT, Primavera LH, Knight EL: Consumer-run service participation, recovery of social functioning, and the mediating role of psychological factors. Psychiatr Serv 52:493–500, 2001

Zhang M, Yan H: Effectiveness of psychoeducation of relatives of schizophrenia patients: a prospective cohort study of five cities of China. Int J Ment Health 22:47–59, 1993

CHAPTER

10

TREATMENT OF CHRONIC SCHIZOPHRENIA

ALEXANDER L. MILLER, M.D.

JOSEPH P. MCEVOY, M.D.

DILIP V. JESTE, M.D.

STEPHEN R. MARDER, M.D.

The advent of new antipsychotics, and of psychosocial interventions that demonstrably improve patient functioning, has made treatment of chronic schizophrenia very different now than it was 20 years ago. Goals of treatment should be loftier than keeping patients out of the hospital and managing side effects. However, few patients become symptom-free and without need for medication or other interventions. Thus, long-term treatment of schizophrenia means long-term efforts to optimize outcomes and minimize morbidity and suffering. Such efforts represent an ongoing problem-solving exercise, in which both patients and treatments change over time.

Our goal in this chapter is to highlight issues that arise repeatedly in chronic schizophrenia and to present evidence to help guide treatment selection. We describe a set of principles for treating the multiple facets of schizophrenia over the course of illness after the first episode and address a series of frequently asked questions faced by psychiatrists in their daily work with patients with schizophrenia.

PRINCIPLES OF LONG-TERM TREATMENT

DIAGNOSIS

The diagnosis of schizophrenia has major implications for treatment and prognosis, as well as for eligibility for public assistance programs. Especially in the early years of illness, diagnosis may be confounded by substance abuse, prominent affective symptoms, denial of symptoms, and the hope that the illness is something other than schizophrenia. Clinicians are understandably reluctant to label patients, but making the correct diagnosis is a critical step. As the course of illness and response to treatment unfold, diagnosis must be updated.

INTEGRATION OF TREATMENTS

The New Freedom Commission on Mental Health (2003) found that mental health care in the United States is fragmented. Patients with chronic schizophrenia must deal with multiple different providers of care and resources, while experiencing some degree of cognitive impairment and disorganization (Palmer et al. 1997). Thus, the treatment plan must be integrative, not compartmentalized. Because physician time is costly, the task of integrating care often falls to nonphysicians, with physicians in the role of prescribing medications and supervising other members of the treatment team. However, prescribing cannot occur in a vacuum of knowledge about living environment, resources, and social circumstances, which can hugely affect prescribing decisions. Conversely, psychotropic medications, and their side effects, can profoundly affect progress toward other goals, such as work and independent living.

DOCUMENTATION

A review of medical record documentation of psychotic symptoms and medication side effects in patients with schizophrenia found that symptom documentation was incomplete 55% of the time and that side-effect documentation was incomplete 85% of the time, when chart documentation was compared with direct patient observations made by trained investigators (Cradock et al. 2001). In mental health clinics, physician turnover is often high and unscheduled visits are common. Under these conditions, if the chart does not convey the information needed to make rational prescribing decisions, the potential for erratic and inconsistent decision making is enormous, and physician time is inefficiently spent trying to extract historical treatment details from patients and their families.

Although documentation is an individual responsibility, much of the care of patients with chronic schizophrenia occurs in organizations such as hospitals and clinics. There is an organizational responsibility to work with practitioners to identify which critical elements of information are needed (and how often) and then to structure paper or electronic record keeping to facilitate documentation of these elements.

CONTEXT

Patients with schizophrenia are affected by physical environment and by family and social environments. Many of these contextual factors can be improved (or made less stressful) by proven therapeutic interventions that change the patient's family, work, or physical environment (e.g., Drake et al. 1996; Pitschel-Walz et al. 2001; Velligan et al. 2000). In addition, the patient's own view and understanding of his or her illness is important. Denial of illness is a strong predictor of medication nonadherence and of relapse (Perkins 2002; Zygmunt et al. 2002). Thus, the treatment team should evaluate and, as indicated, work to change the context within which the patient operates, including patient understanding and perceptions.

COMMON CLINICAL QUESTIONS

WHAT ARE THE OPTIONS FOR ANTIPSYCHOTIC TREATMENT FAILURES?

In an illness that, for most patients, needs treatment for decades, decisions about how to handle treatment failures are far more frequent than decisions about what to start at the outset of the illness. Moreover, even though a large majority of patients with chronic schizophrenia in the United States are now taking second-generation antipsychotics, many have had one or more trials of first-generation antipsychotics in the past. Thus, the most common clinical

decision about what to do next is for the patient who has failed or been intol-
erant of at least one first-generation antipsychotic and at least one second-
generation antipsychotic.

Most of the literature on randomized controlled trials of antipsychotics in
chronic schizophrenia consists of parallel-group studies comparing antipsychotics with one another or with placebo. This study design yields no information about how to treat those who do poorly on their assigned treatment.
By far, the highest-quality evidence for how to treat antipsychotic medication
failures comes from multiple studies of clozapine that showed its unique
value for treatment-refractory schizophrenia (Kane et al. 1988, 2001).

Findings from several studies of switching between antipsychotics have
been published and typically show that patients do better on a new antipsychotic
(Casey et al. 2003a; C.T. Lee et al. 2002; Weiden et al. 1997, 2003). Unfortunately, most of these studies are designed to address the question of how
best to switch from current medications to a new one rather than quantifying
the benefits of switching. To answer the latter question, the study needs to
include a group that is not switched so that the effects of time and natural
variation in illness severity can be controlled for. Published switch studies that
lack this comparison group do not inform us if improved outcomes after
switching are a result of the new medication or other factors. However, a secondary analysis of the Clinical Antipsychotic Trials of Intervention Effectiveness (CATIE) results showed that patients who were taking olanzapine or risperidone and were randomly assigned to stay on that drug stayed on it longer
than they stayed on a new drug if they were randomly assigned to start a different antipsychotic (Essock et al. 2006).

Various expert consensus guidelines and algorithms have attempted to
guide clinicians in selecting a rational sequence of medication treatments for
chronic schizophrenia (Altamura et al. 1997; "Canadian Clinical Practice
Guidelines for the Treatment of Schizophrenia" 1998; Frances et al. 1996;
Kane et al. 2003; Lehman et al. 2004; McEvoy et al. 1999; Miller et al. 1999,
2004; Moore et al. 2007; Pearsall et al. 1998; Smith and Docherty 1998;
Stahl 1999). The recommendations in these guidelines and algorithms are
based on a mixture of established evidence and expert opinion. An antipsychotic algorithm based solely on data from two or more methodologically
sound randomized controlled efficacy trials for schizophrenia would have
two recommendations: 1) begin with an antipsychotic that does not carry a
"black box" warning from the U.S. Food and Drug Administration (FDA),
and 2) use clozapine for treatment-refractory schizophrenia. Among the
guidelines, the Schizophrenia Patient Outcomes Research Team (PORT) re-
lies least upon expert opinion. The Schizophrenia PORT recommends any
antipsychotic other than clozapine for treatment of multi-episode schizophre-

nia that is expected to be treatment responsive, and recommends clozapine for patients with refractory symptoms (Buchanan et al. 2010). In all situations, patient preferences and variable risks of adverse effects among antipsychotics are key considerations in making an antipsychotic choice.

WHAT ARE THE OPTIONS FOR PATIENTS WITH TREATMENT-REFRACTORY SCHIZOPHRENIA?

The terms *treatment refractory* and *treatment resistant* usually refer to persistent positive symptoms in a person who has had two or more adequate antipsychotic trials (Buckley et al. 2001). Functional impairment is not specified but implied. That is, residual psychotic symptoms that have little or no effect on day-to-day functioning are not viewed as warranting aggressive changes in therapy to totally eliminate them.

As noted in Chapter 8 ("Pharmacotherapies") in this volume, clozapine should be tried in *every* patient with treatment-refractory schizophrenia who does not have a specific contraindication. However, about half of this group will have an inadequate response to clozapine. Before concluding that clozapine is ineffective, the clinician should use blood levels to verify that an adequate trial has been achieved. Evidence suggests that a plasma clozapine concentration of 350 ng/mL or more is needed for optimal effectiveness (Perry 2001).

There is little to guide clinicians when clozapine does not work. Because the literature is so sparse, most treatment guidelines have no recommendations for treating this population. When expert groups have addressed the issue, clozapine augmentation is the first-choice recommendation for those patients with an inadequate response to clozapine (McEvoy et al. 1999; Miller et al. 1999, 2004; Moore et al. 2007). However, the recent literature on clozapine augmentation has been quite mixed, with no consistent winning combination (see section on combination antipsychotics, later in this chapter).

For patients who refuse clozapine, medication options are to administer an antipsychotic that has not already been used (including a first-generation antipsychotic if the patient has no history of failure to respond to one from this group) or a combination of agents. A patient history of having had a partial response to an earlier antipsychotic trial would suggest that this agent should be one of the components of a trial of combined antipsychotics.

Nonmedication interventions may be very useful for patients with refractory symptoms. For example, there is evidence that cognitive-behavioral therapy can modify problematic behavioral responses to persistent psychosis (Tai and Turkington 2009). Strong evidence shows that family members and other caregivers can benefit from support, support groups, and multiple family therapy (Dixon et al. 2001).

WHAT IS THE EVIDENCE REGARDING POLYPHARMACY?

In the United States, 10%–20% of patients with schizophrenia are simultaneously taking more than one antipsychotic drug, but the prevalence of this practice may well be even higher in some settings (Correll et al. 2007; Miller and Craig 2002). Most combinations have not been systematically studied (Gören et al. 2008). However, studies that added risperidone to clozapine have shown mixed results, with studies of longer duration and lower doses more likely to show benefit for the combination (Kontaxakis et al. 2006). Absence of evidence for efficacy of combination antipsychotics does not mean that they are ineffective for individual patients, but it does mean that clinicians should carefully evaluate the effects of the combination relative to monotherapies, including clozapine, and document their superiority. In addition to the lack of evidence supporting this strategy, reasons for not using combination antipsychotics include added side-effect burden, increased risk of harmful drug–drug interactions, decreased adherence, difficulties in making rational dose adjustments, and increased costs (Miller and Craig 2002).

The 2009 Schizophrenia PORT (Buchanan et al. 2010) concluded that there were insufficient data to support the use of lithium or anticonvulsants as an adjunct for persistent symptoms. However, there is some evidence supporting the combination of clozapine with lamotrigine (Dursun and Deakin 2001; Dursun et al. 1999) although the magnitude of the improvement was quite small (Tiihonen et al. 2003). Augmentation of risperidone or olanzapine with divalproex was found to reduce positive symptoms more than adding placebo to these antipsychotics in the initial weeks of treating acute episodes, but the difference was no longer detectable after 4 weeks (Casey et al. 2003b). Efforts to treat negative symptoms of schizophrenia with antidepressants have produced mixed results, with little evidence of much effect on "core" negative symptoms (R. W. Buchanan et al. 1996, 1998).

WHICH ACUTE PATIENT CHARACTERISTICS INFLUENCE CHOICE OF TREATMENT?

Goals of treatment of an acute psychotic exacerbation include

> To prevent harm, control disturbed behavior, reduce the severity of psychosis and associated symptoms (e.g., agitation, aggression, negative symptoms, affective symptoms), determine and address the factors that led to the occurrence of the acute episode, effect a rapid return to the best level of functioning, develop an alliance with the patient and family, formulate short- and long-term treatment plans, and connect the patient with appropriate aftercare in the community. (Lehman et al. 2004, p. 3)

Once diagnosis is established, treatment with an antipsychotic should begin promptly. The patient's past experiences with antipsychotic medications, in terms of both therapeutic benefit and tolerability, may help in selecting a particular agent. The usual dosage ranges for the available antipsychotics are listed in Chapter 8 ("Pharmacotherapies") in this book. During the first few days of treatment, adjunctive benzodiazepines can be very helpful in decreasing agitation and subjective distress and can improve sleep. Affective features that accompany acute exacerbations frequently clear with antipsychotic treatment alone. However, if depression persists, an antidepressant can be added. Persistent agitation and hostility can be addressed with a mood stabilizer or β-blocker.

Clinicians must immediately assess risk for dangerousness to self or others in patients experiencing an acute exacerbation of psychosis. Prior suicide attempts, depressed mood, hopelessness, and suicidal ideation all elevate the risk for suicide attempts and should lead to heightened monitoring by staff. Prior violence to others, current violent impulses, comorbid substance use disorder, current intoxication, and unmedicated psychosis all predict increased short-term risk for violence (Borum et al. 1996). The goal of risk assessment is to establish any information that should lead to clinical concern; clinical concern should lead directly to clinical intervention (e.g., treatment of psychosis, detoxification, or hospitalization).

Acute psychotic exacerbations occur for a variety of reasons during the long-term course of schizophrenia. Initially, it is useful to determine whether the exacerbation resulted from a period of nonadherence with prescribed antipsychotic medication. Patients whose exacerbations are related to medication nonadherence tend to have low levels of insight and often require involuntary commitment to receive treatment (McEvoy et al. 1984). Recovery may take weeks to months after antipsychotic treatment is reinstituted. As the patient recovers, the clinician should explore with the patient what led him or her to discontinue the prescribed medication (e.g., side effects, cost, felt he or she did not need it), attempt to resolve the issues involved, and develop a collaborative plan.

Patients with acute psychotic exacerbations despite adherence to antipsychotic treatment tend to have higher levels of insight, to be subjectively distressed, and to seek treatment on a voluntary basis. Independent, external stresses often can be identified (e.g., death of a supportive relative), or an episode of substance abuse may have occurred. These patients usually will recover within days in a protected setting if their current antipsychotic is simply continued at its original dose, although a brief temporary increase in dose or the addition of a benzodiazepine for a few days may be helpful. Psychosocial interventions to relieve the external stressors, or referral for substance use treatment, may be indicated (McEvoy et al. 1984).

WHICH LONG-TERM PATIENT CHARACTERISTICS INFLUENCE CHOICE OF TREATMENT?

In the context of treating chronic schizophrenia, long-term patient characteristics refer to demographic or relatively enduring features of the patient that clinicians should attend to in selecting treatments.

In promoting informed decision making and medication adherence, discussion of potential side effects of medication options with patients is a critical step in the medication selection process. Characteristics such as obesity, high blood pressure, family history of sudden death, high sensitivity to side effects, family history of diabetes, and cardiac conditions can help guide choice of antipsychotic medication.

HOW SHOULD MEDICATION ADHERENCE PROBLEMS BE EVALUATED AND TREATED?

Potential causes of relapse in chronic schizophrenia are manifold, but inadequate adherence to prescribed medication regimens always should be considered as a contributing factor. No "gold standard" exists for assessing outpatient oral medication adherence (Velligan et al. 2003). If a patient's illness worsens with no change in the treatment regimen, then careful questioning about the details of medication taking and side effects is warranted. If a patient cannot describe when, where, and what medicines are taken, nonadherence may be the problem. Similarly, if there are no side effects, or if previously reported side effects are suddenly denied or have become more tolerable, the patient may not be taking the medication.

Repeated relapses, with improvements during periods of controlled supervision of medications and worsening when medication administration is not supervised, are strongly suggestive of adherence problems. Many factors can contribute to inadequate medication adherence, but a few deserve special mention here because of their frequency:

- Substance abuse involving drugs and/or alcohol is common in schizophrenia and can result in poor medication adherence. Direct inquiries about substance abuse to patients and those in frequent contact with them can be supplemented with blood and urine testing.
- Problems with side effects can contribute to erratic taking of medications, and patients may incorrectly attribute dysphoric experiences to medication side effects. Exploration of the contribution of side effects, real or perceived, to medication nonadherence is worthwhile.
- Availability of medications can interfere with medication adherence. Sometimes the issue is cost, but often long waits and relatively remote

pharmacies stand in the way of better adherence. For patients with an illness that affects motivation and planning abilities, the role of systemic barriers to obtaining and refilling medication prescriptions is always a consideration.

Several psychosocial interventions to improve medication adherence in schizophrenia have been evaluated. One controlled study of compliance therapy found that identifying patient goals and aspirations and relating them to treatment outcomes affected by medications improved medication adherence (Kemp et al. 1998). However, this finding was not confirmed in a recent replication study (O'Donnell et al. 2003). Both studies began with inpatients, but the earlier study included outpatient follow-up sessions, which may have contributed to the differing results.

Boczkowski et al. (1985) found that behavioral tailoring resulted in significantly greater increases in adherence than did psychoeducation:

> The investigator helped each participant tailor his prescribed regimen so that it was better adapted to his personal habits and routines. This involved identifying a highly visible location for the placement of medications and pairing the daily medication intake with specific routine behavior of the participant. Each participant was given a self-monitoring spiral calendar, which featured a dated slip of paper for each dose of the neuroleptic. The participant was instructed to keep the calendar near his medications and to tear off a slip each time he took a pill. (p. 668)

Supervision of outpatients by family members or friends can enhance compliance (Buchanan 1992; McEvoy et al. 1989b). Case workers and Assertive Community Treatment teams can deliver and oversee taking of medications, as can operators of residential facilities.

Sometimes hospital-based, legally sanctioned coercion is needed to ensure that medications are delivered. Unfortunately, available evidence suggests that the patients who most resist treatment and require coercion show little or no improvement in acknowledgment of illness and need for treatment when they are forcibly treated, even though their psychiatric symptoms diminish significantly (Marder et al. 1984; McEvoy et al. 1989a). Therefore, after discharge, these patients are unlikely to continue with treatment when the choice is again theirs in the outpatient setting. However, outpatient commitment has been shown to improve medication adherence in this group (Swartz et al. 2001).

Depot preparations have the virtues of certainty of administration and immediate knowledge of missed doses. The magnitude of the relapse-prevention advantage of using depot antipsychotics has varied considerably across studies, depending on study design and type of patients enrolled (Adams et al.

2001; Schooler 2003), but outcomes generally have been superior to oral treatment with the same medication. As discussed in Chapter 8 ("Pharmacotherapies"), there are now several depot antipsychotics available in the United States and even more elsewhere.

UNCOMMON SYNDROMES

POLYDIPSIA–HYPONATREMIA

The literature review of De Leon et al. (1994) suggested that more than 20% of chronically hospitalized patients have polydipsia, and one-quarter of these (5% of the total) also have hyponatremia. In a subsequent prospective epidemiological study of a state hospital, De Leon et al. (1996) found that 26% of the total chronically hospitalized population had polydipsia and that 5% also had hyponatremia. Nursing and other clinical staff can often identify patients who are drinking excessive amounts of water. A urine-specific gravity less than 1.009 is suggestive of polydipsia. Patients with polydipsia who have developed hyponatremia should have their weights checked several times daily. A gain of 10% or more of their baseline weight (first morning weight after voiding) should lead to fluid restriction.

Clozapine is the one pharmacological treatment that has shown consistent therapeutic benefit for patients with polydipsia–hyponatremia (H.S. Lee et al. 1991; Spears et al. 1996; Verghese et al. 1998). Clozapine produces decreased fluid intake and urine volume and increased serum sodium and osmolality. Other pharmacological agents, including other second-generation antipsychotics, angiotensin-converting enzyme inhibitors, clonidine, β-blockers, naloxone, and demeclocycline, have been tried but have not shown replicable benefit (Delva et al. 2002). Patients who develop severe hyponatremia need medical treatment in an intensive care unit. The serum sodium levels should be raised gradually over several days to avoid risk of osmotic demyelination syndrome (Edoute et al. 2003).

CATATONIA

Catatonia is a syndrome of motor and behavioral abnormalities that may accompany a wide range of psychotic, mood, or medical disorders (Rosebush and Mazurek 1999). Examination for catatonia is not a part of the routine mental status or physical examinations, and catatonia can be missed. The Catatonia Rating Scale has been developed and tested for this purpose (Braunig et al. 2000). In patients with schizophrenia, catatonia is predominantly characterized by grimacing, jerky movements, mannerisms, rituals, exaggerated responsiveness, and posturing.

It is important to correctly recognize catatonic hypomotility because hypomotility is associated with considerable morbidity, including dehydration, infection, malnutrition, and thromboembolism (Rosebush and Mazurek 1999). Intramuscular or intravenous benzodiazepines usually will relieve catatonic hypomotility within minutes and preclude or limit the need for maintenance intravenous or nasogastric tube feeding and catheterization. Electroconvulsive therapy can benefit those patients with hypomotility not relieved by benzodiazepines.

INTEGRATING PHARMACOTHERAPY AND PSYCHOSOCIAL TREATMENT

Long-term treatment in chronic schizophrenia should be based on a recovery model that seeks to optimize an individual's overall well-being. The recovery orientation focuses on improving functional outcomes, including vocational, social, and educational outcomes, and quality of life. Because improvements in these outcomes almost always require both psychosocial treatments or rehabilitation and pharmacotherapy, these two modalities of treatment should be integrated in long-term strategies. The recent Schizophrenia PORT guidelines (Kreyenbuhl et al. 2010) document several evidence-based psychosocial treatments that are effective in schizophrenia.

The treatment literature provides some guidance regarding approaches to combining treatments. Psychosocial treatments are most likely to be effective when symptoms have been adequately treated with drugs. A large multicenter study found that psychosocial treatments could actually lead to a worse outcome when outpatients with schizophrenia were given a placebo (Hogarty et al. 1974). In addition, psychosocial treatments are more effective when medication adherence is ensured by a long-acting injectable antipsychotic (Hogarty et al. 1979). Another study with social skills training found that patients who received a type of pharmacotherapy that minimized the proportion of time that they were in a psychotic state also showed the greatest improvements in social adjustment (Marder et al. 1996).

TREATMENT OF CHRONIC SCHIZOPHRENIA IN OLDER PATIENTS

The number of older people with schizophrenia is expected to more than double over the next three decades (Palmer et al. 1999). Several unique clinical features associated with aging make treatment in older patients a challenge as well as an opportunity to help improve their functioning and quality of life.

DIAGNOSIS

A little more than 20% of the patients with schizophrenia manifest symptoms of the illness for the first time in middle or old age (Harris and Jeste 1988). Inconsistencies in nosology and a tendency to attribute late-onset psychoses to "organic" factors or to mood disorders have led to diagnostic confusion in these cases.

The International Late-Onset Schizophrenia Group (Howard et al. 2000) concluded that two separate categories had face validity and clinical utility: 1) late-onset schizophrenia (mostly middle-age onset—i.e., during the fifth, sixth, or seventh decade of life) and 2) very-late-onset schizophrenia-like psychosis (onset during or after the seventh decade). Patients with late-onset schizophrenia are similar to those with early-onset schizophrenia in clinical symptomatology, family history, cognitive deficits, nonspecific brain imaging abnormalities, course of illness, and treatment response and do not manifest mood disorders or dementia when followed up over several years (Vahia et al. 2010). Differences between early- and late-onset schizophrenia include a much higher prevalence of late-onset schizophrenia in women, its association with paranoid subtype, less severe negative symptoms and cognitive impairment, and a need for lower doses of antipsychotics.

Very-late-onset schizophrenia-like psychosis, a heterogeneous group of disorders, differs from both early- and late-onset schizophrenia in that it is associated with sensory impairment, social isolation, visual hallucinations, and, usually, progressive cognitive decline but is not characterized by formal thought disorder, affective blunting, or family history of schizophrenia.

COURSE

Whereas a small minority of older patients experience complete or nearly complete remission of symptoms, and a small minority worsen to the level of dementia, most patients have a relatively stable course, with significant improvement in psychotic symptoms (Auslander and Jeste 2004; Bleuler 1972/1978; Cohen et al. 2000; Folsom et al. 2009). The rate of aging-associated cognitive decline in older community-dwelling schizophrenic patients is similar to that in age-comparable nonschizophrenic individuals (Eyler Zorrilla et al. 2000). However, because patients with schizophrenia generally have a greater degree of premorbid cognitive deficits, they continue to be more impaired than nonschizophrenic subjects in later life as well.

USE OF ANTIPSYCHOTICS

Physical comorbidity and polypharmacy (including the use of prescribed and over-the-counter medications, nutritional supplements, and herbal supplements) frequently complicate treatment in older patients. Cognitive and sensory deficits may interfere with adherence to prescribed medication regimens. Older patients show greater variability of response and greater sensitivity to medications than do younger adults (Jeste et al. 2005).

In terms of choosing among different antipsychotics, no studies show greater efficacy of one over the others in older patients. Therefore, the selection is determined primarily by the side-effect profiles of individual antipsychotics in the context of a given patient's medical status, other pharmacological regimen, and relevant psychosocial considerations including medication costs. Because the risk of EPS and tardive dyskinesia in older persons is high, medications with low risk of EPS are preferred in this population. The risk of developing tardive dyskinesia has been shown to be significantly lower for patients taking second-generation antipsychotics than for those taking first-generation antipsychotic medications (Dolder and Jeste 2003). An additional reason to avoid EPS in older patients is that the anticholinergic medications used to treat EPS have adverse effects on cognition.

In addition to EPS, side effects of antipsychotics that are of concern in older persons include sedation, orthostatic hypotension, weight gain, and type 2 diabetes mellitus. Recently, the FDA issued a "black box" warning regarding increased mortality with antipsychotics in older patients with dementia who have serious behavioral problems. There is a similar black box warning regarding aripiprazole, olanzapine, and risperidone for strokes in dementia patients. Whether these increased risks extend to older patients with schizophrenia is unknown. Given the elevated risk of most side effects, older patients should be assessed more frequently than younger adults are. Older patients would be considered to be in the high-risk category for the recommended monitoring of most side effects listed in Chapter 8 ("Pharmacotherapies").

The "start low and go slow" approach to starting new medications is often appropriate for older patients. The starting dose in older patients generally should be one-quarter to one-half of the usual starting dose for younger adults. The required dose of an antipsychotic for an older patient tends to correlate inversely with current age and with age at onset of illness. Thus, a good guideline is the older a patient is, the lower the recommended dose should be. Patients with late-onset schizophrenia typically require a lower dose than comparably aged early-onset patients; for patients with very-late-onset schizophrenia-like psychosis, even lower doses may be warranted (Howard et al. 2000). Occasionally, however, an older patient with refractory symptoms may need amounts comparable to those given to younger adults. As chronically ill

TABLE 10–1. Recommended average dosage ranges (mg/day) for older patients with schizophrenia

Medication	Initial dosage	Maintenance dosage
Risperidone	0.5–1	1.5–3
Olanzapine	5–7.5	7.5–12.5
Quetiapine	25–50	100–300
Clozapine	25–50	75–200
Aripiprazole	5–15	15–25

patients who have been taking antipsychotics for many years continue to age, their dose requirements often decrease. Doses should, therefore, be monitored according to the clinical needs of a given patient at a given time. The length of treatment trial in an older patient should generally be longer (6–10 weeks) than that in a younger adult, with slower dose increases.

The recommended average dosage ranges for older patients with schizophrenia are shown in Table 10–1.

SWITCHING MEDICATIONS

When switching antipsychotics is indicated, it should be done gradually and over a much longer period than in younger adults (except in the instance of life-threatening adverse events). The dose of the antipsychotic to be discontinued should be slowly decreased while the new agent is slowly titrated up (Jeste et al. 1999). Generally, the dose should be reduced by no more than 25% at a time, with further dose reductions staggered over a period of several weeks. During the time of dose reduction of an older drug, the new agent should be started at a low dose and increased slowly. The lowest effective maintenance dose should be used once the patient is clinically stable.

PSYCHOSOCIAL MANAGEMENT

The notion that psychotherapeutic treatments do not work in older people is wrong and must be discarded. Psychosocial management is at least as useful in older people with schizophrenia as it is in younger adults. Several randomized controlled trials have demonstrated the efficacy of specific manualized interventions targeted toward older individuals with schizophrenia. Recent work has shown the benefits of integrated cognitive-behavioral social skills training (Granholm et al. 2007) and of functional adaptation skills training (Patterson et al. 2006) in improving daily functioning in older persons with schizophrenia. Whereas medications are usually needed for improving psychotic symptoms and preventing relapse, psychosocial interventions should be a regular part of management of older people with schizophrenia in order to enhance their subjective quality of life as well as objective everyday functioning.

REFERENCES

Adams CE, Fenton MKP, Quraishi S, et al: Systematic meta-review of depot antipsychotic drugs for people with schizophrenia. Br J Psychiatry 179:290–299, 2001

Altamura AC, Barnas C, Bitter I, et al: Treatment of schizophrenic disorders: algorithms for acute pharmacotherapy. International Journal of Psychiatry in Clinical Practice 1 (suppl 1):S25–S30, 1997

Auslander LA, Jeste DV: Sustained remission of schizophrenia among community-dwelling older outpatients. Am J Psychiatry 161:1490–1493, 2004

Bleuler M: The Schizophrenic Disorders: Long-Term Patient and Family Studies (1972). Translated by Clemens SM. New Haven, CT, Yale University Press, 1978

Boczkowski JA, Zeichner A, DeSanto N: Neuroleptic compliance among chronic schizophrenic outpatients: an intervention outcome report. J Consult Clin Psychol 53:666–671, 1985

Borum R, Swartz M, Swanson J: Assessing and managing violence risk in clinical practice. Journal of Practical Psychiatry and Behavioral Health 4:205–215, 1996

Braunig P, Kruger S, Shugar G, et al: The Catatonia Rating Scale, I: development, reliability, and use. Compr Psychiatry 41:147–158, 2000

Buchanan A: A two-year prospective study of treatment compliance in patients with schizophrenia. Psychol Med 22:787–797, 1992

Buchanan RW, Kirkpatrick B, Bryant N, et al: Fluoxetine augmentation of clozapine treatment in patients with schizophrenia. Am J Psychiatry 153:1625–1627, 1996

Buchanan RW, Breier A, Kirkpatrick B, et al: Positive and negative symptom response to clozapine in schizophrenic patients with and without the deficit syndrome. Am J Psychiatry 155:751–760, 1998

Buchanan RW, Kreyenbuhl J, Kelly DL, et al: Schizophrenia Patient Outcomes Research Team (PORT): the 2009 Schizophrenia PORT psychopharmacological treatment recommendations and summary statements. Schizophr Bull 36:71–93, 2010

Buckley P, Miller AL, Olsen J, et al: When symptoms persist: clozapine augmentation strategies. Schizophr Bull 27:615–628, 2001

Canadian Clinical Practice Guidelines for the Treatment of Schizophrenia. The Canadian Psychiatric Association. Can J Psychiatry 43 (suppl 2):25S–40S, 1998

Casey DE, Carson WH, Saha AR: Switching patients to aripiprazole from other antipsychotic agents: a multicenter randomized study. Psychopharmacology 166:391–399, 2003a

Casey DE, Daniel DG, Wassef AA, et al: Effect of divalproex combined with olanzapine or risperidone in patients with an acute exacerbation of schizophrenia. Neuropsychopharmacology 28:182–192, 2003b

Cohen CI, Cohen GD, Blank K, et al: Schizophrenia and older adults: an overview: directions for research and policy. Am J Geriatr Psychiatry 8:19–28, 2000

Correll CU, Frederickson AM, Kane JM, et al: Does antispsychotic polypharmacy increase the risk for metabolic syndrome? Schizophr Res 89:91–100, 2007

Cradock J, Young AS, Sullivan G: The accuracy of medical record documentation in schizophrenia. J Behav Health Serv Res 28:456–465, 2001

De Leon J, Verghese C, Tracy JI, et al: Polydipsia and water intoxication in psychiatric patients: a review of the epidemiological literature. Biol Psychiatry 35:408–419, 1994

De Leon J, Dadvand M, Canuso C, et al: Polydipsia and water intoxication in a long-term psychiatric hospital. Biol Psychiatry 40:28–34, 1996

Delva NH, Chang A, Hawken ER, et al: Effects of clonidine in schizophrenic patients with primary polydipsia: three single case studies. Prog Neuropsychopharmacol Biol Psychiatry 26:387–392, 2002

Dixon LB, McFarlane WR, Lefley H, et al: Evidence-based practices for services to families of people with psychiatric disabilities. Psychiatr Serv 52:903–910, 2001

Dolder CR, Jeste DV: Incidence of tardive dyskinesia with typical versus atypical antipsychotics in very high risk patients. Biol Psychiatry 53:1142–1145, 2003

Drake RE, McHugo GJ, Becker DR, et al: The New Hampshire study of supported employment for people with severe mental illness. J Consult Clin Psychol 64:391–399, 1996

Dursun SM, Deakin JFW: Augmenting antipsychotic treatment with lamotrigine or topiramate in patients with treatment-resistant schizophrenia: a naturalistic case-series outcome study. J Psychopharmacol 15:297–301, 2001

Dursun SM, McIntosh D, Milliken H: Clozapine plus lamotrigine in treatment-resistant schizophrenia. Arch Gen Psychiatry 56:950, 1999

Edoute Y, Davids MR, Johnston C, et al: An integrative physiological approach to polyuria and hyponatremia: a "double-take" on the diagnosis and therapy in a patient with schizophrenia. Q J Med 96:531–540, 2003

Essock SM, Covell NH, Davis SM, et al: Effectiveness of switching antipsychotic medications. Am J Psychiatry 163:2090–2095, 2006

Eyler Zorrilla LT, Heaton RK, McAdams LA, et al: Cross-sectional study of older outpatients with schizophrenia and healthy comparison subjects: no differences in age-related cognitive decline. Am J Psychiatry 157:1324–1326, 2000

Folsom DP, Depp C, Palmer BW, et al: Physical and mental health-related quality of life among older people with schizophrenia. Schizophr Res 108:207–213, 2009

Frances A, Docherty JP, Kahn DA, et al: Expert Consensus Guidelines Series: Treatment of schizophrenia. J Clin Psychiatry 57 (suppl 12B):5–58, 1996

Gören JL, Parks JJ, Ghinassi FA, et al: When is antipsychotic polypharmacy supported by research evidence? Implications for QI. The Joint Commission Journal on Quality and Patient Safety 34:571–582, 2008

Granholm E, McQuaid JR, McClure FS, et al: Randomized controlled trial of cognitive behavioral social skills training for older people with schizophrenia: 12-month follow-up. J Clin Psychiatry 68:730–737, 2007

Harris MJ, Jeste DV: Late onset schizophrenia: an overview. Schizophr Bull 14:39–55, 1988

Hogarty GE, Goldberg SC, Schooler NR: Drug and sociotherapy in the aftercare of schizophrenia patients. Arch Gen Psychiatry 31:609–618, 1974

Hogarty GE, Schooler NR, Ulrich R, et al: Fluphenazine and social therapy in the aftercare of schizophrenic patients: relapse analyses of a two-year controlled study of fluphenazine decanoate and fluphenazine hydrochloride. Arch Gen Psychiatry 36:1283–1294, 1979

Howard R, Rabins PV, Seeman MV, et al: Late-onset schizophrenia and very-late-onset schizophrenia-like psychosis: an international consensus. Am J Psychiatry 157:172–178, 2000

Jeste DV, Rockwell E, Harris MJ, et al: Conventional versus newer antipsychotics in elderly patients. Am J Geriatr Psychiatry 7:70–76, 1999

Jeste DV, Dolder CR, Nayak GV, et al: Atypical antipsychotics in elderly patients with dementia or schizophrenia: review of recent literature. Harv Rev Psychiatry 13(6):340–351, 2005

Kane J, Honigfeld G, Singer J, et al: Clozapine for the treatment-resistant schizophrenic: a double-blind comparison versus chlorpromazine/benztropine. Arch Gen Psychiatry 45:789–796, 1988

Kane JM, Marder SR, Schooler NR, et al: Clozapine and haloperidol in moderately refractory schizophrenia: a 6-month randomized and double-blind comparison. Arch Gen Psychiatry 58:965–972, 2001

Kane JM, Leucht S, Carpenter D, et al: Expert Consensus Guidelines Series: Optimizing pharmacologic treatment of psychotic disorders, introduction: methods, commentary, and summary. J Clin Psychiatry 64 (suppl 12):1–100, 2003

Kemp R, Kirov G, Everitt B, et al: Randomized controlled trial of compliance therapy: 18 month follow-up. Br J Psychiatry 172:413–419, 1998

Kontaxakis VP, Ferentinos PP, Havaki-Kontaxakis BJ, et al: Risperidone augmentation of clozapine: a critical review. Eur Arch Psychiatry Clin Neurosci 256:350–355, 2006

Kreyenbuhl J, Buchanan RW, Dickerson FB, et al: The Schizophrenia Patient Outcomes Research Team (PORT): updated treatment recommendations 2009. Schizophr Bull 36:94–103, 2010

Lee CT, Conde BJ, Mazlan M, et al: Switching to olanzapine from previous antipsychotics: a regional collaborative multicenter trial assessing 2 switching techniques in Asia Pacific. J Clin Psychiatry 63:569–576, 2002

Lee HS, Kwon KY, Alphs LD, et al: Effect of clozapine on psychogenic polydipsia in chronic schizophrenia. J Clin Psychopharmacol 11:222–223, 1991

Lehman AF, Lieberman JA, Dixon LB, et al: Practice guideline for the treatment of patients with schizophrenia, second edition. Am J Psychiatry 161 (2 suppl):1–56, 2004

Marder SR, Swann E, Winsdale WJ, et al: A study of medication refusal by involuntary patients. Hosp Community Psychiatry 35:724–726, 1984

Marder SR, Wirshing WC, Mintz J, et al: Two-year outcome of social skills training and group psychotherapy for outpatients with schizophrenia. Am J Psychiatry 153:1585–1592, 1996

McEvoy JP, Howe AC, Hogarty GE: Differences in the nature of relapse and subsequent inpatient course between medication compliant and noncompliant schizophrenic patients. J Nerv Ment Dis 172:412–416, 1984

McEvoy JP, Appelbaum PS, Apperson LJ, et al: Why must some schizophrenic patients be involuntarily committed? The role of insight. Compr Psychiatry 30:13–17, 1989a

McEvoy JP, Freter S, Everett G, et al: Insight and the clinical outcome of schizophrenic patients. J Nerv Ment Dis 177:48–51, 1989b

McEvoy JP, Scheifler PI, Frances A: Expert Consensus Guideline Series: Treatment of schizophrenia 1999. J Clin Psychiatry 60 (suppl 11):1–80, 1999

Miller AL, Craig CS: Combination antipsychotics: pros, cons, and questions. Schizophr Bull 28:105–109, 2002

Miller AL, Chiles JA, Chiles JK, et al: The Texas Medication Algorithm Project (TMAP) Schizophrenia Algorithms. J Clin Psychiatry 60:649–657, 1999

Miller AL, Hall CS, Buchanan RW, et al: The Texas Medication Algorithm Project antipsychotic algorithm for schizophrenia: 2003 update. J Clin Psychiatry 65:500–508, 2004

Moore TA, Buchanan RW, Buckley PF, et al: The Texas Medication Algorithm Project antipsychotic algorithm for schizophrenia: 2006 update. J Clin Psychiatry 68:1751–1762, 2007

New Freedom Commission on Mental Health: Achieving the promise: transforming mental health care in America. 2003. Available at: http://www.mentalhealthcommission.gov.

O'Donnell C, Donohoe G, Sharkey L, et al: Compliance therapy: a randomised controlled trial in schizophrenia. BMJ 327 (7419):834, 2003

Palmer BW, Heaton RK, Paulsen JS, et al: Is it possible to be schizophrenic yet neuropsychologically normal? Neuropsychology 11:437–446, 1997

Palmer BW, Heaton SC, Jeste DV: Older patients with schizophrenia: challenges in the coming decades. Psychiatr Serv 50:1178–1183, 1999

Patterson TL, McKibbin C, Mausbach BT, et al: Functional Adaptation Skills Training (FAST): a randomized trial of a psychosocial intervention for middle-aged and older patients with chronic psychotic disorders. Schizophr Res 86:291–299, 2006

Pearsall R, Glick ID, Pickar D, et al: A new algorithm for treating schizophrenia. Psychopharmacol Bull 34:349–353, 1998

Perkins DO: Predictors of noncompliance in patients with schizophrenia. J Clin Psychiatry 63:1121–1128, 2002

Perry PJ: Therapeutic drug monitoring of antipsychotics. Psychopharmacol Bull 35:19–29, 2001

Pitschel-Walz G, Leucht S, Bauml J, et al: The effect of family interventions on relapse and rehospitalization in schizophrenia—a meta-analysis. Schizophr Bull 27:73–92, 2001

Rosebush PI, Mazurek MF: Catatonia: re-awakening to a forgotten disorder. Mov Disord 14:395–397, 1999

Schooler NR: Relapse and rehospitalization: comparing oral and depot antipsychotics. J Clin Psychiatry 64 (suppl 16):14–17, 2003

Smith TE, Docherty JP: Standards of care and clinical algorithms for treating schizophrenia. Psychiatr Clin North Am 21:203–220, 1998

Spears NM, Leadbetter RA, Shutty MS: Clozapine treatment in polydipsia and intermittent hyponatremia. J Clin Psychiatry 57:123–128, 1996

Stahl SM: Selecting an atypical antipsychotic by combining clinical experience with guidelines from clinical trials. J Clin Psychiatry 60 (suppl 10):31–41, 1999

Swartz MS, Swanson JW, Hiday VA, et al: A randomized controlled trial of outpatient commitment in North Carolina. Psychiatr Serv 52:325–329, 2001

Tai S, Turkington D: The evolution of cognitive behavior therapy for schizophrenia: current practice and recent developments. Schizophr Bull 35:865–873, 2009

Tiihonen J, Hallikainen T, Ryynanen OP, et al: Lamotrigine in treatment-resistant schizophrenia: a randomized placebo-controlled crossover trial. Biol Psychiatry 54:1241–1248, 2003

Vahia IV, Palmer BW, Depp C, et al: Late-onset schizophrenia: a subtype of schizophrenia? Acta Psychiatr Scand March 20, 2010 [Epub ahead of print]

Velligan DI, Bow-Thomas CC, Huntzinger D, et al: Randomized controlled trial of the use of compensatory strategies to enhance adaptive functioning in outpatients with schizophrenia. Am J Psychiatry 157:1317–1323, 2000

Velligan DI, DiCocco M, Castillo DA, et al: Obstacles in assessing adherence to oral antipsychotic medications (abstract). Schizophr Res 60:330, 2003

Verghese C, Abraham G, Nair C, et al: Absence of changes in antidiuretic hormone, angiotensin II, and atrial natriuretic peptide with clozapine treatment of polydipsia-hyponatremia: 2 case reports. J Clin Psychiatry 59:415–419, 1998

Weiden PJ, Aquila R, Dalheim L, et al: Switching antipsychotic medications. J Clin Psychiatry 58 (suppl 10):63–72, 1997

Weiden PJ, Simpson GM, Potkin SG, et al: Effectiveness of switching to ziprasidone for stable but symptomatic outpatients with schizophrenia. J Clin Psychiatry 64:580–588, 2003

Zygmunt A, Olfson M, Boyer CA, et al: Interventions to improve medication adherence in schizophrenia. Am J Psychiatry 159:1653–1664, 2002

INDEX

*Page numbers printed in **boldface** type refer to tables or figures.*

Hostility, 16, 18, 33–35, 174. *See also*
  Aggressive behavior
Huntington's disease, 42
9-Hydroxy-risperidone. *See* Paliperidone
Hygiene, 28
Hyperglycemia, 161, 189. *See also* Diabetes
  mellitus; Glucose dysregulation
Hyperprolactinemia, antipsychotic-induced,
  163, **177,** 179, 180, 181, 182, 190
  monitoring for, 190
  osteoporosis and, 190
  symptoms of, 190
  treatment of, 190
Hypersalivation, clozapine-induced, 179
Hypertension, 161, 191
Hyperthermia, in neuroleptic malignant
  syndrome, 184
Hypnotic drugs, 198
Hypochondriasis, 21
Hyponatremia, 164, 234
Hypotension, antipsychotic-induced,
  176–178, **177,** 179, 180, 181, 182
  in older adults, 237

ICD-10 (International Classification of
  Diseases), 13, 14, 37
  schizophrenia subtypes in, **44–45**
Illness management and recovery resource
  tool kit, 211
Illness self-management skills, 99
Illogicality, 31
Iloperidone, 175, **177,** 182
Imipramine
  for comorbid schizophrenia and cocaine
    use, 135
  for obsessive-compulsive symptoms,
    144
  for panic disorder, 140
Immigrant populations, 2, 3
Impersistence at work or school, 28
Implementing Evidence-Based Practices
  Project, 211, 213
Impulse-control problems of childhood and
  adolescence, 94
Impulsivity, 16, 33

mood stabilizers for, 64
suicide and, 138
Incidence of schizophrenia, 1, 2
Incoherence, 13, 31
Independent living, 95, 96, 100
Individual Placement and Support (IPS)
  model of supported employment,
  102–105, **103, 104,** 216–217
Infectious diseases, 160
  HIV/AIDS, 162
  prenatal exposure to, 3, 7
  risk reduction strategies for, 167–168
  viral hepatitis, 163
Information processing speed, 76
Insomnia
  aripiprazole-induced, 181
  quetiapine for patients with, 180
Insulin resistance, 160, 189
Insulin therapy, 162
Integrated Dual Disorder Treatment, 134,
  134
Integrated psychological treatment, 215
Intelligence, 75. *See also* Neurocognitive
  impairment
  theory-of-mind deficits and, 108
International Classification of Diseases
  (ICD-10), 13, 14, 37
  schizophrenia subtypes in, **44–45**
International Late-Onset Schizophrenia
  Group, 236
Intoxication. *See also* Substance use disorders
  and schizophrenia
  aggressive behavior and, 34, 35
  psychosis and, 43
IPS (Individual Placement and Support)
  model of supported employment,
  102–105, **103, 104,** 216–217
Irritability, 34
  in prodrome, 58

Jealousy, delusions of, 18
Jumping to conclusions, 112

Kinesthetic hallucinations, 23
  somatic delusions and, 21